For James
With Best Wishes
for much Success

The Managed Care Contracting Handbook

Second Edition

The Managed Care Contracting Handbook

Second Edition

Planning and Negotiating
the Managed Care Relationship

Maria K. Todd

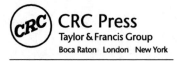

CRC Press
Taylor & Francis Group
Boca Raton London New York

CRC Press is an imprint of the
Taylor & Francis Group, an **informa** business
A PRODUCTIVITY PRESS BOOK

Productivity Press
Taylor & Francis Group
270 Madison Avenue
New York, NY 10016

© 2009 by Maria K. Todd
Productivity Press is an imprint of Taylor & Francis Group, an Informa business

No claim to original U.S. Government works

International Standard Book Number-13: 978-1-56327-369-8 (0)

Library of Congress Cataloging-in-Publication Data

Todd, Maria K.
    The managed care contracting handbook : planning & negotiating the managed
care relationship / Maria K. Todd. -- 2nd ed.
        p. ; cm.
    Includes bibliographical references and index.
    ISBN 978-1-56327-369-8 (alk. paper)
    1. Managed care plans (Medical care)--United States--Handbooks, manuals, etc. 2.
Negotiation in business--United States--Handbooks, manuals, etc. I. Title.
    [DNLM: 1. Managed Care Programs--United States--Handbooks. 2.
Contracts--United States--Handbooks. 3. Negotiating--United States--Handbooks. W
49 T635m 2009]

    RA413.5.U5T63 2009
    362.1'04258--dc22   2009000765

Visit the Taylor & Francis Web site at
http://www.taylorandfrancis.com

and the Productivity Press Web site at
http://www.productivitypress.com

Contents

Acknowledgments

Many people contributed to bringing this manuscript to closure. To my colleagues, clients, students, and friends who have served as resources, sounding boards, and friends, namely, attorneys Paul DeMuro and Ellen Stewart; fellow consultants David Samuels, Fellow of the Healthcare Financial Management Association (FHFMA); Mickey Duke; Bill DeMarco; Bill Phillips; David Hammer, FHFMA; and the many students, colleagues, and clients with whom I have exchanged counsel along the development of this manuscript. The insights, applications, and issues raised by my colleagues, clients, and students helped stimulate much of the thinking brought to this book.

To Kristine Rynne-Mednansky goes a debt of gratitude for her understanding and that of Taylor & Francis, my publishers. Collectively, you were patient with me through life's little surprises that kept demanding my attention.

I wish to acknowledge my capable assistant Mark Dragotta, MFA, who assisted in the completion in the manuscript by performing an initial proofread for continuity and assisting with the writing of the "Introduction." His dependability enabled me to delegate certain tasks to him so that I could focus on writing without interruption, and his journalism skills are an invaluable bonus.

To Alan Burch I owe a debt of appreciation for his encouragement, support, and tolerance. He always thought he would fall in love with an English major; instead he ended up with an author, speaker, and consultant in this "Kafkaesque" business of health administration. Maybe now I can take time out and read a novel … and plan a wedding!

Maria K. Todd

Introduction

The most efficient approach to making your hospital or practice more financially responsible is just plugging the often invisible leaks that payers poke in your financial bottom line. Throughout this book you will learn tried-and-true tricks, tools, shortcuts, and techniques that you can use to evaluate current and future agreements with an eye toward clarifying and negotiating better contracts before they get the best of your hospital or practice.

Having trouble with Employee Retirement Income Security Act (ERISA) loopholes? Are silent preferred provider organizations (PPOs) eating up your revenue? Did you sign an evergreen contract without negotiating automatic capitation increases? Do you even know what these potential problems *really* mean? Identify and eliminate these and other contracting cancers by examining the hands-on advice found in these pages.

Managed care contracting is a complex process that can frustrate your best lawyers, hospital decision makers, and consultants. Know what questions to ask, terms to clarify, clauses to watch for and then make *certain* all that planning, clarification, and hard work is locked into the contract. (Trust me; it is not as easy as it sounds.) This handbook is an all-access guide to saving money by avoiding the pitfalls and reimbursement "gotchas" draining untold amounts of provider revenue each year.

This book is intended for decision makers such as chief financial officers (CFOs), revenue managers, contract analysts, business office managers, and hospital finance officers who have the daunting task of negotiating contracts for hospitals, medical groups, and physical therapy and other alternative site providers. Find facts and resources on everything from health maintenance organizations (HMOs) and PPOs to Consumer Driven Health Plans (CDHP), reimbursement methods, single and continuous discount agreements, self-funded ERISA payers, contract law basics, Medicaid managed care, and contract negotiating strategies.

Taken separately, these resources are an important dissection and discussion of managed care in its many complex forms. However, taken together, these chapters rise to the higher purpose of first decoding and then evaluating almost every reimbursement problem, loophole, and managed care contract agreement. With a fuller understanding of these practical components, this book's "Evaluating a Managed Care Agreement—Step-by-Step" (Chapter 15) is a detailed guide to examining and negotiating all future contracting. In addition, the "Insurance and Managed Care Glossary" (Appendix) is virtually its own guidebook/dictionary, explaining hundreds of acronyms, terms, and general managed care language.

The beauty of this book is that you can read it in any order you please. Skip to a section or chapter that holds particular interest to you or read it cover to cover. Start with those things affecting you directly, or gain a well-rounded understanding of managed care by examining all the unknowns that *could* affect your contracting and revenue. It is up to you. If there is an acronym or word you need clarified, just flip to the glossary. It is all here.

Whether you find yourself contracting for the first time or you are a veteran of many contracting wars, this book is an opportunity to gain an advantage over the often complicated language and uneven practices tipping the scale in the payer's direction. Do not let frustration and naivety guide important and *binding* contract decisions. Do not let your overburdened and often unprepared lawyer take on contracting challenges alone. Do not pay thousands of dollars for consulting when this contracting guide is as good (and a tenth of the price) of most fly-by-night consultants.

And if you *do* need more help, you are welcome to all the resources on my Web site, *www.askmariatodd.com*. Finally, if you still feel hopelessly lost, give me a call at 800-209-7263, and we can set up a complimentary 45-minute consultation that focuses specifically on your unique needs. Good luck and happy reading.

Chapter 1

What Is Managed Care?

"Managed care" is a term used to describe a system and method designed to control the utilization of health care services. Optimally, in order for it to work, a great deal of effort must be spent to perform reviews of medical necessity, gain preauthorization to carry out the necessary treatment, manage the case, and obtain the care from the medically appropriate type of provider. The system often involves financial incentives to use certain providers, as well as denials by persons not directly examining the patient or involved in the patient's treatment. The decisions are often made by administrators and insurance plan personnel who have little, if any, medical training, who use decision-tree software and algorithms to determine medical treatment appropriateness, combined with actuarial analyses that predict risk of the cost of treatment and the likelihood that the plan making the decisions might be called to task to spend its assets on care instead of margin. If that statement makes me sound cynical, it is because, after more than 20 years in the business that is more than 30 years old, I have witnessed all kinds of operations described as managed care, and most of them that take away the independent clinical decision making of the attending physician are not involved in "managed care," they are involved in "managed cost."

The colloquial reference to managed care in the United States includes the clinical, financial, and organizational activities assumed to be designed to ensure the provision of appropriate health care services in a cost-efficient manner. Managed care activities are most often conducted by insurance plans, health plans, and a variety of industry professionals that assume risk for a defined population such as health maintenance organizations, but managed care is often used as a broader term and encompasses many different types of organizations, payment mechanisms, review mechanisms and sometimes, provider collaborations. Sometimes the term is used more generically, as a term for the activity of organizing doctors, hospitals, and other providers into groups in order to enhance the quality and cost-effectiveness of health care.

Managed care has its own language of acronyms and nomenclature, its own mathematical calculations and formulae tied to creative (dizzying) techniques in reimbursement. When one refers to a managed care organization (MCO), one often refers to the entity that manages insurance risk for the cost of care, contracts with providers, is paid by employers or patient groups, or handles claims processing.

Managed care has, in essence, formed a third-party arrangement by sometimes operating as the gatekeeper between payers and providers and patients. This has faced lots of backlash from providers and patients alike. In response, the market has formed new consumer driven health plans, designed to give the patient more flexibility in decision making with regards to provider access and assumption of financial responsibility, and inappropriately (in this author's professional, learned opinion) has conjoined these consumer driven health plans to the reimbursement agreements and rates to existing managed care participation agreements, despite their antithetical objectives.

As such, the term "managed care" is used generally as a synonym for any arrangement for which a discounted contractual reimbursement arrangement has been undertaken, as it refers to many facets of health care management, payment, and organization.

The term "managed care" can be used to describe a system of health payment or delivery arrangements where the plan attempts to control or coordinate use of health services by its enrolled members in order to contain health expenditures, improve quality, or both. These arrangements often involve a defined delivery system of providers with some form of contractual arrangement with the plan and, with that, you have the focus of this handbook.

Chapter 2

Managed Care Organizations

In 2001, Paul Ellwood, who is often credited with coining the term "health maintenance organizations," said:

> If managed care means organizations that combine health insurance and health care competing on price and quality to serve informed consumers with the primary goal of enhancing health, managed care is over in most of the country. In fact, it barely got started.

Managed care is usually delivered through health care organizations of various shapes and structures that, on the surface, appear very similar. The truth is that they are very different, although most resemble a blended entity capable of providing care and the insurance component to protect the enrollee from financial exposure for claims arising from incurred covered expenses. It is no surprise to the intended audience of this book that most Americans have little to no understanding of what kind of coverage they have and do not think to take the time to understand the nature of their coverage until they have to use it.

True managed care organizations limit the enrollees' choice and access to designated, participating providers within the system, other than primary care physicians (PCPs) and ob-gyns in many cases. These limitations were the subject of much backlash in the 1990s, which brought about the change to permit direct access to ob-gyns as PCPs for women and for access by annual standing referrals to specialists for certain patients with particular diseases as part of many states' patient protection acts. The systems often also limit their ability to self-refer throughout the system of fixed panels of physicians, facilities, and other contracted providers, a methodology known as a "gatekeeper" approach.

The managed care delivery system usually emphasizes preventive care and is often associated with alternative delivery systems such as health maintenance organizations (HMOs), preferred provider organizations (PPOs), exclusive provider organizations (EPOs), independent practice associations (IPAs), physician–hospital organizations (PHOs), and management services organizations (MSOs), utilizing a capitated or discounted fee-for-service reimbursement system. In this chapter, we will study the structure and functional differences of each system.

HMOs—Health Maintenance Organizations

Originally, HMOs were the fastest growing type of managed care plans as far as the number of covered enrollees. This trend has not continued in the advent of the consumer driven health plan movement, but the jury is still out as far as if the trend for HMO replacement will continue.

The health maintenance organization is a health plan that may be for profit or not for profit. HMOs may seek federal qualification on a voluntary basis by the Centers for Medicare & Medicaid Services (CMS) in accordance with the HMO Act of 1973, as amended in 1988. Federal qualification status may be designated by CMS after conducting an extensive evaluation of an HMO's organization and operations. An organization must be federally qualified or be designated as a competitive medical plan (CMP) to be eligible to participate in Medicare and cost and risk contracts. This federal designation allows an organization to participate in certain Medicare cost and risk contracts including Medicare Advantage. A federally qualified HMO is also eligible for loans and loan guarantees not available to nonqualified plans. Additionally, HMOs must pass state licensure requirements, which vary state by state. The basic regulatory model is that a state insurance department or corporations department reviews rates, policy documents, and compliance with state financial reserve and surplus requirements in the amount necessary to cover all covered expenses up to the minute that they are incurred. HMOs may also receive a Certificate of Authority for each county in which they are permitted to sell their product.

Federally Qualified HMOs

As a federally qualified HMO, a plan is required to offer an extensive basic benefits package that includes inpatient and outpatient services, home care benefits, specified drug abuse treatments, and outpatient mental health services. The plan must also enroll individuals in a contracting group on a "come-as-you-are" basis, without regard to preexisting health status and must establish prepayment charges on a community-rated basis for most groups. The plan must provide evidence of fiscal solvency and provide for patient "hold harmless" provisions. Federally qualified HMOs may enroll Medicare and Federal Health Benefit Plan (FEHBP) members as well.

Under the Medicare risk models (also known as TEFRA risk plans), Medicare contractors receive capitated payments from CMS. Capitation is a per-member, fixed, monthly payment to the plan that covers contracted services and that is paid in advance of the delivery of the care. It is usually expressed in units of per-member, per-month (PMPM). In essence, the health plan agrees to provide specific services to Medicare beneficiaries enrolled in the health plan for this fixed, predetermined payment for a specified time, regardless of how many times the member uses the service. The rate can be fixed for all members and is known as the adjusted average per capita cost (AAPCC).

Tax Equity and Fiscal Responsibility Act of 1982 (TEFRA)

The Tax Equity and Fiscal Responsibility Act of 1982 is a federal law that created the current risk and cost contract provisions under which health plans contract with CMS (formerly HCFA). The legislation created the target rate of increase cost-based limits on reimbursements for inpatient operating costs. These limits are considered per Medicare discharges total amounts. A facility's target amount is derived from costs in its base year (first full fiscal year of operation with application to CMS as same) updated to the current fiscal year by the annual allowable rate of increase. Medicare payments for operating costs generally may not exceed the facility's target amount and still be paid by CMS. These provisions apply to hospitals and units excluded from prospective payment system (PPS) and diagnosis-related group (DRG). When cost reports fall short of the TEFRA limit, certain paybacks are provided. If costs exceed TEFRA, facilities can submit an exception report and may or may not be provided additional payment. Many facilities that established TEFRA limits in the early 1980s are finding they consistently exceed their TEFRA limits.

CMS pays 95% of the AAPCC to the plan in exchange for arranging Medicare-covered services for their enrollees. The other 5% is retained by CMS for plan oversight and administration. The AAPCC is the best estimate, from CMS, of the amount of money it costs to care for Medicare recipients under fee-for-service Medicare on a countywide basis. The AAPCC is made up of 122 different rate cells; 120 of them are factored for age, gender, Medicaid eligibility, institutional status, and whether a person has both Part A and Part B

Medicare. The two remaining cells are for individuals with end stage renal disease (ESRD).

Two other financial terms used in conjunction with Medicare risk models are *adjusted community rate* (ACR) and *average payment rate* (APR). The ACR is used by HMOs and CMPs. A competitive medical plan (CMP) is a type of managed care organization created by the 1982 TEFRA to facilitate the enrollment of Medicare beneficiaries into managed care plans. Competitive medical plans are organized and financed much like HMOs, but are not bound by all the regulatory requirements facing HMOs. A health plan can be eligible for a Medicare risk contract if it meets specified requirements for service provision, capital, risk protection, and financial solvency. CMP designation is established in the TEFRA and granted by the federal government to an organization that meets specific requirements enabling that organization to obtain a Medicare risk or cost-based contract. This is different from a federally qualified HMO.

The ACR is a calculation of what premium the plan would charge for providing exactly the Medicare-covered benefits to a group account adjusted to allow for the greater intensity and frequency of utilization by Medicare patients. The ACR includes the normal profit margin for a for-profit HMO or CMP. It may be equal to or lower than the APR, but can never exceed it.

The APR is the amount of money that CMS could conceivably pay an HMO or CMP for services to Medicare recipients under a risk contract. The figure is derived from the AAPCC for the service area, adjusted for the enrollment characteristics that the plan would expect to have. The payment to the plan, the ACR, can never be higher than the APR, but it may be less.

HMO Premium Rate Setting

HMOs may have considerable flexibility in establishing their premium rates to remain competitive. Typically, an HMO sells a policy to an insured and is thereby in the "business of insurance" but not necessarily an insurance company. Statutory definitions further explain state by state what constitutes an insurance company, an HMO, a health insuring organization (HIO), or a health services corporation (HSC). Essentially, the premium is paid in exchange for a policy that is a formal contractual agreement between the insured and the payer and that warranties and guaranties that expenses for covered services shall be paid as long as the payer pays premiums. Both enrollees and providers should review the summary plan description(s) (SPDs) to determine what the premium pays for in covered services, identify specific exclusions, and gain a better understanding and more clear expectations regarding payment for services under a reimbursement agreement.

Some states now have regulations in accordance with then-state health care reform initiatives, which require health plans such as HMOs to abide by community rating policies. A community-rated premium is based on the HMO's average cost of providing health care benefits to its entire population of beneficiaries, as opposed to experience rating, which estimates expected costs for individuals and groups with identified preexisting medical conditions or occupations. States may also have requirements that HMOs require physicians and other health care providers to hold the enrollee "harmless" in the event that the HMO does not pay for services as agreed. These agreements or statutory provisions restrict a provider's ability to bill an enrollee for covered services that the HMO owes moneys for, even in the event of HMO insolvency. Other insolvency protection methods may include reserves or deposits, insolvency insurance or reinsurance provisions, or contractual insurance provisions that require physicians to continue to provide services or arrange for alternative suitable coverage for a period following the insolvency.

HMO Models

The main models of HMO delivery systems include the IPA, staff, group, and network models. The IPA model included independent practice associations that contracted with the health plan. The physicians were independent contractors to the IPA, and the IPA then had a contractual relationship with the health plan to provide services to the HMO's members on an exclusive basis. If your physician was not a member of the IPA, your services would be considered "out of network" and might be subject to reduced benefits or no benefits at all, depending on the reason for your out-of-network services. A variation on this theme was the PHO model, where providers joined a physician–hospital organization (PHO) as independent contractors or employees and the PHO contracted with the health plan as the provider of medical and hospital services. In some cases, the health plan sponsored the IPA, (among others, some CIGNA plans were structured this way), while other IPAs were sponsored by the members themselves, or by a select group of the members (for example the PCPs), and the balance of the membership were nonshareholder participants.

The main reason for forming these alliances was to share risk and entertain capitated contracts with HMOs. Many across the country failed miserably, went bankrupt, and were abandoned. As a consultant, I designed about 150 of these alliances nationwide and assisted in their strategic development, business rules adoption, and contract negotiations. While many have disbanded or been rendered inactive, some that I designed are still successful and in business today because the models used for their design matched the market need at the time and have since adapted to changes in the market, with reliance on good medical management, disease management, and physician leadership.

An HMO is premised, in part, on the idea that aligning incentives between the managed care organization (MCO) and the provider can keep costs down. Studies have shown that HMOs can be successful in reducing the costs and preserving measurable quality in many instances. Few plans actually collaborate with physicians, and many keep costs down using several tactics, including cost-fixing the cost of care through capitated reimbursement, denying claims that the health plan deems medically unnecessary, or not including certain medically necessary services, drugs, and technology in the plan design. There are some forward-thinking HMOs that are working collaboratively with their physicians and financially rewarding efforts to keep quality high and costs down, but these are still the exception rather than the rule.

The staff model is often mislabeled as the "Kaiser" model. In most cases, this is incorrect because the staff model implies that the physicians rendering most of the care in the network are on staff at the same company that owns the HMO and those physicians are employed in a W-2 employment relationship, rather than contracted as an independent contractor with the plan. There are some remaining staff-model HMOs, but in the late 1990s many of those operating staff models chose to shut them down or redesign them. Essentially, it became quite apparent that the "bricks and mortar" clinic model of staff-model HMO was much more expensive to maintain in comparison with the IPA model. Furthermore, the public came to affectionately refer to the staff model as "take a number" health care because of the delivery model permitting a walk-in system of access to PCPs and midlevel providers that entailed long waits in some cases.

The group model was more of an accurate description of the Kaiser model. In the group model, the physicians were employed by a medical group that contracted with the health plan to render care to its members. Those physicians rarely, if ever, saw patients with health plan or insurance coverage outside the designated health plan. For example, Colorado Permanente Medical Group saw few outside patients other than those that were cardholders of the Kaiser Health Plan. In the group model, an HMO contracts with a group practice that provides medical services to the HMO enrollees at their medical group's facility, owned or operated by the HMO. Usually there are two types of group model HMOs: (1) the closed panel plan, in which the medical services are delivered in the HMO-owned health center or satellite clinic by physicians who belong to a specially formed but legally separate medical group that only serves the HMOs customers or (2) the plan in which the HMO contracts with an existing, independent group of physicians to deliver medical care. In the last few years, even these models have changed their strategy, and the model is not as insular anymore.

In a network-model HMO the physicians come from more than one group. Network-model HMOs are organizational models in which the HMO contracts for medical services with a network of medical groups.

HMO Products

HMOs offer different products. An HMO typically has a lock-in feature that provides payment for covered medical expenses if the enrollee uses the system in accordance with plan provisions, and that exposes the enrollee to financial responsibility for services rendered outside the plan provisions. HMOs differ from traditional indemnity health insurance, known as sickness and accident policies, because they have plan limitations on coverage. When an employer or individual purchases coverage from an HMO, they are agreeing to the plan's terms, policies, and conditions of coverage for covered medical, dental, or psychiatric services.

HMO Provider Contracts

Services from certain types of practitioners may be specifically excluded in the plan's evidence of coverage (EOC) or plan handbook. Often, these practitioners include chiropractors, optometrists, opticians, podiatrists, and alternative healing arts practitioners such as massage therapists, acupuncturists, nutritionists, Reiki therapists, biofeedback therapists, therapeutic touch specialists, and so on. Certain treatment modalities may also be specifically or nonspecifically excluded as unaccepted or experimental standards of practice.

Most HMOs contract with an average of over 2000 physicians, of which about 30% are PCPs. Typically, more than 75% of the PCPs, but significantly fewer specialists, are empanelled on HMO participation rosters.

Point-of-Service Products in HMOs

Another product in the marketplace is the point-of-service (POS) product. Here, we hear references to dual-option and triple-option packages. In a POS product, the member of the plan has a choice of provider at the time health care service is required. The member can remain within the plan's panel of providers and receive maximum coverage benefits or choose to go outside the system but pay higher out-of-pocket expenses. POS plans were offered by a majority of the HMOs in the mid 1990s and have seen stability in the marketplace, because employees want options and are willing to pay more to see the physician of their choosing. The term "dual choice" refers to an HMO-like plan with an additional indemnity plan, and "triple choice" refers to the addition of a PPO to the dual-choice option. Many POS programs require the enrollee to select a participating primary care physician to authorize referrals to any specialist. Also, preadmission certification is often required for admission to both participating and nonparticipating hospitals.

Transferring Risk to Providers in the HMO Setting

Many state laws permit the transfer of financial risk from the HMO to contracting providers selected by the HMO. In an HMO setting, the role of the primary care physician expands to primary care coordinator. There are issues of ostensible agency theory of liability on behalf of the PCP, because he or she directs patients to specialty or ancillary providers and facilities from within a restricted list of providers credentialed by another entity. Most HMOs require that the PCP guide the patient through the system and discourage the PCP from directing the patient to a provider outside the fixed panel of providers chosen by the HMO. This often places a PCP in a dilemma if he or she feels that the clinical needs of the patient may not be appropriately met by the available panel of providers and that the patient's needs might be better served outside the panel. In an HMO setting, for covered services, if the physician argues the case as patient ombudsman, the cost of the time and any resources spent to argue the case is a cost risk, because that time is uncompensated.

The use of physician extenders provides another exposure to risk. Nurse practitioners and physician assistants have been used to augment a short supply of PCPs to help provide care. On a state-by-state basis, the physician extenders may provide a great deal of care under the direct supervision and protocol of a physician, but the physician will be held accountable for their actions. Lack of supervision, improper delegation, and lack of due diligence in credentialing may lead to malpractice claims. From a patient-satisfaction standpoint, many patients resist care provided from someone who appears to have less training, and they may be quite critical in their evaluation of the care provided. They often cite beliefs that their physician might have picked up on subtle or elusive symptoms that went undiagnosed or misdiagnosed.

Another risk in HMO settings is that of utilization management decisions. Often, practitioners are genuinely concerned with keeping within normal utilization patterns. Outliers are often sanctioned financially through withhold mechanisms tied to increased utilization. When withholds do not produce corrected behavior, the practitioner may be expelled from the panel. Other times, when utilization is determined to be too low, perhaps causing jeopardy to the health of a patient, the practitioner may also be terminated from a network for a quality issue, usually patient endangerment. Within this monitored and managed utilization system, referrals and testing are controlled; this creates greater exposure to risks. This is because, when there is a less-than-favorable outcome, patients are likely to think that the decision was financially motivated, which could lead to punitive damages if proven. Cases have been tried in many jurisdictions to establish case law in these matters.

Other instances of risk may come in the number of treatments or days of hospitalization coverage one can access as a coverage limitation. Take, for example, borrowing from the area of physical therapy, a benefit limitation of "20 visits or 2 months of physical therapy treatments per acute condition." In this example, once the patient has reached a maintenance level of care and fails to continue to improve, the limitation may be declared within the first week of treatment if the patient is no longer deemed or documented to be in an acute phase of rehabilitation. Strict monitoring of utilization and documentation might well defend the position of the payer that the care no longer falls under the guidelines of what is covered. By comparison, unmanaged "indemnity" insurance policies may allow physical therapy benefits for as long as the attending physician deems necessary. Thus, the attending physician may continue to prescribe therapy without a limitation of 20 visits or two months, and the indemnity carrier must pay. This is why indemnity coverage premiums are so much higher than managed care premiums. By choosing a managed care plan, the buyer is betting against the need for coverage in excess of the stated benefit limitation.

Preferred Provider Organizations (PPOs)

PPOs are networks of providers brought together by some sort of corporation, group, or marketer to contract with providers at a discount for health care services. A PPO is usually a non-risk-bearing marketing entity that markets itself to insurance companies and self-funded ERISA (Employee Retirement Income Security Act of 1974) plans via an access fee. The network is actually rented or leased to the payer(s).

PPOs now expand their presence beyond health plan coverage purchased by individuals and employers, to workers' compensation products, motor vehicle accident reparations coverage, and unaffiliated employers involved in health care purchasing coalitions. The panel is often limited in size and may have some utilization review system associated with it. The benefit design of PPOs encourages the covered individual to choose a contracted provider to access the discounted fee-for-service reimbursement system. Typical out-of-pocket expenses, such as coinsurance and deductibles, are less expensive to the member when they utilize in-network preferred providers compared to out-of-network providers. Health care providers usually agree to accept payments below their full charges, in accordance with a contractual negotiation that pays the lesser of the provider's actual billed charges or the network's negotiated fee schedule. The provider also usually agrees not to balance-bill the patient, with the exception of deductibles, coinsurance, and noncovered services.

Risk-sharing arrangements such as capitation are not encountered in PPO plans, because most PPOs are not regulated and do not have a license to engage in the business of "insurance." (At the time of this writing, only a few states regulate and license PPOs to do business.) As such, they cannot transfer the risk of the cost of claims to the providers in the form of capitation. Instead, many times providers are offered a chance to participate in the network if they are willing to negotiate per diem or case rates with the hospital, and ancillary levels and discounted fees-for-service with the physician. Per diem and case rates are flat fees for a daily package of services or an episode of care from beginning to end, with specific inclusions and exclusions concerning payment. Most PPOs reimburse participating physicians under a contract, using a maximum allowable fee or fee cap. Services provided by PPOs vary greatly from plan to plan. Almost all PPOs contract with managed pharmacy plans, catastrophic case management firms, wellness firms, and long-term care providers.

Many PPO plans charge prospective provider applicants a credentialing fee and retain a portion of the net payment as a marketing fee or withhold. A provider who agrees to withhold with no hope of reclaiming the payment at some later date should call a withhold more appropriately a "discount." Many providers join PPOs in hopes that they will be sent patients to care for in exchange for negotiating the discount. Providers must remember that PPO participation merely makes one accessible to the stream of patients in the system. The PPO does not "send" or steer patients to any provider with any measurable significance. The essential marketing that takes place is the inclusion of the providers' names in a directory.

In most cases, PPOs utilize third-party administrators (TPAs) to process claims. TPAs are organizations outside an insuring organization that handle the administrative duties and sometimes utilization review. TPAs are used by organizations that actually fund the health care benefits but do not find it cost-effective to administer the plan themselves. Usually, when a TPA performs the utilization review and management function for a payer, the TPA is accredited through the Utilization Review Accreditation Commission (URAC). In the event that the payer is a self-funded ERISA plan, coverage decisions and utilization management may be outsourced to one of these agencies, but the self-funded plan is still held liable for the utilization/payment actions and decisions of the TPA.

As the PPO may rent or lease the network to a myriad of payers, self-insureds, and other sources of funding, the number of fee schedules, repricing schedules, and TPAs multiply. In essence, one PPO could have this scenario replicated hundreds of times, with claims going in hundreds of different directions at the same time. This brokering and marketing has led to a new phenomenon called the silent PPO.

Silent PPOs

The silent PPO can mean losses of thousands of dollars for providers. Silent PPOs are PPOs that are not really specified in a contract, but the provider is paid at a PPO-discounted fee anyway. The key to the silent PPO is that there is no valid contract to entitle the payer to any discount. Usually the patient is identified as a policyholder of an indemnity plan, because he or she prefers to have no restrictions on choice of provider. When the preverification is performed at the provider office, it is confirmed that the patient is in an indemnity plan and has 80% coverage for the first $5000 in charges and 100% thereafter. The patient is treated and released. The practice sends a bill to the insurance company, billing at full usual and customary fee, with no discount. The payer, preferring not to pay full price, calls a broker or TPA who has access to all the lists of providers and discount levels for several legitimate PPOs. The broker searches its rosters and discovers that the physician has a contract with a certain PPO that calls for a 20% discount. The broker sends a fax to the payer with that information. The payer then recalculates the physician's bill and discounts the fee 20% from the original price, citing that the reason for the lower price is because of a contract with the PPO that the physician already is contracted with. The billing and collections clerk, upon receiving the explanation of benefits (EOB) citing the discount, deducts the discount from the amount owed. Only if the staff members search the patient's intake sheet, and photocopy of the insurance card, and peruse the list of PPO participating groups, will they realize that the deduction is cited in error, as the patient is not a member of the PPO. Silent PPOs happen when TPAs obtain lists of providers who have PPO contracts in their locality. Anytime the indemnity beneficiary happens to use a physician who is a PPO provider, the TPA tries to claim the discount. While the American Medical Association (AMA) has received complaints and calls the practice fraudulent, no official investigator has done so. There is nothing illegal about this because, if the provider fights the discount, the payers simply back down and pay the difference. When the error is not caught, the TPA and the silent PPO split the profit. There is no clause on many contracts prohibiting the broker or TPA from leasing out contractual information to others.

Technically, these unfair business practices are accepted as legal as long as the physician's contract does not specifically prohibit them. Some states have taken steps to outlaw these practices, but the majority of the states look to the provider contracts to determine the appropriateness of each party's actions according to the specifications of the contract rather than create more regulation that requires additional oversight. The crux of the issue is informed contracting with the PPOs. A silent PPO will anger providers. In the long run, this issue, along with all the layering of intermediaries within the discount system, is causing the PPOs to lose popularity and transfer the growth rate to IPAs, PHOs, MSOs, and concierge practices that choose to use more prudent contracting terms rather than simply accept what the market tries to get away with.

Exclusive Provider Organizations (EPOs)

EPOs are similar in purpose and organization to PPOs, but many have the lock-in feature of HMOs. EPOs allow members to go outside the network, but the member must pay the full cost of the services. An EPO is similar to the HMO in that it uses a PCP as a gatekeeper, has a limited provider panel, uses an authorization system, and so forth. The main difference between an EPO and an HMO is that EPOs are generally nonregulated. EPOs are not allowed in some states, because they too closely resemble HMOs, but do not have to obtain and maintain a state HMO license and demonstrate fiscal soundness.

Physician Organizations

Over the last twenty years, and through the various phases of managed care that have evolved, the American physician has witnessed the evolution and demise of various organizations for the purposes of contracting with health plans and employers.

For some time, medical groups and independent practice associations (IPAs) held fast to dreams of displacing health plans only to face insolvency and an inability to manage financial risk for the cost of care to patients. Many have retrenched to their original geographic areas and have abandoned contracts that require participation in capitated plans, financial risk for drug benefits and hospital services, and abandoning other organization forms such as physician–hospital organizations (PHOs) and clinics without walls (CWWs).

As before, many independent physicians and medical groups have recently rejoined with hospitals in collaborative efforts that enable both the hospital and physicians to take advantage of gainsharing on certain care delivery projects, negotiate higher case rates from insurers and employers, and find new ways to create branded identities with their chosen hospital partners.

Before we become too philosophical, let us examine some of the organizational structures that are still popular throughout the nation. Keep in mind, however, that the old adage in this industry is "If you've seen one [IPA, PHO,

MSO], you've seen one." The other is "It's not what you call it, but instead what it's doing that makes a difference."

Independent Practice Associations (IPAs)

An IPA is a legal entity organized and directed by physicians in private practice to negotiate contracts with insurance companies on their behalf. Participating physicians are usually paid on a capitated or discounted fee-for-service basis and may also continue to care for patients not covered by the insurers with whom the IPA contracts. Perhaps the most significant function of an IPA is to exert influence on behalf of its members to counterbalance the leverage of health care insurers when done properly in the eyes of the law with regard to antitrust concerns.

IPAs can present a significant antitrust risk. Antitrust laws prohibit a range of behaviors designed to restrain trade. Among the most serious of antitrust violations are price-fixing, group boycotts, and monopolization or attempts to monopolize. Price-fixing occurs when competitors such as independent physicians and groups of physicians not economically integrated agree on a common fee schedule or discount without sharing any risk for the collaborative business activities. Group boycotts occur when a group of competitors conspire not to deal with a third party, such as a managed care organization. Monopolization or attempts to monopolize reflect an overinclusive network that controls the availability of health care services, forcing purchasers to pay higher prices. Because an IPA is often simply a loose combination of otherwise competing physicians, it can raise all three types of problems. When physicians or other providers form an IPA, careful attention must be paid to federal and state antitrust laws and their associated exceptions.

While some IPAs are simply formed as a *"commiseration club,"* others organize the delivery of care by the IPA's administrative staff. The IPA often negotiates contracts with insurance companies; assembles documentation of physician credentials, vets the credentials, and manages participation by member physicians, institutions, and services; constructs authorization and referral processes; establishes primary care provider and specialist responsibilities; disburses payment to physicians; conducts utilization review and quality assurance; and ensures the fiscal integrity of the IPA itself. Sometimes these duties are performed by a management services organization (MSO) either codeveloped or owned by the physicians or another entity.

Depending on the business knowledge of the physician and IPA administration, one generally sees variables in business and operational sophistication. IPAs are usually capable of assuming greater degrees of financial risks than individual physicians. They offer their members the advantage of strong physician leadership with the drive to develop progressively more mature organizations. IPAs wield far greater bargaining power than individual physicians or networks, and they are usually able to undertake administrative functions that reduce health care costs.

IPAs are often formed by single-specialty physicians, but many are successful as primary care only. Still others are formed as multispecialty groups that are fully inclusive of primary care, medical subspecialists, surgeons, and hospital-based physicians of all types. The best design is dictated by the market, and there truly is no single best design. One simply needs to match the model to market needs.

Physician–Hospital Organizations (PHOs)

A PHO is a joint venture between one or more hospitals and a group of physicians. It acts as the single agent for managed care contracting, presenting a united front to payers. In some cases, the PHO provides administrative services, credentials physicians, and monitors utilization. There are at least three different models of physician–hospital arrangements that are popular throughout the United States.

PHOs have been around since the early 1990s and were popular through the first term of the Clinton administration. According to the 1995 Report of the Physician Payment Review Commission, 15% to 20% of all hospitals had a PHO in 1994, and most others reported plans for a PHO. PHOs were popular because they allowed hospitals and physicians to join forces for managed care contracts, while maintaining separate lines of business.

PHOs often concurrently develop or hire a management services organization (MSO) that may be a freestanding corporation that is owned by a hospital or PHO. It is capable of providing management services to one or more medical practices and serves as a framework for joint planning and decision making for the physician medical staff as an IPA alone or together with the hospital as a PHO.

Often, the MSO employs all administrative and clerical staff and provides administrative systems, in exchange for either a flat fee or a set percentage of group revenues.

Another model seen frequently in the 1990s tied to many not-for-profit hospitals was the foundation-model PHO. The foundation model was a corporation, usually nonprofit, that was either a subsidiary of a hospital or an affiliate with a common parent organization. The foundation owned and operated medical practices, including facilities, equipment, and supplies. The foundation employed all nonphysician personnel and contracted with a physician-owned entity such as the IPA to provide medical services for the practice.

Still another model, the integrated health organization (IHO) is a single legal entity with three subsidiaries: a hospital corporation, a medical services corporation, and an educational and research foundation. Typically, the IHO and its subsidiaries are all tax exempt and nonprofit. The medical subsidiary has a physician-controlled board and employs physicians to provide patient services.

A key feature of many PHOs is that the PHO attempts to align the interests of hospitals and physicians, but it does not always turn out that way.

Prominent models that have seen success throughout the nation are few and far between. While the two parties can exert greater bargaining leverage and respond to purchaser preferences for a single, bundled price, many are not actually able to collaboratively decide how to divide the pie. This becomes even more difficult when the hospital is not-for-profit and the physicians are either unorganized into an IPA or are in a for-profit equity-model IPA. The difficulty arises because of the inurement or private benefit issues that arise when two disparate entities are paired together in a PHO. The doctors do a good job, offer discounts, act as conscientious team players working diligently to manage utilization, and work efficiently, only to be told that any margins realized need to stay with the PHO and not be distributed to the physicians. Other issues arise with percentage of ownership and voting power. Often, the hospital requires that it be majority owner of the PHO, as opposed to an equal partner.

To be seen as cost-effective by purchasers, the PHO must have active utilization management, sophisticated information systems, and intensive involvement of physicians in developing standards of care. Many PHOs across the country have never developed this infrastructure.

To avoid concerns of antitrust, the PHO must entail significant elements of risk sharing for the both parties. Because of lack of infrastructure and agreement on operations and distributions, many PHOs fell apart long before the ink was dry on the antitrust compliance initiatives and had to be dismantled or were abandoned.

A Google search of the term "Physician Hospital Organization" yields greater than 40 million hits on the term, many of which are Web sites of existing PHOs, while some lead nowhere. The PHO structure has been all but abandoned in some markets, while others still function and create margins within the contracts they hold with payers. In the new era of consumerism, the PHO that keeps matching the model to the market will find ways to develop pricing transparency, a cobranded name identity with their hospital partner, and loyalty products and service lines that will engage their community regardless of any payer antics to create narrow networks and create acrimony between select hospitals and groups of physicians.

Management Services Organizations (MSOs)

MSOs provide a means for community physicians to establish relationships with organizations planning to develop integrated delivery systems. A properly managed MSO focuses on managing and retaining covered lives for its partner PHO or IPA. The crucial areas of MSO development, specifically, affiliation relationships, capital acquisition, and implementation, can make or break an MSO's success within the world of managed care contracting and operations.

MSOs are most valuable if they are not viewed as stand-alone moneymakers but as a way to increase a health care system's ability to contract for covered lives by tying a greater number of physicians to the system and thereby increasing patient volume. Revenue generated by additional managed care contracts far outweighs any attempt to create a hospital-based MSO that is a vendor of services in competition with for-profit physician practice management companies. That may have been popular in the early 1990s, but has since been abandoned, as hospital-based MSOs that attempted to purchase physician practices, employ the physicians, and control their admissions and utilization habits failed miserably in most parts of the country.

MSO affiliations are best accomplished when spearheaded by groups of savvy physicians who perceive a need to organize and affiliate. Strong physician interest, trust, and leadership can be far more effective catalysts for integration than any combination of economic enticements or fancy and complicated implementation plans. Physician leadership within the management of the group is the most significant success element of the MSO model—particularly if the MSO is owned and governed by physicians. Economic and implementation details often are less important to physicians contemplating affiliation than the credibility and reputation of their prospective partners. It takes time to build trust and agree on a shared vision, to outline guiding principles, and to mutually agree on goals and objectives. The organization and community physicians must share definite economic incentives.

In order to run a successful MSO, the MSO needs operating capital. Those organizations that were leadership rich but cash poor never really made it. Too often, new MSO management and governance focus only on cost. But it is the revenue earned and its equitable division among the partners that ultimately determine the enterprise's success or failure. Revenue distribution and payment rates for institutional services were not always properly compared to the market rates, and shared risk arrangements among the parties were often not spelled out in enough detail. Many physician organizations failed to plan for excess loss in capitated deals, and the capital went away in a few short months. Without necessary reinsurance, there was no money left to pay MSO staff or to pay physicians, and many MSOs deteriorated to a state of insolvency and were unable to complete the initial terms of contracts they had negotiated with large payers in their communities.

Today, the market has noticed a resurgence of IPAs, PHOs, and MSOs, but with a different agenda that often does not include capitation. This may be shortsighted, but if the infrastructure can be developed properly and adequate capitalization achieved, there may be creative ways that these organizations may see a renaissance under the consumer driven health plan system.

It is interesting that while many MSOs, IPAs, and PHOs have gone dormant, faced demise and bankruptcy, or been abandoned and their corporations ended, some are still functioning profitably, contracting, and finding new ways to meet the marketplace. In addition, these models are being adapted for the new trend in medical tourism by organized medical providers abroad. As a consultant, I am engaged by several of these international provider networks, and though they may not entertain capitation, they will aspire to the quality metrics, disease management, and continuity of care that these organizational structures can provide, as well as collectively contract with health plans and employers with a branded identity and operational infrastructure.

It would be remiss of me to not repeat that in America the group may not engage in certain activities that could be construed as anticompetitive behavior, unless the group receives advice from a competent health law attorney that they have the right conditions to engage in these activities for the purpose of contracting with payers. This is not always the same in foreign integrated delivery systems, where the laws may be different with regards to both anticompetitive behaviors, as set forth in U.S. laws, and inurement and private benefit issues, in conformity with U.S. tax laws when not-for-profit and for-profit entities work collaboratively.

Chapter 3

All-Products Contracts

All-products contracts are a problem for health care providers and a solution for managed care health plans and preferred provider organization (PPO) networks. Historically, most insurers offered a limited menu of flavors: traditional fee-for-service/indemnity, preferred provider (discounted fee-for-service) and health maintenance organization (HMO), and before managed care became widespread many physicians signed up with every plan that came their way.

Managed care plans cannot sell policies without having a sufficient number and variety of physicians under contract to meet the needs of subscribers. While developing this network the provider really has leverage, as the plan cannot go to market with a certificate of authority until it can prove to regulators that it has an appropriate group of credentialed physicians and other health care providers sufficient to meet the need of its subscribers in the network. Without this group of providers empanelled, it would be difficult for the plan to require the use of the in-network (INET) provider roster in order to access prenegotiated discounts and create a disincentive to avoid the use of out-of-network (ONET) providers who have not agreed by contract to uphold health plan utilization and quality parameters and performance requirements. Once a network is in place, the only real leverage or power an individual physician or hospital may have in negotiations with a managed care company is the power to say "no" to contract terms that are unacceptable for clinical, financial, or other market-driven reasons. The insurance and payer industries recognize this power and have begun to implement and enforce "all-products" clauses, a controversial technique to limit providers' ability to pick and choose whether to participate in the many types of plans each company offers.

All-Products Language Example

The language often appears in contracts as follows:

> Health Plan contracts directly or indirectly with Payers, employers, individuals, insurers, sponsors and others, to provide, insure, arrange for or administer the provision of Covered Services.

First, what exactly does this recital mean to contract "directly or indirectly"? If one has a direct contract and there is a breach of any materiality, then the parties will likely have standing in order to cite the breach and request remedy. What about in the case of an indirect contract? What is an indirect contract, anyway? (Only the author of the contract knows for sure!) Take a moment to pull out any number of sample contracts from your files and see if this language or something similar is not present. Unless you have taken steps to eliminate this, it is lurking somewhere in there.

Second, who are all these entities? "Payers" generally means those who pay claims. Employers and individuals are self-explanatory, right? If one purchases an individual health care coverage plan, it might not be the same benefit levels as the group up the road at the local hardware store, and it might not cover the same service lines or supplies, drugs, and equipment, but the card has the logo on it. Employers and unions both often either sponsor ERISA (Employee Retirement Income Security Act of 1974) plans with totally different rules than "insurance" or "health plans" unless they are functioning in one state or are so small that paying premiums is more prudent than establishing their own self-funded health care coverage arrangement through ERISA or a self-insured program under a certificate from the state.

Sponsors can be PPOs, health care purchasing coalitions, and so forth. Chambers of commerce have been known to "sponsor" plans and establish virtual groups through membership channels in some communities.

Third, who are these "others"? How many "others" are there? How will you recognize them? Do you already have contracts with them under other agreements? If so, which ones will access under this contract exclusively, and how will you control the potential conflict in rates and pricing? Also, if they already access through a different program or contract, in the event of a breach which contract will you argue the breach? If that is not enough to dizzy you, if you cancel one contract because of a bad actor payer, can they come back under a different contract and still access a discount even though you do not want them as a business associate anymore? This can be reminiscent of playing "Whac-a-Mole," the popular arcade redemption game (Aaron Fechter, Creative Engineering, Inc., 1971). In Whac-a-Mole, once the game starts, the moles will begin to pop up from their holes at random. The object of the game is to force the individual moles back into their holes by hitting them directly on the head with the mallet, thereby adding to the player's score. If the player does not strike a mole within a certain time or with enough force, it will eventually sink back into its hole with no score. Although gameplay starts out slow enough for most people to hit all of the moles that rise, it gradually increases in speed, with each mole spending less time above the hole and with more moles outside of their holes at the same time. After a designated time limit, the game ends, regardless of the skill of the player. The final score is based upon the number of moles that the player struck. I am sure you get the picture, and at the next carnival or fair you attend, you will never look at that game the same! I am a firm believer that most managed care administrators and contract negotiators should have one of these games in their office just like many executives have little putting greens for stress relief!

The next part of the sentence discusses "*to provide, insure, arrange for or administer.*" These words each have meaning in the context of "all-product" contracts.

For example: to "provide" refers to HMO arrangements only whereby both the provision of services and the financial exposure protection is delivered in one arrangement as part of the coverage for which the premium is paid.

To insure refers to "insurance" or indemnity coverage, as compared with a health plan or HMO arrangement where indemnification is not always offered and the need for appropriate medically necessary services may exceed the defined benefit levels for services that are considered "covered" under the policy. Those services may be covered only to a specific benefit level stipulated in the summary plan description (SPD) or evidence of coverage (EOC), and exhaustion of those benefits might not get the person to a health status where he or she is "made whole." Therein lies the main difference between HMO and "insurance." One makes the claimant "whole," while the other only provides benefits up to a specific benefit level, and the indemnification must come from the claimant for any remaining coverage necessary to get to the point of maximum medical improvement (MMI).

To arrange for or administer implies access by third-party administrators, employee benefits administrators, PPOs, or administrative service organizations. These entities are not responsible for the cost of claims, only their administration.

Incongruence and Inconsistency

As one can imagine, these payment sources all have different regulatory requirements, participation schemes, utilization profiles, and access habits. To commingle them all in one contract with one set of rules of engagement is poor practice on the part of the provider, but this sometimes is done with full consideration as part of a business strategy when there is no alternative means to be included into the panel of participating providers. Usually, these contracts default to the most stringent set of rules of the bunch, those of the regulated HMO requirements. Many HMO regulations, such as plan insolvency and patient indemnification rules, are not seen in any of the other arrangements, but commingling these payers means that those who did not pay for the financial protection through the HMO arrangement obtain similar discounts and courtesies just for being on the paper with the HMO contract.

Sitting in the concierge lounge of the Marriott Hotel in East Lansing, Michigan, one day, I overheard a contracting representative from a large national health plan outlining a strategy to force the all-products issue on local providers by saying that if they would not take their worst-paying business, they could not have any of it. I can imagine that this conversation is repeated routinely at many health plans, as it is a common tact for many plans who want to increase their revenue portfolios and charge a fee to those other payers who would otherwise have to build their own at a much greater expense than the access fees exchanged for network "leasing" of existing panels of providers who have agreed to discounts off their fees and whose credentials have been vetted in accordance with network accreditation standards.

This aggressive use of all-products clauses in managed care participation agreements is becoming the focus of increased scrutiny as insurers use them more coercively to build and retain their physician networks across product lines. Do not think for a minute that the conception of consumer driven health plan (CDHP) products was not done with this clause in mind, as the health plans frequently market on their Web sites that a participant will not have to pay any more than an HMO or PPO preferred rate, and that, just like their PPO and HMO counterparts, the Web sites tout that the participant will not have to pay any monies until after adjudication of the claim.

These clauses, which require providers to accept all present and future insurance products and payment methods or "funding methods," as CDHPs are commonly referred to in this argument, are offered by a particular insurer as a condition of participating in any of the insurer's products and have drawn fire on a national scale. A number of states have outlawed them, and authorities have insisted that one national insurer drop the provisions as a condition of settling litigation. The American Medical Association (AMA) has developed a position statement against the practice of requiring all-products clauses in contracts, and the Department of Justice (DOJ) has realized that this is one of many factors that can lead to an "uneven playing field" in bargaining power between individual providers, who are prohibited from acting collectively by the antitrust laws, and large insurers, who by sheer numbers of subscribers control patients' access to health care and control health care providers' access to patients. This problem is examined under the concept of monopsony in certain markets. Monopsony can be most simplistically described as when the buyer sets pricing instead of the seller, and when, but for access to customers through this one essential market force, there would be no other business to be had that would be significant to sustain the life of the business otherwise. Monopsony power is the power a dominant purchaser has to artificially drive down prices for the purchase of goods or services when negotiating with sellers that wield less bargaining power. A dominant health insurer may be in a position to set terms of participation for physicians that those physicians would be commercially unable to reject without turning away a large percentage of their patient base. The Department of Justice has agreed that it will investigate accusations of this power play in health care and did so in Dallas, Texas, in the 1990s when Aetna and Prudential were about to merge in that market. They have also investigated other situations across the nation and have forced several deals to be redesigned in order to move forward. Your attorney will be familiar with this concept, because it has been around for as long as the Sherman and Clayton Acts, but has newfound meaning in the face of all-products clauses in managed care participation agreements. Health insurance contracts have routinely included all-products clauses with little attention being directed to their potential anticompetitive effect until recent years. These contractual provisions may be used to force providers to contract with networks that include plans that may be unacceptable on a stand-alone basis, not just because of low reimbursements, but also because of poor financial risk, limited significant service line coverage exclusions, burdensome referral requirements, limited drug formularies, or previous relationships that involve a history of the payer as a "bad actor."

In addition to the power play created with monopsony, there is a distinct effect on the marketplace because all-products clauses can distort the market for physician services if the physician or hospital declines the all-products arrangement or is forced to close its doors, which may result in reduced patient access to the health care providers of their choice. This direct effect on the market is where the DOJ draws the line.

A health plan with monopsony power might violate the federal antitrust laws if it engages in activity that makes it more difficult for providers to abandon business dealings with that insurer in favor of providing services to competing insurers, or if it engages in actions that serve to protect and maintain the insurer's monopsony power. Forensic economists are often called in to evaluate the market conditions to determine if the health plan's contractual requirements or actions would violate Section 1 of the Sherman Antitrust Act, unless the insurer could demonstrate that they resulted in procompetitive effects or increased efficiencies. In addition, these activities may violate Section 2 of the Sherman Antitrust Act if they constitute predatory conduct.

Medicare and Medicaid Concerns

If the contract also includes Medicare Advantage or Medicaid program participation, the plan might incur potential violation of the Medicare and Medicaid antikickback law by demanding a price concession in exchange for access to other lines of business, because of the potential for interpretation as an inducement in exchange for referring any business reimbursable under the Medicare or Medicaid systems. The Office of Inspector General (OIG) has warned managed care companies that, by forcing physicians to provide services at below-market rates in exchange for access to their other health care programs, those compulsory discounts may be the equivalent of the extortion of prohibited kickbacks which may result in civil and criminal penalties. It also means that the government is probably not getting the best rate from the provider. In the compliance guidance for Medicare + Choice organizations published on November 15, 1999, the OIG stated:

> We are concerned that a managed care organization or contractor may offer (or be offered) a reduced rate for its items or services in the federal capitated arrangement in order to have the opportunity to participate in other product lines that do not have stringent payment or utilization constraints. This practice is a form of a practice known as "swapping," in the case of managed care arrangements, low capitation rates could be traded for access for additional fee-for-service lines of business. We are concerned when these discounts are in exchange for access to fee-for-service lines of business, where there is an incentive to overutilize services provided to federal health care program beneficiaries.

State regulators and legislatures are beginning to take notice of the impact of all-products clauses. In 1998, Nevada's Commissioner of Insurance declared all-products clauses to be a violation of the state Unfair Trade Practices Act, which prohibits acts of boycott, coercion, or intimidation that would result in the unreasonable restraint of any business of insurance. According to the commissioner, the coercion occurs when the insurer cancels the provider's PPO contract as a consequence of his not signing an HMO contract. Such termination unfairly prevents the provider from continuing to furnish PPO discounted medical care to the insured marketplace, which restrains the business of insurance.

Kentucky's General Assembly passed legislation outlawing all-products clauses. Virginia's governor signed a bill allowing health care providers to refuse to participate in an insurer's other products or plans without affecting the provider's status as a member in the plans in which he or she wished to participate, effective July 1, 2000. Responding to efforts from the physician community, including one dermatologist who held a symbolic public burning of his HMO contracts, Maryland's legislature has enacted a similar statute, which is awaiting the signature of the governor. Texas has also seen activity on this front in a 1998 lawsuit against Aetna U.S. Healthcare for various abusive practices. Among the terms of the settlement is a promise by Aetna U.S. Healthcare to discontinue using an all-products clause and to give physicians the option to care for patients who are enrolled in some or all of Aetna products.

Chapter 4

Dealing with Self-Funded ERISA Payers in Managed Care: Employee Retirement Income Security Act (ERISA) of 1974

ERISA has been around for more than 30 years, and the problems with health benefit administration have been around for just as long. When an employer has several hundred employees working in multiple states or countries, it is difficult to administrate health benefit plans in accordance with each state's regulations. Therefore, those employers (most in the Fortune 1000 category) opt to establish an ERISA health benefit plan for their eligible employees and dependents that permits them to be preempted from state-by-state insurance laws in favor of Department of Labor (DOL) regulations.

The Department of Labor released the first regulations governing claims procedures in 1977. In the 1990s, the DOL looked at regulatory changes that would give claimants more rights, better notice, and quicker turnaround on decisions under managed care. In 1997, an advisory panel established by the administration recommended certain patient protections that were enacted into current law. The Clinton administration then ordered federal agencies with control over ERISA employer-sponsored health benefit plans to enforce patient protections to the greatest extent possible under current law. This has had an excellent financial impact for those who are aware of the changes and how they affect denials and appeals activities, and the arguments raised under those denials. In my case, it has benefitted my clients greatly to have insight into exactly how to wage these little battles in a way that most often has been met with success and full payment of benefits due under the plan.

In January 2003, the Department of Labor made all ERISA plans subject to new claims regulations. (This is available for review in the *Federal Register,* Tuesday, November 21, 2000, Vol. 65, No. 225, pages 70246–70271. The citation for the effective date of the regulation is *Federal Register,* Monday, July 9, 2001, Vol. 66, No. 131, pages 35886–35888.)

Plans to Which These Claims Procedures Apply

The new claims procedures apply to all private employer-sponsored group health plans regulated under ERISA, regardless of the size of the employer's workforce. This should make it easier for provider administrative staff to work with, since the rules apply to all types of ERISA plans, whether fully insured or self-funded.

ERISA does not cover plans sponsored by state or local government entities (for example, plans sponsored by the State of Washington or the City of New York) or so-called "church plans," plans sponsored by religious organizations that meet certain IRS requirements. In addition, individual or other nongroup plans are not subject to ERISA. In order for you as a reader to discern which plans under ERISA access your services under preferred provider organization (PPO) or health maintenance organization (HMO) networks, simply ask for a list from the provider relations department or claims management department from the health plan in question. They must know this in order to administrate claims properly. Contrary to popular myth, it is not a mystery.

Issues outside the ERISA Claims Rules

The daunting task as a revenue manager at the provider billing and collections office, as well as for contractors, is that there are some very specific areas to which the ERISA claims regulations do not apply. These include:

■ Decisions regarding eligibility for benefits (whether the person is a current member of the plan and eligible for all benefits listed in the Summary Plan Description [SPD]).

■ Requests for preapproval where the plan does not require it—for example, a patient does not need to seek preapproval for surgery (however expensive) in order to have the surgery covered if the plan does not require preapproval. This presents a problem in PPO and HMO network agreements when the contract requires preapproval of the HMO or PPO, but the preapproval is not acknowledged or honored by the ERISA payer within the network. It creates a dilemma with the legal concept of promissory estoppels if the contractor for the provider requires by contract that the payer honor all preapprovals it issues once the case has commenced. This is because, even though the plan may agree to the provision to honor those approvals, the ERISA payer can and will likely disavow responsibility for such guarantees, since to do so may not be a requirement under the plan description. This frustration that arises for contractors and revenue management staff is described in legal terms as the concept of Privity of Contract. You do not have a contract with the ERISA payer in most cases, but only with the HMO, PPO, administrative services organization (ASO), or third-party administrator (TPA) that has included them in their network access agreements. Therefore, you may not be able to enforce your contract with the ERISA plan, but may be limited only to enforce your contract with the network, which may not have the leverage or power to cause the ERISA payer to act in accordance with the contract you negotiated. While there are certain very specific contracting provisions to work through this, you may not always have the leverage to get them included into your contract and will need the assistance of a skilled attorney or a cum laude diploma from the *School of Hard Knocks* to effect a good work around. I offer these in a very focused class several times each year.

■ Casual inquiries about whether a benefit is covered—for example, if a doctor asks the plan whether a treatment like Botox® for a therapeutic purpose might be covered, the ERISA payer's response is not subject to these regulations.

■ Time frames in which a claim has to be paid—however, this will be addressed in more detail later.

■ Decisions by an HMO or PPO network pharmacist or pharmacy benefit manager (PBM) or specialty pharmacy plan (SPP) regarding coverage for prescription drugs that ERISA payers have discretion to mandate whether and to what extent denials would be covered under the rules.

Regulation Expands Claimants' Rights and Access to Information

The revised ERISA regulations greatly expand the information that a claimant can receive from a health plan. This reduces some of the frustration that was typical of years prior, where everything seemed to be secret and accessing useful information for the purpose of denials, appeals, and case management was essentially unavailable to providers or plan participants. The summary of the regulations contains a detailed list and explanation of the documentation that claimants must receive or can request from their health plans.

As a best practice, this should be requested by the contract analyst for the five to ten ERISA employer-sponsored plans having the greatest impact on revenues. From a practical standpoint, every time I suggest this in a training session or coaching session with contract analyst, I meet with a response that the employer information is missing or unavailable. This little data detail is crucial to contract analysts for many reasons, one of which is to determine the tendency for denials and the potential success for appeals, and also for the purpose of revenue modeling. Suffice it to say, if your best reimbursement margins are for procedures that you offer and have contracted for through an HMO or PPO, but which are not covered by the top five to ten employers in your service area who sponsor ERISA benefit plans, the margins are illusory, and the modeling will be flawed if tied to projected utilization when assessing the potential profitability from a particular contract. It can be very frustrating if your negotiation yields a great rate for services for which a large number of your plan participants have no coverage, and therefore have no expectation of plan reimbursement.

Plan Participants' Right to Sue under ERISA

The 2003 regulations allow claimants to sue their plan sponsor in federal court faster. One goal in developing new regulations was to provide improved access for claimants to get to the external review process or to federal court. Both self-insured and fully insured plans can be sued under ERISA. The snag here is that in most cases, the claimant has to pay as they go, and often may not work with an attorney on a contingency basis. It also means that they must sue their employer. These three details often serve as a deterrent for most claimants.

Generally, they must also exhaust all administrative processes. This alone can be frustrating and daunting, as no one generally knows what "all" really means for all practical intents and purposes. In fact, the subject of exhaustion of internal process has been controversial. Under the final rule, claimants (or their *authorized representatives*) can go directly to external review or to court without exhausting the internal claims process if the plan has failed to comply with the rule's requirements. This again creates a dilemma for the contractor, as in many cases, the contract terms stipulate that this exhaustion is a requirement for a matter to be set for dispute resolution by the provider. In cases where the provider has been officially designated in writing as the authorized representative of the plan participant, this creates a further dilemma if the provider contract stipulates that all administrative processes must be exhausted, and yet, when stepping in the shoes of the participant, the authorized representative is not required to do so to appeal plan decisions on behalf of the participant. Ask your attorney if it would be wise to apply special allowances and set aside the requirement for exhaustion of all administrative remedies in matters involving ERISA plan participants in your contracts, especially when you are designated in writing as the authorized representative of the plan participant in the case of denials and appeals or benefit determinations and requesting access to specific details in the summary plan description.

Interpretive guidance from DOL clarified that this exception to the exhaustion rule would only apply if the plan failed to follow the plan rules. As discussed above, unless you are designated as the authorized representative, you will not know what those rules are or were at the time the claim was incurred, and you will not have the right to request this information without such designation. The failure must be substantial and must adversely affect the claimant's individual rights to receive coverage or reimbursement from plan funds. Keep in mind that, if a plan can rectify its failure to follow the rules in the appeal process, the claimant or authorized representative has to proceed with the internal process before going to federal court. When the courts review a challenge to the plan's actions, the interpretive guidance published states that the courts should generally defer to the plan's judgment as to whether a violation was substantial. In this way, the interpretive guidance appears to give the plan the benefit of the doubt. My advice is this: establish and follow a strategic work plan when acting as authorized representative. Determine a dollar threshold above which you will act on claims, and develop a list of those egregious violations where litigation or formal dispute or external review might be considered as an option, and establish a secondary list of those violations that should be pursued through internal processes. Situations that arise that do not fall into either category should be reviewed to determine if they are insufficient to produce much of a financial impact and warrant further action. Make sure that you do track their frequency to improve your knowledge base and know the root cause of the problem. If possible and worthwhile, refine your contract language to address them in the future, and establish materiality to be reported as a data element in your payer report cards.

Preemption and Interaction of ERISA with State Law

Many physicians and their staff are unfamiliar with how ERISA's relationship to state law works. Often, they are told, "We are an ERISA plan, and we do not have to follow state law." That is not always such a simple case, and definitely not as simple as the plan might try to lead a physician or revenue management staffer to believe. Under the final claims rule, ERISA is considered the floor for regulation. States can provide greater rights for members of plans subject to state laws—that is, fully insured plans—to the extent that such laws do not conflict with ERISA's claims rules and remedial scheme. This generally occurs in matters involving:

- *Formulary*—Inclusions and exclusions must be specified in the plan documents including matters related to off-label restrictions, if any.
- *Preexisting conditions*—Any exclusions must be specifically detailed in plan documents. (See 29 CFR § 2590.701-3(e) for prescribed requirements.)
- *State mandated benefits*—Any exceptions to state law must be specifically cited in plan documents.
- *Medical necessity*—Any exceptions to state law must be specifically cited in plan documents.
- *Prudent layperson issues and the definition of emergency*—Definition must be specifically cited in plan documents.

While it is generally accepted that self-funded ERISA plans are never subject to state regulation, if there is (1) no additional benefit to the ERISA participant, (2) no conflict in the plan documents, and (3) if the state has attempted to regulate insurance on the point in question, the ERISA payer may have to adhere to state law and may not be able to substantiate their right to preempt state laws. While the matter is for an experienced lawyer to sort out, contract analysts and revenue management staff should never simply assume that the two do not intersect at some points. To facilitate your review and research, direct your general counsel to review 20 USC 1132 (c)(1)(B) to guide you on how to access plan documents as an authorized representative to research if there is a conflict as mentioned in (2) above. Also, see 29 CFR 2560.503-1(K)(1) which states that "Nothing in this section shall be construed to supersede any State law that regulates insurance, except to the extent that such law prevents the application of this section (claim procedure)."

Key Concept: If a state seeks to regulate claims payment and is not more restrictive, then state law may apply.

Tip

As best practices,

1. Keep abreast of legislative changes in your service area for recently enacted updates to patient protection acts enacted by your state and those states that may be nearby and in your service area.
2. Create a plan data dictionary that highlights which ERISA plans do not follow those patient protection acts by specific exclusion, to save you time in future denials and appeals with these plans.
3. Keep it up to date on an intranet where anyone coming into contact with this information can update the dictionary with new findings.
4. Do not accept oral or written plan denials as the final word where you have not personally verified the written summary plan description (SPD) that was in effect on the date of service to determine if there was indeed a plan conflict that limited application of the benefits under the patient protection act(s).

ERISA and State External Review Laws

While these regulations provide no new federal external review protections, they do clarify that states' internal and external review laws are NOT preempted and are valid unless they conflict with the regulations' requirements or ERISA's corrective requirements. This interpretation of ERISA's preemption of state external review laws was generally validated by the Supreme Court in its decision in *Rush Prudential HMO, Inc. v. Moran*. In *Rush*, the court held that ERISA did not preempt Illinois's external review law. States can add protections, but states cannot do away with a claimant's federal right to an internal appeal or to the right to sue under ERISA.

Timing of Decisions on Claims and Appeals

ERISA regulations have very specific requirements that plans must follow in notifying a claimant of a denial. Since plans are required to answer urgent care claims within 72 hours, if plans do not meet that time frame, the claimant might investigate a temporary restraining order or preliminary injunction through their attorney. That is between the plan and the participant, but knowledge of this as an option to discuss with the patient in limited circumstances would be handy for a social worker to possess, combined with familiarity with attorneys skilled in this body of law that can assist the patient if the matter warrants and is requested by the patient.

The Role of the Authorized Representative

As discussed previously, the authorized representative is able to *step in the shoes of* the plan participant or claimant or beneficiary. In ERISA, the term "beneficiary" means a person designated by a participant, or by the terms of an employee benefit plan, who is or may become entitled to a benefit thereunder. (29 U.S.C. 1002 (7)(8)). Only the authorized representative can discuss matters with the plan administrator or its agent. The ERISA plan administrator or its agent does not owe any duty to discuss claims, benefits, short paid claims, etc., with someone not designated as such. Plans can prescribe specific procedures a claimant must follow or forms a claimant must submit to name a representative. Keep in mind that these specifics are dictated by the ERISA plan and are not always consistent with ASO or TPA procedures (and may actually be simpler).

This means that, once authorized in writing, a case worker, revenue management staffer, or other person may assist the plan participant in exercising their rights and privileges under the plan.

Once named the authorized representative, that individual has all rights, including the notice rights, so the patient may not receive notice directly from the plan. Physicians or their staff must be appointed as the authorized representative to merely speak to the plan about denials and appeals. See the model letter (Figure 4.1) for an example of the text for such a letter.

In order to ensure that the patient receives all information from the plan, the authorized representative should write to the plan to request that all notices go to the patient as well as the authorized representative. Once that request has been sent, the plan administrator has 30 days to comply with the request, or fines accumulate at the rate of $110 per day, payable to the authorized representative. For more information on this, see 20 USC 1132 (c)(1)(B) and ask your attorney for guidance. If the plan administrator does not comply, at the discretion of the court, the plan administrator may be personally liable for up to $100/day to the plaintiff (or his or her authorized representative) until he complies (29 USC 1132(c)(1)(B) or (c)(3)). This is not a penalty, but "statutory damages."

ERISA AUTHORIZATION

Name of Patient:

Subscriber Identification Number:

Group Number:

For good and valuable consideration, I _____, do hereby designate, authorize, and convey to _____ to the full extent permissible under law and under any applicable insurance policy and/or employee health care benefit plan: (a) the right and ability to act on my behalf in connection with any claim, right, or choice in action that I may have under such insurance policy and/or any employee health care benefit plan; and (b) the right and ability to act on my behalf to pursue such claim, right, or choice in action in connection with said insurance policy and/or employee health care benefit plan (including, but not limited to, the right to act in my behalf in respect to an employee health care benefit plan governed by the provisions of the Employee Retirement Income Security Act of 1974 as provided in 29 CFR §2560.5031(b)(4)) with respect to any medical or other health care expense incurred as a result of the services I received from the above-named doctor and, to the extent permissible under the law, to claim on my behalf, such medical or other health care service benefits, insurance, or health care benefit plan reimbursement and any other applicable remedy.

_____
Patient's Signature   Date

Note: It is also important to check with the plan to determine if it has its own authorization form for enrollee/beneficiary use.

Figure 4.1   An ERISA authorization letter.

Form **5500** Department of the Treasury Internal Revenue Service Department of Labor Employee Benefits Security Administration Pension Benefit Guaranty Corporation	**Annual Return/Report of Employee Benefit Plan** **This form is required to be filed under sections 104 and 4065 of the Employee Retirement Income Security Act of 1974 (ERISA) and sections 6039D, 6047(e), 6057(b), and 6058(a) of the Internal Revenue Code (the Code).** **Complete all entries in accordance with the instructions to the Form 5500.**	Official Use Only OMB Nos. 1210 - 0110 1210 - 0089 **2006** **This Form is Open to Public Inspection**

Part I | **Annual Report Identification Information**

For the calendar plan year 2006 or fiscal plan year beginning January 01, 2006, **and ending** December 31, 2006

A This return/report is for:
  (1) ☐ a multiemployer plan;
  (2) ☒ a single-employer plan (other than a multiple-employer plan);
  (3) ☐ a multiple-employer plan;
  (4) ☐ a DFE (specify)

B This return/report is:
  (1) ☐ the first return/report filed for the plan;
  (2) ☐ the amended return/report;
  (3) ☐ the final return/report filed for the plan;
  (4) ☐ a short plan year return/report (less than 12 months).

C If the plan is a collectively-bargained plan, check here ☐

D If you filed for an extension of time to file, check the box and attach a copy of the extension application ☐

Part II | **Basic Plan Information -- enter all requested information.**

1a Name of plan

MARRIOTT INTERNATIONAL, INC. MEDICAL BENEFITS PLAN

1b Three-digit plan number (PN) | 501

1c Effective date of plan (mo., day, yr.)
October 08, 1993

2a Plan sponsor's name and address (employer, if for a single-employer plan)
(Address should include room or suite no.)

MARRIOTT INTERNATIONAL, INC.
1 MARRIOTT DRIVE, DEPT 52-935.62
WASHINGTON, DC 20058-

2b Employer Identification Number (EIN)
52-2055918

2c Sponsor's telephone number
301-380-6073

2d Business code (see instructions)
721110

Caution: A penalty for the late or incomplete filing of this return/report will be assessed unless reasonable cause is established

---

Figure 4.2   Form 5500. Annual return/report of employee benefit plan.

The request must be addressed to "Plan Administrator," and not the PPO, ASO, TPA, or other entity. The IRS Form 5500 (Figure 4.2) details the name, address, and telephone number of the plan administrator to facilitate this communication.

The maximum daily penalty was increased in 1997 to $110, per 29 CFR 2575.502c-3. It may have been raised since then. Always have your attorney check to be sure.

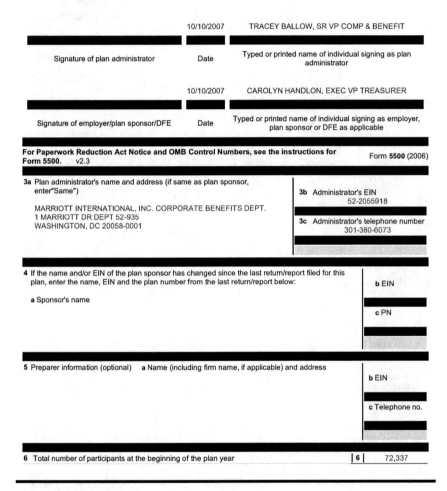

Under penalties of perjury and other penalties set forth in the instructions, I declare that I have examined this return/report, including accompanying schedules, statements and attachments, and to the best of my knowledge and belief, it is true, correct, and complete.

	10/10/2007	TRACEY BALLOW, SR VP COMP & BENEFIT
Signature of plan administrator	Date	Typed or printed name of individual signing as plan administrator
	10/10/2007	CAROLYN HANDLON, EXEC VP TREASURER
Signature of employer/plan sponsor/DFE	Date	Typed or printed name of individual signing as employer, plan sponsor or DFE as applicable

For Paperwork Reduction Act Notice and OMB Control Numbers, see the instructions for Form 5500. v2.3

Form **5500** (2006)

3a Plan administrator's name and address (if same as plan sponsor, enter"Same")

MARRIOTT INTERNATIONAL, INC. CORPORATE BENEFITS DEPT.
1 MARRIOTT DR DEPT 52-935
WASHINGTON, DC 20058-0001

3b Administrator's EIN
52-2055918

3c Administrator's telephone number
301-380-6073

4 If the name and/or EIN of the plan sponsor has changed since the last return/report filed for this plan, enter the name, EIN and the plan number from the last return/report below:

a Sponsor's name

b EIN

c PN

5 Preparer information (optional)   **a** Name (including firm name, if applicable) and address

b EIN

c Telephone no.

6 Total number of participants at the beginning of the plan year | **6** | 72,337

Figure 4.2   (continued)

ERISA Myths and Realities

How can a provider become an authorized representative under ERISA to appeal on member's behalf? Does this provider have to be a participating provider with a PPO contract or HMO contract with the plan, network, or TPA?

a Active participants	a		70,870
b Retired or separated participants receiving benefits	b		1,390
c Other retired or separated participants entitled to future benefits	c		
d Subtotal. Add lines **7a, 7b,** and **7c**	d		72,260
e Deceased participants whose beneficiaries are receiving or are entitled to receive benefits	e		
f Total. Add lines **7d** and **7e**	f		
g Number of participants with account balances as of the end of the plan year (only defined contribution plans complete this item)	g		
h Number of participants that terminated employment during the plan year with accrued benefits that were less than 100% vested	h		
i If any participant(s) separated from service with a deferred vested benefit, enter the number of separated participants required to be reported on a Schedule SSA (Form 5500)	i		

8 Benefits provided under the plan (complete 8a through 8c, as applicable)

a ☐ Pension benefits (check this box if the plan provides pension benefits and enter the applicable pension feature codes from the List of Plan Characteristics Codes (printed in the instructions)):

b ☒ Welfare benefits (check this box if the plan provides welfare benefits and enter the applicable welfare feature codes from the List of Plan Characteristics Codes (printed in the instructions)):

4A	4L									

9a Plan funding arrangement (check all that apply)	9b Plan benefit arrangement (check all that apply)
(1) ☒ Insurance	**(1)** ☒ Insurance
(2) ☐ Section 412(i) insurance contracts	**(2)** ☐ Section 412(i) insurance contracts
(3) ☒ Trust	**(3)** ☒ Trust
(4) ☐ General assets of the sponsor	**(4)** ☐ General assets of the sponsor

10 Schedules attached (Check all applicable boxes and, where indicated, enter the number attached. See instructions.)

a **Pension Benefit Schedules**	b **Financial Schedules**
(1) ☐ R (Retirement Plan Information)	**(1)** ☒ H (Financial Information)
(2) ☐ T (Qualified Pension Plan Coverage Information)	**(2)** ☐ I (Financial Information -- Small Plan)
If a Schedule T is not attached because the plan is relying on coverage testing information for a prior year, enter the year	**(3)** ☒ 56 A (Insurance Information)
	(4) ☒ C (Service Provider Information)
	(5) ☐ D (DFE/Participating Plan Information)
(3) ☐ B (Actuarial Information)	**(6)** ☐ G (Financial Transaction Schedules)
(4) ☐ E (ESOP Annual Information)	
(5) ☐ SSA (Separated Vested participant Information)	

Figure 4.2 (continued)

This is a very popular question and mostly misunderstood, as many providers mistakenly believed that, as a participating provider with a managed-care contracting with a TPA, a network, or the plan directly, such provider will be automatically eligible or recognized as an authorized representative under ERISA to appeal and that, if a provider is not contracting with the payer, or network, this provider cannot appeal under ERISA on behalf of the patient even with ERISA recognized authorized representative designation form.

This is wrong. First, whether a claim is governed by ERISA is determined by the plan sponsor and type of the plan under federal law. In general, if the patient obtained health insurance or benefits from the employment in the private sector, this claim may be an ERISA claim, especially if the employer paid 100% of the employee's premium. In this regard, ERISA law equally applies to either a self-insured plan or a fully insured plan where the employer purchased an insurance policy from an insurance company.

The traditional assignment of benefits form used by most of us since the first passage of ERISA in 1974, and traditionally used in HMO, PPO, or "all-products" network participation instances does not grant an authority to the provider to appeal on a patient's behalf under ERISA, except for receiving benefits directly from the plan, if they are payable.*

A PPO participation contract has nothing to do with ERISA authorized representative designation, except that the PPO or other managed care or reimbursement contract will create a contractual right between the provider and PPO network, but not between the provider and an ERISA plan (see the discussion on *Privity* above), which may establish some rights for the provider to dispute with plan payment of PPO discount only, but and unless entitlement of an ERISA benefits claim or denial is completely resolved, or there is no genuine dispute over benefits claim, a provider PPO contracting right cannot be triggered, because any dispute or lawsuit concerning remedy of benefits denial from an ERISA-regulated, private employer-sponsored health plan falls completely under ERISA, and the PPO dispute or state law claim is completely preempted by ERISA, according to the U.S. Supreme Court unanimous ruling on June 20, 2004, in *Aetna v. Davila*. Therefore, in a simple explanation, if the dispute is about money, or ultimately about a claims payment from an ERISA plan, the physician is disputing under ERISA, not a PPO. Regardless if the physician is participating or nonparticipating, even there is no benefits or coverage, under ERISA new claim regulation, a patient may freely designate his or her authorized representative to appeal a claim denial. While an ERISA plan may verify such designation and authorization, the plan may not interfere or prohibit such free designation from an ERISA participant or beneficiary.

---

* DOL FAQs (B2).

Threats Regarding Payment Circumvention to Nonparticipating Providers

Although it was a past industry practice for some insurers not to send payment checks to nonparticipating providers prior to ERISA claim regulations taking effect on January 1, 2003, a plan must recognize, and may not prohibit, regardless of benefits coverage or provider participation, a patient, plan participant, or beneficiary from freely designating a health care provider as his or her authorized representative under ERISA to appeal, again even if there is no benefits coverage at all (it is called a colorable claim under ERISA) or provider does not participate in the network.[*]

Once a provider has appropriately obtained sufficient authorization (see Figure 4.1) to become an authorized representative on behalf of a patient, the plan must treat the authorized representative as the agent of the patient, recognize his or her authority to act on behalf of the patient, including providing whatever the patient is legally entitled to, such as receiving payments, plan coverage information, notification, and appealing, for the purpose of ERISA claim regulation (see Figure 4.3).[†]

It is important to understand that ERISA, as a federal law, completely governs and regulates any dispute or lawsuit as long as the physician wants money from an ERISA plan, health insurance, or benefits from employment in the private sector, and ERISA preempts and invalidates most state laws, PPO contracts, HMO contracts, and any third-party contracts, as long as your dispute is about money from an ERISA plan, according to U.S. Supreme Court unanimous ruling on June 20, 2004, in *Aetna v. Davila,* and as recent as a California class-action lawsuit, Ninth Circuit, ruling regarding California state law in reference to an ERISA plan.[‡]

Finally, if a physician or his billing company disputes money payment with and from an ERISA plan, regardless of its shape, PPO, HMO, POS, EPO, or P4P (pay for performance), and despite provider's participation, the provider must understand ERISA regulation and become an authorized representative under ERISA. However, if your dispute is only about PPO discount or HMO capitation and there is no ERISA dispute at all, your PPO and HMO contracts will be the governing document, and your applicable state law will be the choice of law for your dispute.[§]

---

[*] § 2560.503-1(b)(4).

[†] DOL FAQs B3.

[‡] *Cleghorn v. Blue Shield of California.*

[§] *Pascack Valley Hospital, Inc. v. Local 464A UFCW Welfare Reimbursement Plan* (3rd Cir. 11/01/2004).

ERISA Authorization and Initial Request for Appeal

Plan Administrator
123 Main Street
(Town), (State) (Zip)

RE: (Name of Patient)
    (Claim Number)

To Whom It May Concern:

Please accept this letter as notification of my authorization as representative to act on behalf of (insert name of patient) in the above-referenced claim matter. Attached is a copy of the authorization for your records. This is also notification and request for an appeal of the recent benefit denial (specify the denial dates of services and attached related denial materials) as further outlined in the attached materials. This authorization and request for an appeal is submitted pursuant to 29 USC §1133 governing health benefit plan subject to the Employee Retirement Income Security Act of 1974 (ERISA), and requiring ERISA plans to:

1. Provide adequate notice in writing to any participant or beneficiary whose claims for benefits under the plan has been denied, setting forth the specific reasons for such denial, written in a manner calculated to be understood by the participant
2. Afford a reasonable opportunity to any participant whose claim for benefits has been denied for a full and fair review by the appropriate named fiduciary of the decision denying the claim

Therefore, in connection with the above-referenced statute and the related claims regulations codified at 29 CFR §2560.503-1, I request as authorized representative the following:

1. Plans, policy, and procedures for filing an appeal and obtaining a review of the above-referenced denied services
2. Any additional requirements you may have for representative authorization
3. All internal rules, guidelines, protocol, or similar criteria relied upon in making the adverse benefit termination
4. The identification of medical or chiropractic experts whose advice was obtained on behalf of the plan in connection with the adverse benefits termination
5. Copies to all documents, records, and other information relevant to the adverse benefit decision. Such relevant documents to include that the document:
    a. Was relied upon in making the benefit determination
    b. Was submitted, considered, or generated in the course of making the benefit determination, without regard of whether it was relied upon
    c. Demonstrates compliance with the plan's administrative processes and safeguards for ensuring consistent decision making
    d. Constitutes a statement of policy or guidance with respect to the group health plan concerning the denied treatment option or benefit for the claimant's diagnosis without regard to whether it was relied upon in making the benefit determination. See Section 2560.503-1(h)(2)(iii) and Section 2560.503-1(m)(8) of the above-referenced claims regulation.

Finally, I would request on behalf of my patient a copy of the summary plan description required to be maintained by the plan and provided upon request to the plan beneficiary under ERISA. Thank you for your cooperation. I look forward to receiving the requested materials and pursuing the appeal of the adverse benefit determination[s].

         Sincerely,

         (Name of Doctor)

CC: (Name of Patient)

Figure 4.3 An ERISA authorization and initial request for appeal.

In order to determine who should receive this notice and letter, it will be necessary to ascertain who the plan administrator is. This is available by obtaining IRS Form 5500 from the health plan itself. Each Form 5500 that is filed by an ERISA plan is available for public review under the Freedom of Information Act (FOIA).

Figure 4.2 shows the top section of the Form 5500, which contains the information that the physician must obtain in order to properly submit the Authorized Representative form.

Chapter 5

Medicaid Managed Care

In moves throughout the country, state welfare and programs for the medically needy have made the change to managed Medicaid. In the early to mid-1990s, much of the transition had to do with research and demonstration projects in the form of Section 1115(a) and 1915(b) and 1915(c) waivers. Presently, at least 45 states use some form of managed care in their Medicaid programs. Some have delegated the entire delivery system to vendor HMOs and pharmacy benefit managers.

Health care providers have shown a growing concern over trends and transitions in the Medicaid programs nationally as capitation has proven to be the reimbursement methodology of choice, thereby transferring risk to the providers. Imagine, if you want to win the proposal in a competitive bid process, you need to be competitive as to price. One way to do this would be to lowball the proposal and then deal with the aftermath of low provider reimbursement on a fee-for-service basis and pay strict attention to utilization, if possible. The other way to bring in the deal within budget is to capitate the reimbursement to providers and transfer the risk of the cost of care to the providers after carving out whatever you need as a company to operate the plan and carve your profit off the top. (I have never been accused of being a politician!) It is the latter than I have more frequently witnessed as a consultant to many provider groups entertaining participation agreements for the provision of managed Medicaid services in different states.

Each time I review the typical 450-page request for proposal (RFP) from the state to the payer vendors vying for the lucrative contract award, I cringe because I know how the answers will be worded and what will take place later in reality. No crystal ball is needed.

In Georgia, as in many states before and since, the request for proposal was sent out along with data that was flawed. The state admitted the flaw and cited a computer conversion as the reason that the data files were corrupted. These data files were the files that enabled any requesting party to evaluate utilization of the past and risk of the future.

Without reliance upon their accuracy, capitation and utilization history were a crapshoot at best. This is often the case, and reliance upon some aspect of information is always precarious. Nonetheless, you have to get the job done as a provider to the system, so that you can be paid for rendering services. That being said, let us start at the beginning.

So you say your state wants to convert to a managed Medicaid system? Okay, this is a contracting handbook, so let us think this through in some organized fashion.

Some Basic Facts

Medicaid is a joint federal and state program that helps with medical costs for some people with low incomes and limited resources through independent providers such as physicians and hospitals and others, as well as a system of federally qualified health care centers (FQHCs). FQHCs, which were formerly paid on the basis of reasonable cost reimbursement, are now facing capitation and competing with county health department managed care initiatives for third-party payer reimbursement and capitation dollars. As such, Medicaid serves the poor, blind, aged, disabled, or members of families with dependent children (AFDC). Each state has its own standards for qualification. Originally, this program was a state-operated and administered program that provided medical benefits for certain indigent or low-income persons in need of health and medical care. The program, authorized by Title XIX of the Social Security Act, is basically for the poor. It does not cover all of the poor, however, but only persons who meet specified eligibility criteria. Subject to broad federal guidelines, states determine the benefits covered, program eligibility, rates of payment for providers, and methods of administering the program. Medicaid programs vary from state to state, but most health care costs are covered for citizens who qualify for both Medicare and Medicaid.

All states but Arizona have Medicaid programs. The Arizona Health Care Cost Containment System (AHCCCS) is Arizona's Medicaid program, designed to deliver quality health care under innovative and new concepts of managed care. As a model program, independent evaluations have repeatedly praised the program's effectiveness, and it has received national acclaim as a model for other Medicaid programs, and the approach has been recommended to other states by the Centers for Medicare and Medicaid Services, the federal agency that oversees Medicaid. AHCCCS contracts with health plans and other program contractors, paying them a monthly capitation amount prospectively for each enrolled member. The plan or contractor is then "at risk" to deliver the necessary services within that amount. AHCCCS receives federal, state, and county funds to operate, including some money from Arizona's tobacco tax. Eligibility is not performed under one roof, but by various agencies, depending on the category. For example, pregnant women, families, and children generally enter AHCCCS by way of the state's Department of Economic Security. The blind, aged, or disabled who receive Supplemental Security Income enter through the Social Security Administration. Eligibility for programs like KidsCare, long-term care, and Medicare Cost Sharing is handled by AHCCCS itself. Each eligibility group has its own income and resource criteria.

When a Medicaid program operates at the state level, it buys lots of drugs. As such, the pharmacy benefit programs and Big Pharma negotiate rebates for steering certain drugs into preferential status in the formulary. These rebates go back into the general fund and are used to fund additional reimbursement for care. Millions of dollars are at stake in this economy of scale purchasing relationship. Stick with me here, as this will become important in just a bit. When the managed Medicaid program starts to parcel out the care management to others as vendors, the single-sourcing purchasing goes with it, as in most cases, each vendor is then responsible for their own pharmacy budget and purchasing.

One of the main reasons for abandoning state managed Medicaid is that they cannot afford to both pay for needed medical care and administrate the program with the cost of the state's employee benefit and retirement programs, as well as the staggering cost of care. When economic downturns occur, and more citizens become medically indigent, or a disaster such as a hurricane, tornado, or terrorist attack occurs, more citizens often need more services. People experience manifestations of emotional trauma as somatic disorders such as hypertension, irritable bowel disease, and fibromyalgia, and these in turn escalate the need for more pharmacology and medical care, as well as an increase in the frequency of both psychological and somatic disorders, so claims cost increases. Nothing new to you as a reader, just think basic epidemiology.

If the state cannot handle the expense with what the federal government and the state contribute, along with the pharmacy rebates, one has to think that the administrative redundancy of outsourcing Medicaid program management to multiple health plans, with their executive compensation budgets, employee benefit programs, and the typical 5% reserved for Wall Street performance, leaves little to compensate providers, no matter how collaborative or innovative both plan and provider are willing to be. In addition, if the single sourcing for drugs goes away, the purchasing power is not the same, and the rebates either get cut or done away with altogether. So now we have less cash in the system to feed potentially more claims and more claims and program administrators—and Wall Street. And, if I were the author of the state's RFP, I would try to get those competing for my business to do a better job of processing Medicaid claims than I did in the past, so I would add in all the things that I was supposed to do, but could never get around to, like improved disease management, community outreach, plan communications, claims turnaround time, and faster enrollment. It was interesting to note that in all the RFPs I read for the transition to commercially managed Medicaid, that is exactly what was in there. Those state folks are smart!

Okay, so now we have an RFP disseminated to the competitors, less than adequate reporting, and numbers that have questionable reliability as to utilization and enrollment statistics. We have a population that is not used to managed care, as well as cultural issues in some states and parts of states where people have always done home doctoring, have a fear of organized health care, may have limited English proficiency or illiteracy issues, and not enough of a critical mass for the commercial payers to have ventured into some of the counties on their own because there were not enough covered lives to sustain risk.

In order for the health plans to submit their completed proposals inclusive of rate bids, they have to produce a roster of participating providers that have confirmed a written intention to participate. This can be done in several ways. Typically, each plan sends out a little packet of information followed by a visit from a provider contracting representative to answer a few standard frequently asked questions (FAQs). Sometimes, the plan refuses to answer questions and stands by their packet, which includes a vaguely worded contract that the state has not even reviewed (because no contract was awarded yet, or as part of its all-products clause). Other times, the provider contracting rep arrives with the best intentions, as long as you do not ask questions that require a firm, reliable answer (because there are none until the deal is inked with the state), and as is the case with many health plans, by the time the bid and award process is over, the staff turnover at the health plan has changed provider contracting people numerous times. Suffice it to say this is a difficult and frustrating time for all concerned.

This is probably the part where you arrived and chose to read this chapter. You have been presented with the "letter of intent" packet, which may or may not have a sample contract in it. It may ask for a letter of intent from you confirming your participation in the program if they win the award, or it may contain a model letter for you to simply sign and return. After all, they want to make it convenient and simple for you, to facilitate their bid process. Not so fast!

Do Your Homework

I have a standard protocol I follow for Medicaid managed care contracting that I will share with you. It contains several components that should all be completed and developed before signing any letter of intent or contract "draft" for Medicaid managed care transition.

First, obtain a copy of the RFP and all the supporting documentation that accompanies the RFP, so that you can see what the health plan is competing for in the bid process. You will see various deliverables that the plan cannot deliver without your cooperation and facilitation, the first of which is care delivery. Unless the heath plan is a staff-model HMO that employs physicians and owns hospitals, it has to obtain these goods and services from you to produce the deliverables which it has agreed to provide to the state for a price. The understanding of these deliverables and how your organization plays a role in it is where you will find your negotiation L-E-V-E-R-A-G-E! Ignorance will cost you!

Each state has an "open records act," and contract awards that involve the use of public funds are all subject to the provision set forth in these acts. So, if an award was already made, you can and should obtain a copy of the contract that was awarded from the state to the vendor. It will show the deliverables, the money paid, the consequences of material breach, and the windows of opportunity for remedy of any breach. Reading this will give you a realistic set of expectations and help you build your contracting policies, business strategy, and business rules.

Next, prepare a questionnaire to perform due diligence on the plan asking you for your hand in participation. The one I use is roughly seven pages long. It is sent to the health plan in question and requests lots of information that I know from my days as a health plan employee and are not only available, they are standard reports that are tendered to the state each quarter and each year to maintain their license as a health plan. They are also Freedom of Information Act (FOIA) available, even though someone from the plan who may be misinformed might tell you that they are proprietary. (Much to my chagrin, while employed at the health plan, my colleagues and I in provider relations told people they were "proprietary," because we were told to give that response, and we really did not know better at the time.) Some of the questions on my questionnaire are listed below:

- Full information for a contact person who can provide reliable information on behalf of the plan; presumably a person of authority.
- Information about organizational management.
  - Their history and ownership summary.
  - An organizational chart.
  - A description of senior management and credentials.
  - The CV of the medical director.

- Their insurance coverage details.
  - Reinsurance and stop-loss coverage.
  - Errors and omissions coverage.
  - Officers and directors coverage.
  - Insolvency protection for inpatient claims.
- Certifications and accreditations.
  - National Committee for Quality Assurance (NCQA), Utilization Review Accreditation Committee (URAC), or others.
  - Certificate of authority from the state you are in.
- Contracting style.
  - Will they take all your physicians and service lines?
  - Are they planning capitation or case rates? If so, obtain details and actuarial assumptions.
  - A sample contract draft.
- Claims management statistics.
  - Description of their claims management and other health care information systems, including the claims payment system, and required Web-based claims verification, filing, and electronic transfer fund/ automated clearing house (EFT/ACH) payment mechanisms.
  - Claims detail statistics (just for their Medicaid claims).
    - Number of claims processed per month.
    - Accuracy rate.
    - Average claims turnaround times, in days.
    - Performance standards for claims processing personnel.
    - Percent retrospective denials for lack of medical necessity.
    - Number of days payer will be able to readjudicate (reconsider) claims after payment.
    - Historical ratio of payment to claims denial (from both the Medicaid and commercial HMO products).
    - Policy regarding retroactive charge backs.
- Marketing and communications.
  - Mock-up of member ID cards.
  - Plan summary descriptions and specific coverage policies for the service lines you are most concerned with or specialty drugs or technology you may need to handle as nonstandard.
  - A description of how they update plan providers to new policies and procedures, coverage decisions, and other medical policies.
  - A summary of how they will communicate updates to members.
- Provider communications and relations.
  - Questions about provider training sessions.
  - Problem solving and joint operating committees.

- Appeals and denials procedures.
- A copy of the provider manual.
- Complete list of other providers in the network upon whose services you will have to rely for lab, radiology, transportation, DME, etc.
- Enrollment and eligibility determination methods and what happens if eligibility information is erroneous from the plan to the provider.

■ Utilization and quality issues.
- Will there be a pay for performance incentive program?
- Can you use your own disease management and utilization management program documents that you published with your accreditation manuals?
- A summary of the experience and training of the nurses in medical management, and their responsibilities.
- Access you will have to the medical director for spot decisions and resource utilization/case management guidance.

■ Financial.
- Audited financial statements for previous reporting period(s).

■ Other questions you want to know.
- Programs that are innovative.
- References from other providers that have done business with them.
- A statement as to why you should partner with them over other competitors in the bid process.

As a consultant, I develop these questions for my clients on the basis of my findings in the RFP. There are things that I know from experience that most payers will be unable to materialize, no matter what they craft in their proposals. I want to go in with eyes open and at least make sure I raise the issue, so that if specific protective language needs to be worded in the contract, I can give the attorney working with me on the contract the specifications of the operational issues that may arise and my preference for a way to handle the matter in case a problem arises.

I ask that the responses to my questionnaire be sent in advance of the meeting with the provider contracting representative. I also ask that they provide three copies of the responses, so that I can immediately distribute them to my C-Suite, contracting and business office managers for review and input. If there is a physician–hospital organization (PHO) or individual practice association (IPA), I also make sure that the executive director receives a copy and is invited to give input. These exercises are always such epiphanies for them.

While waiting for the responses to the questionnaire to gain information from the plan(s), they also serve as an additional useful tool for the strategic planning committee and the board to develop a set of contracting policies.

Together with the observations from the RFP and any known operating issues that have become evident by experience with managed care in general and with Medicaid reimbursement, work together with your leadership and your board to establish a written contracting policy that states the hospital's or medical group's requirements before any valid intent can be expressed to the state on your behalf with their proposal. This is necessary, because all RFPs I have ever reviewed for managed Medicaid state that, if the network of providers substantially changes from the list that accompanied their original proposal, the state reserves the right to rescind the award. This little hook makes them mind their manners if your contingent letter of intent is accompanied by a statement that says that, if their final contract contains conflicts that cannot be resolved, then your letter of intent is null and void and should not be considered by the state to be valid. Tie this to a longer-term contract if you can get all your standards integrated into your contract, so that they cannot use your name to get themselves up and running, and then toss you by the wayside.

The standard contracting model policy I use for Medicaid managed care contracting for my clients has 35 points or business rules that my client's attorney can use to draft ironclad language that gets what I need from a fledgling plan, which may have little or no experience with Medicaid populations, for my client to be successful with the endeavor. In order to get this piece of the project going, I request that the client's leadership team, board, and key business office personnel, as well as key specialists, pediatricians, and representatives from the hospital-based medical staff are in attendance in a working retreat, away from PDAs, cell phones, pagers, and other preoccupations. What gets turned out in 1 to 2 days of a facilitated retreat ends up being a worthwhile contracting policy that is used for much more than just Medicaid contracting, but that can be applied to Medicare Advantage contracting, commercial payer contracts, and also direct-to-employer contracts that begin to eliminate all the middleman interference of contracted reimbursement. The most productive of these meetings have been held in remote locations such as a Florida panhandle beachside cottage, a large house on the beach in Kailua, a remote cabin in North Texas, a ski lodge in Aspen, but never on the campus of the hospital. I do not know if it has any bearing on the outcome, but these meetings almost always seem to be conducted in khakis, socks, or bare feet and with a basket of fruit in the center of the table. It was suggested in one of the meetings in Ohio that the bowl of fruit be replaced by the anxiolytic samples from pharmacy reps once the RFP was explained to the physicians. The point is to relax; get away to where you can study, think, and strategize and return with a publishable work product that will be useful for more than just managed Medicaid.

While I would love to give you an example of the model contracting policy, that document is useless without specific context, and I would be remiss to provide it without an exhaustive review of your specific situation. Instead, below is a list of categorical topics you should consider in your document:

- If you will contract with someone with Medicaid managed care experience and a license in your state, or with a newcomer to the state who has nothing set up yet
- Your stance on retroactive charge backs versus requests for refunds that are mutually agreed upon
- Your tolerance for service line carve-outs of specific services, or specific physicians
- Financial liquidity standards
- Claims payment standards
- Use of your own disease management and utilization standards
- Pay-for-performance incentive program participation
- Their use of Web site for communications tools to you and to participants
- Reliance on their eligibility and advance coverage determinations
- What to do if operating performance and claims payment deteriorates drastically and you do not want to quit, alternative measures that can be implemented such as drawing down on advance funding similar to pre-bankruptcy measures, and a host of others that will be elicited from the review of the RFP

Marketing to and Enrollment of Medicaid Recipients

Marketing methods such as direct mail to encourage enrollees to pick a network and a primary care physician usually end up in the trash. Many beneficiaries are blindly assigned providers too far away to obtain access to care or inconvenient to public transportation. Not enough educational outreach is being done to teach the recipients how to use the system correctly. This fosters persistent, inappropriate use of the system. In addition, in many cases, the recipients are allowed to change health care networks and providers on a 30-day basis. Medical providers who have never worked with this population and still others, who have never dealt with managed care because it was not present in the commercial population in their remote counties, are getting into the act for fear of being left out. There are reports of decreased quality of care, appointment-access issues, and high consumer frustration due to changes in emergency room utilization requirements. Not enough specialty providers are joining the networks, leaving gaps in service coverage, which is especially dangerous for at-risk capitated primary care physicians (PCPs). In many cases, reimbursement is inadequate, forcing many health departments to provide stopgap care without reimbursement.

On the positive side, capitation increases coordination of care and provides the opportunity to build physician–patient relationships with the establishment of the PCP. Perhaps in the future capitation will improve the health status of pregnant mothers, decrease the number of low-birth-weight babies, and increase immunizations and well-child-care compliance ratios. One of the most troublesome diagnoses to manage under managed care Medicaid is asthma. The proof of success in the system is when we can wrangle costs and increase health status of the asthmatic patients in the system.

Another trouble spot in the Medicaid system that shows promise through the transition to managed care Medicaid is emergency room (ER) utilization. Medicaid recipients accounted for a disproportionately higher percentage of new ER patients. According to the General Accounting Office (GAO), more than 50% of the ER patients inappropriately used the ER for diagnoses and conditions that were neither emergent nor urgent. Of these, most cited lack of a relationship or access to a primary care provider. About a third of the population without a PCP is either uninsured or Medicaid recipients who are unable to locate a PCP who will treat them.

It costs more than five times the office visit amount to treat a nonurgent Medicaid recipient in the emergency room. It is estimated that 30% to 40% of the ER visits could and should be rendered in a PCP's office or through 24-hour triage.

Reimbursement Issues

Some of the billing hassles that providers have experienced in the past should bring new meaning to the word *confusion* as commercial risk contractors enter the picture. It will no longer be adequate to learn one set of rules and bill one fiscal intermediary for program expenses. Another concern of Medicaid capitation has to do with eligibility problems, as recipients may switch providers and plans on a monthly basis. Hopefully, the electronic data interchange (EDI) process will assist providers with preverification of eligibility status, and more providers will negotiate retroactive noncoverage denials out of their contracts on a nationwide basis.

Chapter 6

Consumer Driven Health Plans: Contracting Implications

Consumer driven health plan (CDHP) arrangements (also called consumer directed or self-directed) involve a combination of an employer-funded spending or savings account with a high-deductible insurance policy, where the deductible amount equals or exceeds the annual funding of the savings or spending accounts.

Consumer Driven Health Plans Overview

Consumer driven health plan design focuses on the following factors:

1. The provisions and funding level of the employee savings/spending accounts.
2. The amount of the insurance plan primary deductible requirement.
3. The gap (if any) between the funded level of the employee savings/spending accounts and the insurance deductible requirement, or imposition of an up-front employee deductible requirement before funding from the accounts.
4. The benefit provisions of the insurance plan.
5. The carve-out of any insurance benefit to be excluded from being subject to primary deductible requirement.

6. The relationships between the savings/spending accounts, the gap or up-front deductible, the primary insurance plan benefits, and any carved-out benefits.

Payments for health care services are made directly from the spending or savings accounts until the account is exhausted or the insurance deductible requirement is met. If the deductible exceeds the annual spending/savings account funding (as is usually the case) the employee is responsible for payment of this gap before insurance coverage applies. The insurance policies in consumer driven health plans vary greatly in nature in respect to benefit provisions and if managed care features and other components are involved.

There are four types of employee spending or savings accounts that are designated for pretax treatment if properly qualified:

1. *Flexible Spending Accounts (FSAs)*: Employer FSAs, when qualified under the tax code regarding "cafeteria plans" for employees, predate the consumer driven health plan movement. They involve an employer pretax contribution that employees may spend on qualified medical expenses. However, there is a "use-it-or-lose-it" provision so that unspent funds cannot carry over from year to year, other than for a grace period extending 2.5 months after the close of a plan year for FSA claims to be filed.

2. *Health Reimbursement Arrangements (HRAs)*: HRAs refer to an employer funded health care spending account defined by the Internal Revenue Service (IRS) in 2002 that allows for eligible funds unspent in a given plan year to be rolled over from year to year on a pretax basis (as opposed to the use-it-or-lose-it provisions of an FSA).

   Numerous provisions apply according to the IRS revenue ruling regarding requirements for eligibility under such arrangements. The revenue ruling addresses such situations as recognizing and allowing for spending accounts to occur in combination with a high-deductible insurance policy such as the consumer driven plans now in the marketplace, or for the spending accounts to pay for insurance premiums. Furthermore, the ruling allows for group retiree plans to use such arrangements.

3. *Medical Savings Accounts (MSAs)*: MSAs are tax-advantaged savings accounts that include a number of qualifying provisions that limit the growth and desirability of these accounts. The Health Insurance Portability and Accountability Act of 1996 (HIPAA) included provisions creating MSAs (also sometimes called Archer MSAs) as a pilot program, with a series of extensions issued by the IRS. The Working Families Tax Relief Act of 2004 provided a final extension for creation of new MSAs through 12/31/05. New accounts may not be created, but existing account holders

can continue, or may choose to rollover into health savings accounts (discussed next).

4. *Health Savings Accounts (HSAs)*: HSAs refer to the structure created under Title VII, section 1201 of The Medicare Prescription Drug, Improvement and Modernization Act of 2003, which included the following provisions:

 – HSAs may be established January 2004 and thereafter.
 – HSAs must be opened with a companion high-deductible health insurance policy.
 – A high-deductible policy is defined as at least $1000 for singles and $2000 for a family, subject to annual cost-of-living adjustments.
 – A taxpayer must be under 65 when opening an account.
 – The taxpayer may take an annual tax write-off equal to the deductible amount of the companion high-deductible plan.
 – However, the tax write-off cannot exceed $2250 for an individual plan, or $4500 for a family plan, again subject to annual cost-of-living adjustments.
 – Contributions may be made for the previous year through April 15.
 – Eligible tax-free withdrawals from HSAs include expenditures for doctors, dentists and hospitals; artificial limbs; drugs; eyeglasses and contacts; chiropractic; laboratory expenses; nursing home costs; physical therapy; psychoanalysis; X-rays; and nursing home insurance premiums.
 – In January, 2009, the Treasury Department and the IRS issued new guidance on the maximum contribution levels for HSAs and out-of-pocket spending limits for High Deductible Health Plans (HDHPs) that must be used in conjunction with HSAs. These amounts have been indexed for cost-of-living adjustments for 2009, and are included in the Revenue Procedure 2008-29, which announces changes in several indexed amounts for purposes of federal income tax. The new levels are as follows:
   i. New Annual Contribution Levels for HSAs
     • For 2009, the maximum annual HSA contribution for an eligible individual with self-only coverage is $3000.
     • For family coverage, the maximum annual HSA contribution is $5950.
     • Catch-up contributions for individuals who are 55 or older have been increased by statute to $1000 for 2009, and all years going forward.
     • Individuals who are eligible on the first day of the last month of the taxable year (December for most taxpayers) are allowed the full annual contribution (plus catch-up contributions, if 55 or older by year-end), regardless of the number of months

Table 6.1   Comparison of Consumer-Driven Programs

FSA	HSA	HRA
• May be used by any employer and employees • May be funded by employer or employee • Balances may not rollover from year to year (use it or lose it) other than for 2.5-month grace period	• May be used by any taxpayer; must be opened before age 65 • Require companion high-deductible insurance policy • May be funded by employer or employee • Balances may rollover from year to year	• May be used by any employer • May only be funded by employer • Balances may rollover from year to year • More flexibility in plan design than HSA

the individual was eligible during the year. For individuals who are no longer eligible on that date, both the HSA contribution and catch-up contributions apply *pro rata* based on the number of months of the year that a taxpayer is an eligible individual.

ii. New Amounts for Out-of-Pocket Spending on HSA-Compatible HDHPs
   • For 2009, the maximum annual out-of-pocket amounts for HDHP self-coverage increase to $5800 and the maximum annual out-of-pocket amount for HDHP family coverage is twice that, $11,600.

iii. Minimum Deductible Amounts for HSA-Compatible HDHPs
   • For 2009, the minimum deductible for HDHPs increases to $1150 for self-only coverage and $2300 for family coverage.

– In addition, a fiscal year plan that satisfies the requirements for an HDHP on the first day of the first month of its fiscal year may apply that deductible for the entire fiscal year.

Table 6.1 summarizes comparative provisions of the major types of accounts:

The other major coverage element to consumer driven health plans is the companion high-deductible insurance policy that provides coverage once the deductible requirement is met. There are countless variations as to the specific benefit provisions of such policies.

Consumer driven health plans can include multiple spending accounts in the same plan. For example, many plans use an HRA for the employer to fund a portion of the high deductible, and an employee-funded FSA to fund the balance of the high deductible. Consumer driven health plans also have often invested major resources in various components of the plan, including health navigation (consumer-accessible health information, decision-support tools, and plan transactions), claims payment tools (including debit cards), value-added programs, and managed care features.

Payment Cards

Debit and credit payment cards are used to facilitate provider payment transactions from health care spending and savings accounts.

A projected 71% of all FSAs, HSAs, and HRAs will be used in connection with a payment card by 2010.[*] Average settlement per transaction in 2005 was $56. Most frequent transactions were pharmacy 60%, medical 31%, dental/orthodontics 5%, and vision 4%.[†]

Managed Care Contracting Implications

When managed care all-products contracts include CDHP products, the frontier on patient check-in and contract management and administration will change drastically.

Coordination of Benefits

For starters, coordination of benefits provisions and coverage are implicated. With high-deductible health plans (HDHPs), no coordination of benefits with first-dollar coverage is permitted. This means that, even though a spouse or domestic partner may have enrolled the patient in the other plan, if it is an HMO or PPO plan, those benefits may not be used together with the HDHP. The patient (or their employer) may not be aware of this. There is no employer due diligence requirement at this time to ensure that, when the dependent coverage is chosen, the coordinated plan may be incompatible. This means that the front office check-in person must know what the coverage is before assuming that there are benefits that may be coordinated.

---

[*] TowerGroup: Payment Cards and the HSA Revolution: A Check-Up on Issuer Opportunities, August 2005.

[†] http://evolutionbenefits.com/resources/EB_Corporate_Factsheet.pdf.

Stacked Deductibles for Out-of-Network Care

Patients who choose to go out of network may incur separate "stacked" deductibles for noncovered services and reduced benefit levels for covered conditions where care was received from out-of-network providers.

Consider, for a moment, this example where the provider is nonparticipating and out of the contracted provider network, but the patient has seen other physicians in network, and has satisfied the "in-network" $1000 deductible for care for the year by receiving treatment and hospitalization from "in-network" providers. When receiving services from the out-of-network provider, none of the previous satisfaction of deductible for the year applies, and the patient starts all over again having to meet a new deductible of perhaps an even higher than "in-network" amount of $2500, and then only receives 60% coverage of allowable amounts instead of 80% of billed charges.

This would confuse the office staff if they failed to ask the correct questions, and the patient would be livid upon finding out that the coverage is different. Often patients do not understand the coverage that they have, but if the office staff fails to elucidate how it all works and fails to obtain any required advance beneficiary notice for noncovered services, the contract may require that the physician write off the charges and not bill the patient.

Timely/Prompt Pay Statutes May Be Difficult to Enforce

Physicians grant discounts and participate on health plan discount arrangements with the intention that they will be paid sooner by the health plan if they have contracted to participate in the network. Part of the equation in assessing the rates and discount is the time value of money.

If the deductible and patient responsibility for coinsurance is so high, the patient may not have funded their account, or the funds may be depleted for the year and previous years such that the account turns into a "slow-pay" account. While the money from the health plan may be paid timely, in accordance with state law, that amount may be very low by comparison to what the patient owes. The prompt pay laws apply to insurance balances, which in CDHP may be much less than the responsibility due from the patient, especially at the beginning of the plan benefit year. Physicians and their staff should also be aware that not all benefit years run from January to December. Some plans have open enrollment set for July 1, and deductibles start midyear.

Physicians and their staff should never assume that, because it is midyear, most patients' deductibles have been satisfied.

Probate Implications

The laws for HRA unused funds when the employer funds the account may require that unused funds that have not been paid to a provider may revert back to the employer at cessation of employment. This could be construed to mean that, while there were funds in the account, they were not used timely, before the patient's demise, and therefore may not be available to pay for expenses incurred while living. This gets into very complicated tax and benefit law, but physicians and their staff should not assume that the rules are identical to other insurance plans where claims can be filed for services rendered prior to the patient's death and that services are paid based on the date of service. The funds may not be available.

No Preauthorization Required

While most managed care plans require preauthorization and verification of benefits, such is not the case with CDHPs. The patient may access care from anywhere and without preauthorization; the physician no longer can make the argument that they depended on the preauthorization in anticipation of payment. This has long been the basis of appeal on unpaid claims where preauthorization was given and the claim was later unpaid.

Marketing Materials

A visit to any Web site for a health plan offering CDHP products will reveal, in most cases, that the patient is not expected to have to pay any estimated patient responsibility up-front—whether a co-pay or deductible. Even if the physician is savvy enough to require by contract that they may collect estimated co-pays and deductibles up-front, the patient may argue that their materials say otherwise. This could likely lead to many patient satisfaction issues, as well as poor financial performance if the patient responsibility, as large as it could be, is not collected at the time of service. While the contract may prevail because of the entire-agreement provision, the physician's staff may have a tough time actually collecting the money due and may have to remove this discussion away from the front desk to a more private place to avoid embarrassing the patient in front of others in a crowded waiting room. A total front-end redesign may be necessary to accommodate CDHP products.

Web Site Collaboration

As part of the managed care agreements, the contract may state that the plan can use its best efforts to market the practice. This may include Web site listings and pricing information that has not been reviewed by the physician. A cursory review of many of the pricing transparency offerings in the world of CDHPs reveals that pricing is either missing or inaccurate. The physician should require the first right of review and the right to refuse how they are marketed by the plan if the marketing verbiage includes statements that are misleading or inaccurate.

Quality Assumptions

Many CDHP listings now include "Gold Star" rating systems listed by physicians. Arbitrary ratings may have been developed in some unknown, unscientific method, or by economic considerations. These ratings may implicate patient perception of quality and should be reviewed regularly by the physician's staff to ensure that they are accurate and competitive with other physicians in the area, if any.

Most Favored Nations

Extending discounts to patients because of individual economic considerations may cause grief with the way contracts are written, requiring that the health plan get equal or better than the best deal the physician gives to "anybody." Many health plans are following the example of CIGNA and others who plan to use their audit rights to determine if someone else got an equal or better deal than the plan, and they will invoke the contract language that requires that the payer receive a rebate or offset for paying more than another payer.

CDHP contracts should be stand-alone, with their own pricing and terms and conditions. By simple comparison, they are not administrated the same as commercial PPO and HMO health plans, and they require many additional considerations and lots of other follow-up and front-end redesign for the medical practice. They should probably not be rolled in as an additional product or "funding mechanism" as they have been labeled by various health plans around the nation.

Chapter 7

Silent Preferred Provider Organizations (PPOs), Secondary Markets, and White Space Management: Three Terms That Translate to Revenue Erosion and Frustration

A "silent PPO" refers to a situation where, unbeknownst to its contracting health care providers, a managed care organization (MCO) "sells" or "rents" its preferred provider organization network of providers to a third party (typically a third-party administrator, insurance broker, or smaller PPO). The third party gets the advantage of whatever discount the MCO has negotiated with the health care provider. The health care provider becomes aware of this only after he or she provides services to a patient who is not covered by the PPO.

It is often encountered in two situations:

1. Legitimate access to your discount purchased under the assignment clause of another existing contract. Usually this occurs through the "assignment" provision.
2. Bogus reference to a nonexistent contract under which a discount is inappropriately taken, and the provider simply receives a notice like "PPO discount applied" on an EOB, or remittance advice without any specification as to which contract the discount refers.

After filing a claim, the provider receives less than full payment and an explanation of benefits (EOB) referencing the discount with the original MCO PPO. Both the "seller" and the "purchaser" of the discount rely heavily on the fact that a busy provider or hospital reimbursement team will have difficulty spotting this anomaly on an EOB. Many software products have been introduced to model payments to prevent this; however, if the provider's reimbursement team does not model the contract rates in the system in advance of receiving payment, there is little hope of catching the payment variance or deciphering which contract was designated as primary to determine the amount payable.

At the time of writing this manuscript, the practice of using a bogus reference to a nonexistent contract or one that has a prohibition against such an assignment has been rendered illegal in some states, but that does not preclude the provider from permitting the practice by contract. While more states may enact similar laws, no statutory provision will likely ever protect a provider from signing a contract that is not in his or her best interest. Furthermore, some providers in certain markets actually use these provisions to tap populations of patients that they would otherwise be unable to attract for one reason or another, including refusal by a plan to contract directly with them.

Depending on the terms of the contract, silent PPO activity may constitute a breach of contract. Because of the potentially significant sums of money involved, providers should take special precautions to assure that their managed care agreements do not contain "all-payer" clauses that allow the MCO to rent or lease its providers' services to noncontracted entities. This might be construed as a breach of confidentiality, for one thing.

Secondary Discount Markets

Another term that is often used in conjunction with silent PPO is that of "secondary discount markets." This term relates to an unregulated process in the world of both PPO and HMO claims management and is very sophisticated.

Over the last 15 years or so, it has evolved in a part of the health care financing system that lacks transparency, making it nearly impossible for providers to detect or identify inappropriate activity. Worse yet is the potential that the patients may not be able to determine their share of the cost of their health care. As a result, the patient often pays a greater portion of the total bill, and the third-party payer ends up paying less.

Due to the number of intermediary entities involved in the health care claims payment process, the complexity of the payment system gives rise to the potential for the secondary discount market to thrive. Generally, a "rental network PPO" exists to market a provider's contractually discounted rates to third-party payers, such as insurance brokers, third-party administrators, local or regional PPOs, or self-insured employers. Rental network PPOs may also rent their networks and associated discounts to entities such as "network brokers" or "repricers" whose sole purpose is finding and applying the lowest discounted rates, often without provider authorization. It is conceivable that one rental network PPO may have *hundreds* of other payers and affiliates to whom it "sells" or "rents" various provider panels and associated discounts, none of which are identified in any one master document attached to a contract for review or comparison for discrepancies or conflict with other prior executed contracts at different rates with the same payer.

A physician, hospital, or other provider who decides to contract with a single rental network PPO may unknowingly end up with dozens, if not hundreds, of payer arrangements. Under this arrangement, the third-party payers that contract with the rental network PPO have access to any and all discount agreements that the rental network PPO has negotiated with the provider. The payer usually gains this access without the provider's express prior knowledge or permission.

Payers can thus "shop" for this provider's lowest payment rate (i.e., highest discounted rate) because the provider signed a contract with one rental network PPO entity, and then that entity sold its rate information to downstream entities, who sold their information further downstream, etc.

This snowball selling effect allows a third-party payer to look at all of the provider's available discounts and then pay the provider the lowest rate—even if that rate is completely unrelated to the prevailing contract. It is patently unfair for the lowest discount that a provider agrees to in any single PPO agreement to become the ceiling for payment, notwithstanding prevailing contracts or other appropriate payment methodologies. The unilateral decision made by the payer to reimburse the provider at the lowest contracted payment rate available not only renders the underlying contract meaningless, but ultimately impedes a provider's right to freely contract.

Increasingly, the tactics of these discounting entities remove the contracting step altogether.

Nationwide, there are documented examples of these entities simply sending what appear to be solicitations for participation in a PPO network, but which are actually treated as "opt-out" agreements. If a provider fails to affirmatively "opt out," that provider is considered to be a participant. Due to the fact that many providers cannot adequately and appropriately maintain the list of executed contracts or manage them, this is easy to pull off.

For example, one rental PPO faxed a short cover document and W-9 form to numerous Texas medical practices. Health plans routinely request that medical practices complete W-9s. This request stated, "Internal Revenue Service Regulations require that payers maintain a current taxpayer identification number on file for all providers of service." If one continues to read on, the document is actually a contract to sign up for the rental PPO network disguised as a routine request for a W-9. The document also indicated that the rental PPO network "members/payers have reported using your services." The practices were unaware that services had ever been provided to patients through that particular rental PPO.

These unregulated secondary discount entities provide no value whatsoever to the health care system. They thrive in a health care market that lacks transparency and exists solely to traffic in provider discounts. In an era of consumer driven health care, even with traditional plans, patients are assuming greater responsibility for health care decision making and cost sharing. Patients have no means of determining the true cost of their health care when these entities apply discounts under a cloak of secrecy.

How to Work around Them

- Do not permit the assignment to your contractual rates to anyone wishing to pay the fee for access without your written consent.
- Prevent those who have come for direct contracts with you which you have declined to do business with, to come in through an assignment basis.
- Demand the right to deny participation with a payer that does not seem credit-qualified or otherwise suitable to meet your requirements.

One organization among many that is against the practice of silent PPOs is the American Association of PPOs (AAPPO). In July 2000, the board of directors of AAPPO passed a policy opposing silent PPO activity. The policy states that PPOs and providers must disclose all contractual intents and purposes when applying contractually permitted provider discounts. Representatives of the AAPPO say they believe it is in the best interest of the providers and PPOs to pursue contractual relationships based on fair business practices and principles to ensure a mutually satisfactory business association.

The courts have examined this practice as well, and the trial courts held that Employers Health Insurance Company improperly discounted its payments to HCA Health Services of Georgia in *Employers Health Insurance Company v. HCA Health Services, Inc.* No. 99-11241 D (11th Cir.). In this matter, an Employee Retirement Income Security Act (ERISA) case involving the denial of benefits allegedly due a patient under the terms of a group health insurance policy issued and administered by an insurance company, the patient underwent covered outpatient surgery at a medical center. At the time of surgery, the patient assigned to the medical center his right to recover 80% of the costs of the surgery from the insurance company. Accordingly, the medical center billed the insurance company for the costs of the surgery. Although the amount of the bill was consonant with the usual and customary fee charged for such services, the insurance company reduced the bill by 25% and paid the medical center 80% of the reduced bill. The insurance company claims it was entitled to reduce the medical center's bill by virtue of the following series of contracts: the medical center promised a third party that it would charge a discounted fee upon rendering specified medical services; the third party, in turn, "leased" the right to the discounted fee to a fourth party; then, unbeknownst to the patient and the medical center, the fourth party "leased" the right to the discounted fee to the insurance company.

The medical center demanded full payment of its bill, and the insurance company refused. The medical center then brought this lawsuit on behalf of its assignee, the patient, seeking recovery of benefits due the patient under the terms of his health insurance policy. On cross motions for summary judgment, the district court granted the medical center the relief it sought, entering judgment for 80% of the full amount of the medical center's bill for services. The insurance company then appealed that judgment. The judgment of the district court is a masterful and complex economic and legal review of the silent PPO machine and should be read by all. An Internet search of the case may be found by typing "*Employers Health Insurance Company v. HCA Health Services, Inc.* No. 99-11241 D (11th Cir.)." As I reread the affirmation by the Appellate Court in preparation of this manuscript, I continue to find it amazing (and appalling!) how often I meet with naiveté on the part of revenue management and contracting specialists who are still unaware of the phenomenon, this case decision, the appeal, and the impact to their revenues as they scurry to jot down notes in my seminars.

White Space Management

"White space management" is defined in the health care industry as medical expense or billed charge volume incurred by a health plan member outside of the payer's owned, contracted, or leased primary networks. Some plans estimate this amount to be over $65 billion in commercial and Blue Cross and Blue Shield volume combined. It is often mentioned in payer circles as "INET" (in-network) and "ONET" (out-of-network) expense.

Innovative market approaches by several payers and cost containment firms attempted to address white space management in a unique way, providing payers and other at-risk entities such as ERISA self-funded employers with breakthrough savings opportunities and administrative improvements across nearly all claim types. These firms maintain huge data warehouses that catalog provider claims and cost data derived from various sources including information gleaned from remittance summaries and explanations of benefits accompanying coordination of benefits claims where discount rates and "sweet spots" can be extrapolated for market intelligence used at a later date when the need arises.

In an educational program designed for national health plan executives, I was able to listen as case studies were presented by various payers and cost-containment consultant firms to outline this practice of discounting non-contracted claims where no discount is due. The presentations gave me two very distinct impressions: first, a sense that these practices are rampant in the industry, and second, that medical providers are unaware of how robust the information contained in the data warehouses can be. In consulting with clients since the day I attended that meeting, and in speaking with seminar attendees, I have been able to confirm for myself just how deeply these practices are entrenched in the revenue cycles of hospitals and other medical providers and that the industry has underestimated the $65 billion dollar figure. By my calculations, it is much higher!

In order to identify if this is happening in your organization, let us examine the many ways in which the process has been witnessed in action.

Example 1

A hospital sends an invoice to a payer with whom they clearly have no contract by any stretch of the imagination. The state has a timely payment requirement by statute for insurance companies and health plans to issue payment for on clean claims in 22 days. The claim has no defect. On or about the twentieth day, a call is received by a revenue management specialist responsible for that account. An acknowledgement is made by the payer that there is no contract, and that they would like to negotiate a discount and settle the bill. The caller advises that if the hospital will negotiate a rate (usually within one or two percentage points higher than the average of most of the contracts currently in force, what I call the "sweet spot"), the caller will issue payment to the hospital immediately. The caller uses the often intimidating tact that if the negotiated discount is not accepted, the payment will go to the patient and the hospital will have to "chase the patient down" before the patient spends the cash.

The busy revenue management specialist has many accounts to tend to. Rather than research to ensure that all the proper documentation is on file and that the claim was submitted with an acceptance of assignment, (which often requires the payment be sent directly to the provider for the amount up to the maximum fee allowable by the plan per the insured's evidence of coverage), or arguing that the payment should be paid directly to the hospital because of a proper assignment of benefits, the specialist simply elects to use what administrative authority they have in the software to simply adjust the claim in accordance with the spot negotiation. This is often done by adding the payer as a "contracted payer" with a revenue code in the software and adding a second revenue code in the system for the adjustment credit. Often the software in revenue management systems does not have a "one-time use" override, so the next time a bill is presented by that payer, the check is processed as if the payer is contracted, and no variance report is generated. This single-case agreement (SCA) has just morphed into a continuous-discount arrangement (CDA). Slick, huh?

Behind the scenes at the payer's headquarters, an entry is simultaneously made when the SCA is negotiated into the data warehouse that is jointly maintained by that payer's information systems across several states or, worse, entered into a database at a consortium level, and may even involve a "finder's fee" reward to the negotiator for the market intelligence of the rate, the acceptable discount, with whom at the hospital the discount was arranged (by name), and the date and time of the occurrence. It is comparable to the scene in the movie *Independence Day* where Jeff Goldblum's character flies into the alien mothership with the captured spacecraft and uploads a computer virus to bring down all the other ships.

Regrettably, this case example could have had a much different outcome if two things were different: First, the policies of the hospital should have been established to include the following:

1. No SCAs are negotiated by anyone other than a supervisor. If a call is received by a revenue management specialist, the call should be referred to that supervisor who can take the time to research the assignment status and argue the assignment eloquently (this assumes that the supervisor has the training and experience to make the argument, which is not always the case).
2. A second policy establishing that only supervisors may establish new payer identities and revenue management codes in the system to recognize SCAs.

Second, the revenue management software should be programmed to identify SCAs as "one-time use" so that subsequent episodes of care are not extended the same discount without a fully executed contract in place.

Example 2

This is a similar situation to the first example, but in this case, the revenue management specialist receives and executes a "fax confirmation" to memorialize the discussion between the payer and the hospital, and immediately signs and returns the document by fax in order to speed the receipt of the payment. The revenue management specialist does not read or understand the implications of the ambiguous language that essentially states that this and any and all future payments from the plan are to be at the rate discussed. The revenue management specialist cannot understand how anyone would be upset with how quickly they arranged to get the payment in the house at the agreed-upon rate. The fax is tossed in the account file folder, and when payment is received, the remittance summary is paired up with it, and off it goes onto the cart with the other paid-in-full files to be archived away in cold storage.

In this case, a CDA is now in effect, but no one else knows of its existence, and no one would ever know in what file folder the fax is contained, or where it might be located, but the claim is paid and paid timely! Oh joy! It is off the books! Job done, and done well, I might add. Hey, the A/R days are down! What is worse is that the CDA may indeed state that the rate is discounted and that no *quid pro quo* has been exchanged for the discount. Therefore, the next time payment is issued, it arrives late, beyond the statutory timely payment time frame. While the statute provides for full billed charges, plus an implied interest or penalty, the CDA may contain language that exonerates the plan from having to pay either the full billed charges or the penalties or interest, and is only responsible for the discounted rate, whenever they get around to paying it. Even more disappointing is the fact that this information may also get entered into the data warehouse previously described, so that all the subsequent payers accessing the data warehouse or the consortium that sponsors it are aware of the situation, thereby enabling them to make lots of money on not only the savings but also to bank the time value of money on the tardiness of payment.

Example 3

Another payer who has no discount arrangement whatsoever with the hospital receives a bill for a white space claim. They pay a fee to the consortium to have access to the data warehouse and search by tax ID that is contained on the UB-04 or CMS 1500 form. Jackpot! They found an entry or four or five or twenty. They research the best one for their particular situation. In the database there is an indication that the contract rate of the contracted, SCA, or CDA plan is able to be "assigned." This comes about when the contracted payer includes language in the contract that states:

> Payer may assign, delegate, or transfer this Agreement or the rights granted herein without written consent of the other party.

In this case, the noncontracted payer contacts the contracted payer that does have the contract and offers to pay an access fee to "lease" the access to the discount. The lease fee is paid, and a remittance advice is prepared that generically states "PPO discount applied" or may even be more specific and state which PPO's rate is being applied.

Here again, the outcome could be better, but the root cause is the assignment language. Rarely is it a best practice to permit a payer to assign your contract rate and access to another payer without the provider's express written consent. In doing this, the hospital in this case does not even receive a call from the payer seeking the discount. Instead it is all done behind the scene; payment may be made timely per statute or timely per the contract, (more often than not the two time frames differ) at the discounted rate. If it is paid late, there may be no recourse either. If the hospital spends resources to research the claim, the margin erosion is never recovered, so after a few times, the staff becomes desensitized, and again, the bill is paid and the file is off their workload. The A/R days are reduced, and all is well.

Wait! There's more! Now comes now the plan whose contract has within it a provision for a "most-favored nations" (MFN) or preferential rate that provides for that plan to receive the lowest of any rate you accept from a plan. This plan also maintains an active membership in the consortium and has database access.

It finds that an entry has been made as the result of the SCA that was signed by the revenue management specialist, resulting in a rate that equals a minimal discount savings over that at which the MFN payer's rate is set. The revenue management specialist has no idea what an MFN provision is, or that any of the contracts contain one. Why would they? They do not regularly negotiate contracts, so it would be rare that they would be afforded the training to understand the implication of such a provision. And after all, the SCA that they signed or negotiated orally was only a "one-time deal" in their mind. How could it possibly be an issue?

Meanwhile the plan with the MFN calculates the minimal discount savings over the course of all its claims and the little savings calculated at the volume of claims it repeatedly pays to the hospital adds up to over $500,000 in the last year alone. I could write you a letter and tell you that you either need to write me a check or I will take it as an offset from future claims paid, if you do not issue me the check to clear the breach. Do you think that the MFN payer will not "dial for dollars" at that kind of opportunity? Why not? What is there to lose?

Last but not least, a payer with whom you no longer have a contract not only had the MFN provision in their contract with you, but the MFN provision stated at the very end that the "provision shall survive the termination of the Agreement." I have seen various CIGNA and other payer contracts that have that very provision in them. So now, as this terminated payer researches opportunities to maximize the return on investment of the fees paid to participate in the consortium, it performs the necessary calculations to determine that a recovery of hundreds of thousands of dollars is a real potential because its contract was in place with you for years.

I cannot stress enough how important it is to be aware of the phenomenon of white space management and its potential impact on your past and future reimbursement. I am sure you can agree with me that the potential for much more than the estimated $65 billion dollars is a reality as we assess the potential implications of this practice and the need to establish policies and safeguards and provide training to the revenue management staff.

---

16 Suggested Best Practices to Mitigate Silent PPO Discounting

1. Do not permit the assignment to your contractual rates to anyone wishing to pay the fee for access without your written consent.

2. Prevent those who have come for direct contracts with you that you have declined to do business with, to come in through an assignment basis, for some period of time, (e.g., two years or whatever time frame is determined to be strategically prudent for your organization).

3. Demand the right to deny participation with a payer that does not seem credit-qualified or otherwise suitable to meet your requirements.

4. Clearly articulate the premise of the contract: that the provider is offering discounts in exchange for steerage of patient volume.

5. Require different coverage for in-network and out-of-network providers.

6. Require that the PPO's name be included on all member identification cards and that the card be presented at the time of service.

7. Require identification of a payer's use of the PPO network on the EOB. No logo, no discount.

8. Attach a complete payer list to the contract and require the plan to provide notice of changes to the list.

9. Review every definition in the contract carefully to ensure that they reflect the provider's intent of giving discounts only to payers who have PPO plans or policies.

10. Define "payer" clearly to identify the entity obligated to pay, and include a statement that the hospital has a right to take legal action against that entity.

11. Negotiate a provision in the contract requiring the forfeiture of all discounts that do not comply with the PPO agreement.

12. State in the contract that all discounts are confidential and proprietary.

13. Stipulate that the PPO must require all payers to abide by the terms of the PPO agreement.

14. Include a contract clause that allows the provider to audit the PPO's records related to patient activity.

15. Include language restricting the plan, and any claims-paying organization with which the plan is affiliated by ownership or contract, from leasing or selling the payment rates established under the agreement.

16. Force them to pick one contract rate and stick with it, not select a discount from several contracts they have paid access fees for.

Model Language Example

One hospital system I am familiar with has employed the following language to limit their exposure on silent PPO activity with much success nationally. I have shared this with you so that you can discuss a similar approach with your strategy team and attorney to come up with a similar approach if you determine that it is in the best interest of your organization.

The parties acknowledge and agree that the Alternate Rates (the discount as opposed to the billed charges) set forth in Exhibit _____ to this Agreement shall apply only where the following conditions are met:

1. PPO causes Payer to provide Financial Incentives to Beneficiaries to utilize the services of HOSPITAL;
2. PPO causes Payer to provide Direction to Beneficiaries to utilize the services of HOSPITAL;
3. PPO causes Payer to pay claims within a timely manner, in accordance with Section _____ of this Agreement;
4. PPO maintains confidentiality regarding the terms and Alternate Rates set forth in Exhibit _____ to this Agreement in accordance with Section of this Agreement;
5. PPO maintains an active agreement with Payer wherein Payer agrees that PPO shall be that Payer's exclusive preferred provider organization within (Your) County, Your State, except in the event that Payer is a third-party administrator acting on behalf of one or more specific Payer(s). However, Payers represented by a third-party administrator defined as "Payer" in this Agreement cannot access another preferred provider organization in (Your) County, (Your) State; and
6. PPO shall ensure that HOSPITAL is a contracted Participating Provider for all product lines of that Payer; and that:
   a. the Payer does not offer an EPO network that excludes HOSPITAL as a Participating Provider for that EPO network, in (Your) County, (Your) State;
   b. the Payer does not offer a physician EPO network that is structured to admit hospitalizations of Beneficiaries primarily to a hospital network that does not include HOSPITAL;
   c. the Payer does not discourage hospitalizations at HOSPITAL in any way through the Benefits Agreement; and
7. Payer qualifies pursuant to Section _____ of the Agreement.

Where full consideration is lacking, HOSPITAL shall have the option, in its sole discretion, to require prompt payment of full billed charges for the Medical Services rendered.

The hospital that shared this with me asserts that it used this provision to collect a claim that paid more than $77,000.00, where the initial discount would have reduced the payment to a mere $17,000.00, but because it did not follow the letter of the contract, the above terms were enforceable, and the payment was at full billed charges. I find that very promising, indeed!

Chapter 8

Single-Case and Continuous-Discount Arrangements

A continuous-discount arrangement (CDA) creates an ongoing contractual relationship between the provider and a noncontract payer or repricer and saves both parties from negotiating a discount each time the provider sees a plan member out of network. If you treat plan members out of network, a repricer (or other agent of a payer) may have already asked you to sign an agreement that gives the repricer a set discount off of your billed charges on an ongoing basis.

Typically, a CDA sounds like a plan contract, but it is not—it is not made with a plan and does not involve the typical contract requirements. It may be totally enforceable and may ultimately be unilaterally beneficial to the repricer, and not even to the patient. There is often no requirement to participate in quality assurance, credentialing, or similar obligation. Repricers are after a relationship that is strictly financial and discount driven. Since they are not the payer, they are simply negotiating the rate, and not the fact that you might not ever actually receive the payment. That is not their issue. Their deliverable is completed when they lock in the provider for a set price, upon which they often receive a commission as a part of the savings.

Although repricers have typically asked for a one-time discount, also referred to as a single-case agreement (SCA) for a plan member treated out of network, more repricers are offering an ongoing discount agreement, which is called a

CDA. Providers need to be very careful with these documents because, while they may seem innocent enough, they can have far-reaching implications into your revenues and your sanity. In Chapter 7, "Silent Preferred Provider Organizations (PPOs), Secondary Markets, and White Space Management," I visited the implications of CDAs and SCAs and the nightmare they can create if the proper diligence is not taken before signing, or if the document is signed by a staffer who is often unaware and untrained to evaluate the consequences of effecting quick payment and getting the receivable off the books. You will wish that A/R days were the problem!

Keep in mind that as a noncontracted provider, you are owed payment timely per insurance statutes and/or administrative codes; you have no contractual obligation to provide a discount on out-of-network services to a plan member; you may have a valid assignment of benefits so that the plan might be obligated to honor the assignment (check with your attorney, as each state's laws and situations may differ); and you are under no obligation to provide a discount on future business from that repricer.

Assuming that there are no reasons not to sign the deal, it may be financially worthwhile for you and may help you avoid the administrative hassle of regularly negotiating discounts with the repricer for plan members whom you treat out-of-network. The problem is that this is often a huge assumption that requires tight control and detailed knowledge of all your other contracts, as well as contracting policies that include a stance that you have no contracts that may have a "most-favored nations" (MFN) or preferential rate that requires that, if you give someone a better rate, even just once, you have to lower your rate with the MFN payer too.

In many cases, the revenue management department or physician practice manager receives a call asking for the discount and is then asked to memorialize the oral agreement with a fax memo that documents the rate which has been agreed upon. Some are only one to two sentences and ask the provider to sign in a designated space. Sometimes it makes mention that this agreement applies to future encounters with this or another patient from the same plan; sometimes it is mute to that fact.

A problem arises in administration of this deal in that, in order to post the payment, a revenue or posting code must be entered for that payer and also for the adjustment. Once that is in the system, it may be misinterpreted or mishandled by admitting staff who verify whether the payer is in the system at the time of admission or scheduling. If so, the presence of a code may lead that registrar to assume that there is a contract and that precertifications and so forth, are required, and that other familiar managed care policies and procedures are applicable.

On the reimbursement end of the revenue cycle, assumptions may be made about write-offs, late payment penalties, medical records copy fees, and the like.

Silent PPO cannot be argued, as the discount is memorialized in writing, even if it is memorialized by someone with no authority to bind the provider or the hospital. In essence, this simple little memo could cost you much more than the discount, and the risks may not outweigh the benefit of a quick spot discount negotiation.

While some argue that CDAs will increase a provider's business, this is difficult to prove. Since the repricer's deal only comes into play when an out-of-network charge is incurred, one could argue that there is no steerage. While it could, in some circumstances, potentially increase your business, it is nearly impossible to track.

It may increase your administrative hassle factor because, as stated previously, the negotiation is only for the rate, not the performance, of actual payment or accurate payment in a timely manner. While it may save you time on future discount negotiations, one could argue the merits of being selective on the execution of CDAs, keeping their number to a minimum, and requiring full payment for all others who bring no value-added proposition to the deal.

Those repricers and others in favor of CDAs often argue by intimidation, stating that the patient will get paid, or that your staff will be inundated with faxes asking for discounts. I have never seen the situation of a "mountain" of faxes awaiting consideration. It may also be difficult to sort out if you already have an executed CDA with a repricer, and they may often negotiate even higher and higher discounts. If there is no restriction as to the ability to assign the discount, they could infect your other higher-paying CDAs and contract by selling access to their price with you.

Typically, repricers ask for generous discounts of 10% to 30% off of the provider's billed charges in a CDA. Do not be afraid to negotiate smaller discounts if there is nothing in the deal that would be mutually beneficial to you. Remember, they will likely make a commission off of each claim that is paid at the discounted amount. The value to them is in the frequency, and every dollar after the first deal is just passive income. Sweet! For them!

Every contract should have the five basic elements: (1) an identification of the parties, (2) an effective date, (3) an agreement to the obligations of the parties, (4) a discussion of the money to be paid, and (5) a termination date and method by which the deal is terminated. Since these two-sentence faxes may be missing a few of these elements, they may not have a way for you to shut them down if you need to. They should also have contained in them a restriction on the ability to assign them to others without your express written consent.

If you do choose to execute CDAs as part of your business model, you may wish to have your attorney draw up your own CDA that has the required protections for you, instead of signing the form of each repricer.

Ensure that your attorney addresses the fact that, if the patient is found to be a member of a different network through some other arrangement or contract, then the discount will not apply, and you will be entitled to the higher of the rates.

Also, have the attorney include some provision for timely and accurate payment and that, if the account is not paid in full by a certain date, the discount is rescinded and the full amount due.

Finally, have the attorney mention in the document that they may not interfere with your financial relationship with the patient with regard to things like balance billing, compensation for noncovered or nonallowed services, medical necessity denials, and so forth.

As with the CDA, the same admonitions apply to the single-case agreement (SCA). Here the form should have the necessary protections for you, but should also designate that the agreement is case specific, episode specific, and for a specific patient for a specific service, admission, test, or episode of care. It should always have an expiration date and should include in it, just for the record, that it is one-time use only.

If they cannot agree to the terms you need, you probably do not need their discount. Remember, they clearly have little to no leverage with you.

Chapter 9

Quality Issues in Managed Care (Pay for Performance)

First, I would like to explain the point of this chapter. It is not about "quality"; it is not a survey of pay-for-performance (P4P) programs going on at the time of this writing. Instead, since most of the P4P initiatives and demonstration projects currently in existence are just that, initiatives and research and demonstration projects, some will likely succeed and some will demonstrate failure in both methodology and purpose. Because my first book outlasted many of the trends and initiatives of the mid- and late-1990s, my goal here is to include a chapter that addresses the contracting issues surrounding these P4P initiatives and demonstration projects. That being said, let us take a moment for a brief overview of the landscape at present.

Pay for performance is an American health care industry trend toward incentivizing providers, both physicians and hospitals, for more appropriate and evidenced-based, efficient utilization of health care resources, which likely translates to better quality of care. Many providers believe this is just another variant of the incentives that were unsuccessfully implemented in past years under shared-risk relationships, with payers utilizing capitation and withholds to change provider behavior. How long will it take before this incentive system runs its course and we move on as an industry to the next incentive system, and what will it be?

The Medicare program currently has multiple projects underway to examine health care quality and efficiency from many angles. I openly admit my skepticism of the sustainability of these programs and the impact of their associated administrative cost redundancy and will go on record to state that I truly believe that there is no real new money in the system for providers, but merely a reallocation of existing dollars. In fact, I will go further and state that I believe that, because of the administrative redundancies, there is actually less money in the system to pay for the cost of good quality care.

Employers seem to have rallied behind outcomes metrics, the Health Employer Data and Information Set (HEDIS), and the Leapfrog program. Because employers embrace these programs, insurers also need to be on board with them. In addition, episode treatment groups (ETGs) are another metric being used by some payers to give form and substance to their own P4P initiatives, regardless if they utilize the metric system in the manner in which it was intended or deviate so far from the intent of the developers of the system that the only thing in common with the initial system is the name.

Still other systems are being implemented all around the country, and some are put into place without the requisite legal counsel and forethought and may place unsuspecting physicians and hospital administrators with the best of intentions in the crossfire of fraud and abuse, stark self-referral prohibitions, and antitrust and tax issues for tax-exempt hospitals. Attorney Gabe Imperato, a former general counsel to the Office of Inspector General (OIG) once said to me, "If it makes sense in business, it's probably illegal in health care." These networks may try to brand their own initiatives in quality and pay for performance that may run afoul of unfair competition regulations, and state fraud and abuse and self-referral prohibitions, and bylaws violations in order to create sustainable competitive advantages that include strategies to develop barriers to entry by other members of the medical staff. Hospitals and health care organizations have for the most part demonstrated their lack of planning and strategy development and operated in reactive mode for some time. This is evidenced by the haphazard styles of contracted reimbursement that tend to yield unmanageable agreements and an inability to easily and accurately benchmark one contract's performance against another. Thanks, I feel better and will now step down from my soapbox.

My goal in this chapter is not to pass judgment on which system payers and providers choose to employ or how correct or incorrect I believe their application to be. Instead, I have been reviewing the phenomenon of P4P terms and conditions as they relate to reimbursement for health care services which have already been delivered pursuant to a contract and a perceived medical necessity, as ordered by the attending physician and hospital or other facility or provider. I first have to ask, "Is there enough money, prestige, or other recognition or incentive to make a provider care about any particular program over another when they may have forty payer contracts with forty different initiatives and forty sets of different goals and objectives to meet?" Yes, I have heard of some providers receiving checks at larger group practices, in the amount of $125,000 to a radiology group, for example, and $300,000 to a rural ob-gyn group, but those are sensational wins that are highly publicized, just like Powerball wins. I do not hear about those every day from excellent providers that go about the business of providing consistently good quality care each and every day as they care for patients. What will it take to make them "want" to participate? Worse yet, their success in P4P may be compromised by the other providers whose metrics and outcomes may be commingled or codependent on theirs and vice versa. Not an easy system to navigate!

Pay for performance is payment or nonpayment for participation in a process; it is not, nor ever will be "pay for quality." For starters, we would first have to standardize a definition and identification of "quality" in health care. Since medicine is not an exact science, and each human body is unique, that will not be easy to do. Therefore, payers and other interest groups have developed certain guidelines, measureable objectives, and outcomes thought to demonstrate (by their established and accepted metrics) that the appropriate care was rendered at the least expensive, professionally acceptable level, at the appropriate intervention time frame, without waste and without avoidable consequences. Keep in mind that these objectives, standards, and guidelines may or may not be published and may or may not be stated in your form agreement initially offered by the health plan in question.

Some of these metrics evaluate a timeline or cost index, while others measure the management of disease. Some measure the cost of an incident that is repeated and has a lower cost but high frequency that must be abated, while others measure an episode of care and its associated cost, in comparison to other providers rendering similar treatment to similar patients with similar resources available by similarly trained physicians.

Still others evaluate treatment approaches and take into consideration vast bodies of knowledge related to both clinical outcomes and overall cost.

Contractually, you are involved in a P4P program the minute you sign a contract that contains a term that refers to your "participation and compliance in the plan's utilization management, quality management, peer review, and other programs as they exist from time to time." You may have no clue what is being measured, how it is measured, the statistical appropriateness of the source of the metrics or the method of assessment, how large or small the statistical sampling, or anything else related to the process or the measurement, or the targeted outcomes. With that sentence, all you know is that you are expected to "participate" (whatever that verb actually means), together with the erosive effect on any margins you may have negotiated and, additionally, the cost, and also to "comply" with any edicts, assessments, or recommendations set forth by somebody, whenever they set those and as they may change from time to time. The fact that these programs or initiatives may exist from time to time may imply fluidity in the measurement system, the importance of the outcomes, the methodology employed to perform the metrics, the appropriateness and validity of the findings, and a host of other unknown variables. The only thing that you can say you know with any certainty is that this pledge of both participation and compliance can have a tremendous impact on your costs and your reimbursements, if you are paid any. I say that because with that contract term, one could defend not paying you at all, or could likewise ask for all the money ever paid to you as a condition of your participation and compliance.

P4P Contract Terms and Conditions

In 2006, at a Healthcare Financial Management Association (HFMA) conference in San Francisco, I listened to speaker and attorney Paul DeMuro from San Francisco address this topic. I credit him and that particular session with my professional development on this topic and my own process improvement in dealing with this topic. His comments were salient and relevant to the audience of chief financial officers (CFOs) and leaders of health care organizations, and his admonitions were well presented, together with a checklist of points to consider when negotiating contracts that contain these P4P terms. I hope I can do my teacher justice and add a few of my own experiential points and observations in this chapter.

First, the provider must determine what specifically is being measured, how, and the objective of the subject of the measurement. Is the objective to save the health plan claims dollars, improve patients' quality of life, enhance the quality of care, or to jump on the bandwagon of a particular disease process or malady to merely keep up with what everyone else is measuring? For how long will the measurement period last, and what is the sampling size that will be considered statistically relevant? From where will the data be derived? Is it primary or secondary data? Will the data be extrapolated from claims submitted or from physician documentation and the patient's medical chart? What if the data collected is not the whole story?

I can remember an outcomes study conducted by a payer that had a contract with a client pediatrician. She was penalized by the plan because her claims data showed that she did not render "well child" examinations in accordance with Academy of Pediatrics guidelines for children from birth to age one.

When the plan finally provided a list indicating which children did not receive exams according to the claims data, each chart was reviewed. The finding was that the services had indeed been rendered, but because the data collection period included a time increment when the patients were covered by a different plan, although all children had the six visits in accordance with the guidelines, some of the visits were billed to a different payer based on the coverage in effect on the date of service. The appeal took some 20 hours of research to prepare and provide documentation. At the time, the physician was capitated for these patients and had already rendered levels of care that far exceeded the amount she was prepaid at her negotiated capitation rate. She also had a percentage withhold (20%), and the penalty for the alleged nonconformance with Academy standards was retention of the entire withhold, which was tantamount to an additional discount. Other colleagues had simply accepted that they did not perform to standard and did not fight to prevail. They ended up financially ahead. We chose to fight to protect her good name and claim the money owed. The 20% withhold was insufficient to cover the time spent by her and the staff to conduct the review. In addition, once the plan received the argument and defenses together with the documentation, another 6 months passed before the money was actually paid. The time value of money was another cost that further resulted in additional negative integers attributed to this project. The other physicians permitted their reputation to be besmirched all the way to the bank.

This anecdote leads me to the next lesson I learned from Paul DeMuro's talk, and that is that both penalty and bonuses should be paid within a contractual time frame, and if paid late, a specific late payment penalty to encourage the party that owes the money to part with the cash according to mutually negotiated time frames. Otherwise, the value of the bonus (or penalty) diminishes. In addition to this, it would also be prudent to have some formula stated within the contract so that the amount owed is easily discernable by any forum, including litigation or alternative dispute resolution such as mediation or arbitration. To state that a bonus is available or that a penalty may be levied but have no means to identify how much is at issue and when it is payable creates problems of enforceability. Further, to not have this detail readily available in the contract or some attachment and to state that the program is able to be unilaterally modified "from time to time" could give rise to problems with enforceability later on.

One way that health plans avoid allegations of breach of contract against them while preserving their ability to make changes to the contract without the need to provide amendments and notices each time is by avoiding specifics in the language of their form agreements. It takes a trained eye to determine if the language is specific enough to be enforceable. These ambiguities also present a "double-edged sword," as they may also be used to allege your breach or nonperformance, since in most cases the author maintains the prerogative to interpret any ambiguity in the event clarification is required to settle a dispute.

If terms are not clearly defined and consistently interpreted, vague and ambiguous terms leave the definition to the author and present difficulties in enforcement. Further, if there are no consequences, sanctions, or liquidated damages for breach, then the contract is essentially unenforceable. However, in the language example provided above, if the terms "participate" and "comply" are insufficiently defined, the author could later explain (if requested to do so by an arbiter) that the compliance means that if the author would levy a penalty for not meeting the objectives and to comply, the provider must pay that penalty.

The lack of a precise and definitive description of the P4P program terms and contract performance standards for either the payer(s) or provider without clear establishment of the metrics to be met or payment terms for a bonus or penalty enable the payer to delay or even avoid payment on these programs altogether. It also makes progress difficult to monitor for the provider and could result in a total loss of the costs associated with participation in the P4P program if the earned bonus is delayed or remains unpaid.

Since P4P is often a part of the quality management and quality assurance programs of the health plan(s) represented under the contract, if the only language in the contract that refers to the quality management or assurance program states that "the provider shall participate and comply with the health plans' utilization management, quality management, peer review, credentialing, and other programs as they may exist from time to time," lacking any additional clarification that may be annexed to the form agreement incorporated by reference, one could interpret this to imply the tacit approval for responsibility for compliance and required participation in the plans' (plural of "plan" intended) P4P program(s), without benefit of bonus payment or entitlement to useful feedback. What is worse is the fact that this language could set the provider up for notification that the provider failed to meet the unspecified objectives or failed on the basis of statistics with insufficient samplings or whatever else the health plan may allege to support a request for payment of a penalty without limitation as to the amount, and if not otherwise restricted, may be recuperated through an offset or withhold from future claims payable by the plan.

I hope that I now have your attention and that you have some antacids available for the next scenario I will present, as this could happen to you as it did one of my clients. Hospital A executed a form agreement with the health plan that only contained "the paragraph" referred to above in its contract. Hospital B, a competitor/neighbor across the street, realized the insufficiency and, in their negotiations, required additional details and clarifications to be added to their contract. As such they were able to determine that they met the specified goals and objectives set forth in the contract and the P4P attachment in their contract. Therefore, Hospital B was able to claim their reward in the amount of 2% of the gross revenue paid by the plan to their hospital. In comparison, Hospital A met the same objectives and actually exceeded them, but was unaware that they had done so, because the objectives were not stated in their executed form agreement. Therefore, they had no basis of calculation for bonus or penalty established in the contract. Nor did they have any requirement that the plan provide them any feedback or the right to request comparative data or equal treatment. Without this they were unable to defend an argument that they should not be required to pay a penalty for allegedly missing the targeted objectives, and were asked to pay an amount curiously similar to the amount their neighbor was due.

Money is tight, and times are hard. When health plans initiate P4P programs, they rarely hit providers with penalties right away. Instead, these dollars come from a big pot of gold that lies waiting at the end of the rainbow. Not! When health plans budget to have dollars to use for a reward system, they must slice it off the portion of the budget from premiums that is used to pay provider claims, not health plan earnings! Therefore, most plans set the fee schedules and allowable lower overall to create the bonus pool and, as a result, pay providers less initially. Therefore, one could infer that Hospital A already suffered a perfunctory loss because the fees were arbitrarily lowered to all providers, and that the penalty assessed creates a larger insult. If Hospital A had to prepare data, track outcomes, submit reports, provide training for staff to participate with the health plans' requirements, purchase special software, or perform any activity to which a cost could be labeled and attributed solely to that activity for that contract, the unrealized payment of a bonus and the required payment of a penalty actually increase the loss associated with participation in the plan. But that is not all.

Since Hospital A and Hospital B are both community-based, not-for-profit hospitals, this payment of the bonus to Hospital B enabled it to purchase a new piece of technology to provide a sustainable competitive advantage to Hospital B, rather than to distribute the dollars to executives and shareholders as a bonus. As such, Hospital B was able to make a press release to state that the bonus for its demonstrated high quality performance had been paid, and that as a result, Hospital B was making an investment back into the community by making this new technology available. The health plan also made a press release to congratulate the winner(s) and to demonstrate its generosity and a willingness to reward high-quality, high-performance providers by payment of the bonuses in the amount of several million dollars distributed overall. In contrast, what press release could Hospital A make?

Take a moment before we move on to jot down the lessons learned from these last paragraphs. Regardless of where your contracted health plans are in the process of operating P4P programs, it is time that you review your contracts and then inquire of the plans if they are presently operating any such plans or if they have intentions to do so in the near future.

Each P4P program should have a detailed attachment outlining the rationale, the methodology, what is at stake, what the rewards and/or penalties are, appeal methods, dispute resolution terms, and formulae that can explain to an outsider the payment logic and time frames for execution of the agreement to participate and comply. From a generalized contracting standpoint, it is always a best practice to obtain written clarification of what it means to "participate" distilled to a level of detail so that one could perform activity-based cost analyses of the cost of that participation, and likewise the details of the compliance and its associated costs as an additional verb requiring performance on the contract.

What should be included in this P4P attachment are some of the concepts and concerns that I learned from Paul DeMuro's presentation in San Antonio. Below are some of the key points that he shared with us.

Best Practices in P4P Contract Disclosures and Terms

- Ensure that any incentives are in the benefit agreements and reflected in the managed care contracts in some form. If there is some form of an upside, it is clearly set forth in the contract, is understandable, and is attainable. Setting forth examples is a good idea. Often, arbiters and mediators get caught unprepared by our use of jargon and may be required to look to the author of the contract to explain while the dispute is ongoing. This may set the provider at a disadvantage. Do not just set yourself up for another contract dispute or litigation. Managed care contracts are increasingly negotiated by litigators out of the litigation between health plans and providers.
- If what a provider is entitled to depends upon what another provider is entitled to or gets, make sure you have access to all relevant data and information that would permit you to ensure you are getting paid correctly (but be cognizant of potential antitrust considerations). Ensure you have a right to audit or to have an independent third-party audit on your behalf.
- Ensure you have done a flow of funds, sensitivity, or reimbursement analysis of what you may receive.
- Be careful of illusory deals (e.g., there is nothing behind the curtain, except the Wizard).
- Be careful of the multiyear moving target (e.g., we met the target this year, but the bar is raised each successive year).
- Is there a downside risk? If so, can it be quantified? What is the upside risk, if any? Do the parties, particularly the physicians, understand it? How do the physicians communicate it? Are the physicians adequately compensated for what they are doing? How is "adequately" defined? Can the

progress be monitored, or does it just seem like a winner take all at the end of some period? What about adjusting for changes in case mix?

- Are all health plan providers part of the P4P program? Are the metrics and objectives the same for everyone? Consider including examples in all documents.
- If the contract is directly with an intermediate entity, beware if that entity goes bankrupt and does not pay the provider. Unless the contract provides that the health plan will pay you under those circumstances, the provider often will not be paid at all. This raises issues of "privity" and has effect on performance under the contract. If the intermediate entity is supposed to share its proceeds with the provider from monies paid by the health plan, but instead the intermediate squanders the money and never pays out the share to cover the P4P incentive, will the health plan be required to pay it again directly to the providers in the amounts negotiated?
- Include a provision that the failure to pay statutory interest with late payment of both regular claims payments and bonuses is a material breach entitling the provider to terminate the contract. Include an attorneys' fees clause so that, if a party must sue for breach, the prevailing party shall be awarded attorneys' fees and costs.
- If the health plan insists on mandatory arbitration, consider a clause that provides that the loser pays the arbitrator's fees and all costs and expenses associated with the arbitration.
- Include language that the arbitrator in rendering the decision is bound to follow the law and must issue a detailed statement of decision setting forth the legal and factual basis of the decision.
- Health plans may try to shorten the statute of limitations with contract language. A provider should not agree to any provisions that would cause a provider to lose its claim for breach of contract if a suit/arbitration is not filed within the applicable statute of limitations.
- Hospitals should negotiate to receive a bonus if they have a score in the top 20% in quality, as defined in the contract, with higher bonuses for the top 10%.
- All the measures for each quality based system should:
  - Be evidenced-based.
  - Be easy to collect and report.
  - Address process, structures, outcomes, beneficiary experience, efficiency, and overutilization and underutilization of health care.
  - Include a measure of health IT infrastructure and other administrative start-up costs in the first year.
  - Each set of quality measures used for specific categories of providers should reflect possible variances in their application to an individual

or entity depending upon the type, size, scope, and volume of services provided by the individual or entity.

- A third-party source may need to be hired to establish risk adjustment procedures and to control for differences in beneficiaries' health status and characteristics to assign weights, and to measure by each quality system.
- The program should take into account and demonstrate in its example algorithms the variations in physician practice patterns and costs.
- The program document should include details that demonstrate financial incentives that are understandable, calculable, and reasonably limited in duration and amount.

Stating Program Objectives

- Each P4P contract attachment should include some examples that affirm the philosophy that the program supports credible clinical approaches such that quality of care and clinical outcomes are not impaired.
- The program documents should detail threshold amounts for use as necessary components of a P4P plan through example formulae and algorithms that can be mathematically proven.
- Detail the distribution methodology to the participating groups or individual physicians.

I wish to convey my deepest gratitude to Paul DeMuro for his invaluable assistance, review and mentorship with this chapter. He is an exemplary role model for the legal, accounting and health care administration professions. You may reach him at:

Paul R. DeMuro, CPA, FHFMA, JD, MBA
Latham & Watkins LLP
San Francisco and Los Angeles, California
(415) 395-8180
(213) 891-7330
paul.demuro@lw.com

Chapter 10

Reimbursement Methods in Managed Care

In most managed care organizations, covered medical and related services are usually rendered, and payments are based upon a prospective budget allocated as a percentage of the premium collected by the health plan and are often referred to as a "target medical cost index" on a per-member, per-month basis. Usually actuaries assist both managed care payers and providers in the measurement of risk exposure by statistically analyzing historical utilization data supplied by organizations such as the Health Insurance Association of America (HIAA). The data is derived by encounters reported via claims for payment of medical and related services. A problem with this system of measurement is that the data is somewhat skewed for at least three reasons:

1. *Data extrapolation*—Data is prepared into reports by various software programs that organize the data into nonstandard formats.
2. *Data entry errors*—Errors occur either in claims processing or claims submission.
3. *Fraud and abuse*—Coding aberrations are used to manipulate payment for claims that might otherwise go unpaid or be paid at substantially lower rates.

Capitation

In highly managed plans, revenue is allocated using a prospective method of payment known as capitation. Capitation is a system of reimbursement that provides financial incentives and disincentives related to the use of specific providers, services, or service sites. In capitated managed care plans, a contract is negotiated for a specific menu of services, and a fixed amount of money is paid to the provider of care in anticipation of rendering those services to patients who have selected that provider. The money is paid in advance of the need for the services on a per-member, per-month (PMPM) basis and usually only varies by the age and the sex of the patient. It is designed to be independent of the actual volume or cost of the services rendered. This way, the provider assumes all risk for high incidence and inefficient/ineffective medical management (see Figure 10.1).

Capitation Demographics Analysis

The capitation calculation takes the following into account:

- Morbidity
- Mortality
- Lifestyle
- Age
- Gender
- Education
- Occupation
- Socioeconomic status
- Historical utilization of services

The Two Components of Risk: Uncertainty and Consequence

1. Volume of services rendered

2. Inefficiency in case management

3. Lack of coordinated, appropriate care

Figure 10.1 Capitation risks and opportunities. (Source: HealthPro Consulting, Inc.)

In previous years, we studied capitation and came to a comfortable point in predictability of risk using a critical mass of patients from a typical case mix that included both users of services and nonusers. More recently, however, with the advent of consumer driven health plans (CDHPs), the healthier populations are now joining the CDHP programs and are no longer mixed as they were in years past in the health maintenance organization (HMO) managed care risk pools.

This leaves a strange new situation that has not been addressed much in current literature. We used to have the consumption of services offset by those on the roster that did not consume services, by paying into the premium pool but not incurring claims. Therefore they offset the use of claims dollars in the risk pools for those who, for one reason or another, spent more than their share of the dollars.

In current times, those nonusers have been moved to a different funding mechanism, and the HMO managed care population contains more users than in years past. This will undoubtedly change the dynamics of the critical mass needed in order to manage capitation and claims risk to the degree that we were able to in years past. We will have to look to our learned actuaries for guidance and lean on excess loss coverage like never before to bolster us financially as we navigate the learning curve.

Services

The capacity and capability of the providers also impact the capitation. Can the hospital/provider provide all services, or must some of the services be "carved out" or subcontracted? What services beyond office visits are included: lab, physical therapy, in-office surgery, radiology, injections? What are the referral arrangements with subspecialists? What is the mix of family practitioners to general internists?

Dealing with Unpredictable and Unmanageable Risk Reinsurance

In managed care, reinsurance is a type of insurance that holders of risk purchase to guard against unpredictable risk, unmanageable risk, or low enrollment. Industry experts used to concur that groups that accept capitated risks should purchase their own reinsurance when their rosters reach more than 2000 covered lives. The sentiment has not changed, but the minimum critical mass has, and no one has been forthcoming about what the new number is. This author maintains that the reason for this is because of the shift in risk associated with the types of lives that remain in the risk pools, now that the healthier populations have moved to health reimbursement arrangement (HRA) and health service agreement (HSA) accounts not always associated with HMO plans.

One of the ways providers can protect themselves against excess utilization costs is to purchase reinsurance or stop-loss coverage (see Figure 10.2). The reinsurance carrier generally prices its coverage at twice what it expects to pay out over a policy period.

Hospitals generally choose to purchase reinsurance using per diems or some other factors as accumulators. A $25,000 deductible may cost an average of 7% of the hospital capitation. Other providers may elect to cover catastrophic incidences, using charges as accumulators with a deductible of $150,000, paying about 1% of the capitation. Now that the minimum critical mass has changed, all those numbers are meaningless. I have not been able to ascertain from any resources what the new numbers are or will be in the short term.

Reinsurance should be used when the provider has low enrollment, is responsible for costs over which it has little or no control, or is dealing in a large number of unknowns. Since we no longer have an industry standard for what "low" enrollment is, it is difficult to provide resources or guidance in a trade book such as this. My best advice is to find an actuary that you trust and a reinsurance broker that will work with you, demonstrate patience, and guide you through the process using relationship as the source of value instead of just a quick commission for a policy sale. There are many brokers out there who are just waiting to assist their clients through this learning curve. Shop carefully and diligently!

- Employee = 2.5 covered lives.
- The IPA or MSO or PHO purchases its own reinsurance when the enrollment reaches a critical mass of membership, placing the providers' reimbursement in greater than 25% risk for nonpayment or inadequate payment. (42 C.F.R. 417.479(e) and (f))
- Purchase reinsurance for the risk that is unpredictable and unmanageable and for low enrollments.
- Average claims $3500 to $4000 per employee, per year.

Figure 10.2 Reinsurance: The Basics.

Table 10.1 Simple Balanced Scorecard: Health Plan Pay-for-Performance (P4P) Programs

Hospital 40%	Miscellaneous 9% to 12%	Professional 28% to 31%
Acute care	Out-of-area claims	Physicians
Tertiary care	Pharmacy fund	Psychotherapy
Psych hospital	Term life	Podiatry
Outpatient surgery	Optical riders	Chiropractic
Physical therapy		Optometry
Speech therapy		
Occupational therapy		
Subacute		
Hospice		
Dialysis		
Home health		
DME/HME		
TC—Lab/Path		
TC—Radiology		
TC—Anesthesia		
Orthotics/Prosthetics		

Source: HealthPro Consulting, Inc.

Dividing the "Pie"

Managed care plans take into account many snippets of data in order to contemplate and create an offer of a contract for capitated reimbursement to providers. One thing they take into account prior to extending an offer is how not to pay for upside risk, and how not to get caught in too much downside risk, such that there is nothing to return back to Wall Street.

Many plans pay providers on the basis of a percentage of premiums, based on historical expenditures tempered by where they are in the underwriting cycle. The typical arrangement is illustrated in Table 10.1.

Once a premium has been established, a capitation development analysis is prepared by the actuaries. A typical commercial capitation analysis looks like Table 10.2. Through the use of this table, payers and providers alike may forecast utilization and payer cost indices under their fee allowances to estimate capitation equivalencies.

Table 10.2 Capitation Development Analysis

Service	Annual Freq./1000	Avg. Charge	Capitation/ PMPM
Primary Care			
Ambulatory office visits	2.550	$41.00	$8.71
Inpatient visits	0.116	62.00	0.60
Home visits	0.005	65.00	0.03
Pathology	1.536	10.00	1.28
Miscellaneous office services			
Immunizations			
Injects, including allergy	0.600	18.00	0.90
EKG, audiometry, etc.	0.250	38.00	0.79
Office surgery	0.100	75.00	0.63
***Total Primary Care*: $12.94**			
Referral Care/Services			
Ambulatory office visits	0.850	48.00	3.40
Inpatient visits	0.115	75.00	0.72
Home visits	0.003	95.00	0.02
Consultations	0.050	135.00	0.56
Miscellaneous office services	0.500	50.00	2.08
Emergency room visits	0.150	80.00	1.00
Surgery			
Inpatient	0.068	675.00	3.83
1-day surgery	0.045	425.00	1.59
Office surgery	0.150	110.00	1.38
Anesthesia	0.072	372.00	2.23
Maternity	0.072	1640.00	3.01
Radiology	0.580	124.00	5.99
OP psychiatric	0.200	68.00	1.13
Hospital Outpatient Services			
Physical and radiation therapy	0.060	90.00	0.45
Ambulance	0.010	195.00	0.16

Table 10.2   Capitation Development Analysis (continued)

Service	Annual Freq./1000	Avg. Charge	Capitation/ PMPM
Home health care	0.020	58.00	0.10
Durable medical equipment			0.45
Prescription drugs	4.500	27.00	10.13
Total Referral Care: $38.23			
Hospital Services			
Inpatient care	0.350	1100.00	32.08
1-day surgery	0.045	1250.00	4.69
Extended care facility	0.015	225.00	0.28
Emergency room	0.180	190.00	2.85
Total Hospital Care: $39.90			
Total Medical Capitation: $91.07/PMPM			
Reinsurance/Catastrophic Allowance: $4.93/PMPM			
Plan Margin 20%: $24.00/PMPM			
Total: $120.00/PMPM			
How to Use This Table			
• Primary Care Ambulatory Visits: 2.550 visits per year • Average Cost to HMO per Visit: $41.00 per visit • Calculation: 2.550% $41.00 = $104.55, divided by 12 = $8.71			

Note: The numbers in this table are fictitious. They are simply there to walk you through the arithmetic modeling.

The utilization numbers must be provided by an actuary by having the information required at the beginning of the capitation section of this chapter. Next, the numbers in the middle column need to either be based on the provider's target reimbursement or the plan's reimbursement as set forth in their fee-for-service equivalent.

In essence, multiply the real number you are provided or can historically derive on the left column of Table 10.2 by the number you establish as correct in the middle column, divide by 12, and you should come up with the needed capitation to meet the projected utilization to cover prepayment of those services at the target reimbursement rate. If either number is off, you have risk, or you will find yourself "in the money" (more frequently the former than the latter).

The significance of correct age, enrollment size, health status, covered services, and gender weighting of capitation cannot be overemphasized. Without these specifics, readers are cautioned not to use this table to negotiate capitation rates.

Fee Schedules

For covered medically necessary services that are not included in the capitation budget, a fee schedule may be utilized to determine reimbursement. Fee schedules are usually a product of the multiplication of one of a variety of reference systems of relative value units by a conversion factor represented by dollars which, when multiplied together, determine the price to be paid for a specific service.

Fee schedules are sometimes manipulated by payers using "cost-fixed" or self-authored codes to represent hybridized bundled services that have no value units established. These are troublesome to coders and actuaries because of their nonconformity to traditional calculations in comparison with established procedure code nomenclature relative value units.

Many hospitals are asked to consider reimbursement based on diagnostic-related groups or DRGs. At the time of this manuscript, the final Inpatient Prospective Payment System reimbursement has just been released. A cursory review led me to some immediate key observations for hospitals that currently have contracts with Evergreen clauses ("rollover features") that do not escalate rates or keep them contemporary with current regulatory recalculations, and this one will be significant.

Providers should revisit existing contracts as well as remodel new proposals with the following questions in mind:

- You will need to consider the continued transition from charge-based to cost-based reimbursement: How will this translate into modeled reality for your existing contracts that are tied to Medicare rates prior to the new DRG system?
- The new 745 "Medicare Severity" DRGs (MS-DRGs) replacing the current 538 DRGs: What will they mean to existing rollover contracts currently in effect with HMOs and PPOs? Have you modeled according to these 745 instead of the current ones you presently have in effect for this new contract?
- How will Health America tie their reimbursement in the current proposal to the Deficit Reduction Act of 2005 (DRA) that prevents your hospital from receiving reimbursement for the additional costs of treating a patient who acquires a condition during a hospital stay? How long will you have to rescind and resubmit a corrected documentation? It looks like 60 days on other things, but this is not specifically addressed.
- I have not seen current proposals and rate sheets that permit many fees to be modeled to address the new methodologies for calculating outlier payments and capital cost reimbursement. Be sure to address those in detail

with your health plan contracting representatives and obtain all explanations and model arithmetic in writing, which can be attached to the contract to prevent an argument of hearsay in accordance with the "entire agreement" provision of your contract.

■ Many contracts state little in the way of specifics of any quality measures that your hospital would need to report in calendar year 2008 in order to qualify for the full market basket update in FY 2009—it typically alludes to the fact that the hospital will participate and comply with the plan's committee decisions and edicts, whatever they may turn out to be.

■ Treatment of recalled medical services and devices, as well as replacement surgeries/procedures were not addressed at all in any of the recent contracts reviewed by me.

Case Rates

A variation on a theme of DRGs is case rate reimbursement. Based on my experience in reviewing contracts for many years, I have come to the conclusion that most providers in the nation have no clue how to negotiate a proper case rate with a health plan or any other payer, and the odds are most often loaded in favor of the plan, not the physicians or hospital.

What defies all logic to me is how the state departments of insurance permit these reimbursement arrangements without requiring that the providers obtain a license to be in the business of insurance without the necessary data, reinsurance or excess loss coverage, and cash reserves. My guess is that they simply are unaware of the existence of the deals because they are in service to premium payers, and the premium payers are not complaining if the hospitals and providers lose money or are underpaid. They will if the providers close up shop and close the doors!

To begin, case rates generally are designed to provide reimbursement for an "episode of care." The very term "episode" means an occurrence, incident, or event. Seems simple enough. So when one is asked to reimburse a provider to cover an episode of care, when is the specific moment that the episode begins and ends? If it is ill-defined or ambiguous, it could be the point in time where care is delivered.

I can think of several examples that I witness in contract proposals time and time again to name just a few:

■ Maternity cases
■ Outpatient surgical cases
■ Rehabilitation cases

What is worse is that the entire concept of pricing transparency surrounding consumer driven health plan expenditures and personal accountability for health care expenditures is woven around online arguments of case pricing. I have a real problem with published pricing and gold stars that are "irresponsibly" posted on a Web site by a health plan or its agent for the purpose of steering consumers to one provider over another. Many of the postings are inaccurate, out of date, and, for the most part, subjective and not exact comparisons of case rates from provider to provider as a standard. Most contracts provide for no first right of review or the right to refuse to be marketed inaccurately, or to besmirch one provider in favor of another on the basis of price. Furthermore, most of the Web sites, industry articles, and speakers coming from industry tend to use a misnomer of "cost comparison" instead of a more accurate term of price comparison. Until we can know our costs in this industry, which is wishful at best, it is impossible to label a case cost, let alone explain that cost to a consumer so that they can understand what it takes to keep a medical group's doors or a hospital open for business. But alas, I digress. Let us get back on target. (Yes, I feel better now!)

So, we were in the beginning of the discussion on case rates and episodes of care as they relate to contracted reimbursement methods. In order to establish a case rate, we first need to define an episode of care, where it begins and where it ends. Some cases should never begin, and some cases never seem to end with managed care. Take, for example, an outpatient surgery set for case rate reimbursement where the patient is a hemophiliac and will require Factor K, a very high-cost biological. If no carve out is stated for the Factor K, the case rate will likely be in the red before it has been scheduled by the surgical scheduler.

As a best practice, both hospital and physician should take a moment together to jointly determine which cases they will entertain as a case rate and then, case by case, determine when the case rate should not be applied in favor of an alternate reimbursement methodology. Start with just five cases. Determine the case by the current procedural terminology (CPT) code, taking into account instrumentation, supplies, surgical approach, operating room (OR) and anesthesia time, recovery time, and potential for adverse events during surgery and afterwards.

As a former OR tech, we can take five categorical cases in outpatient orthopedic surgery—"categorical" because that is how I repeatedly see them presented in contracts for case rates. At worse, they are categorically described as "outpatient surgery–orthopedics," "outpatient knee surgery," etc. At best, they are often only described by ambulatory surgical center (ASC) groupers (there are nine) and then arbitrarily parked into some reimbursement schema.

Let us examine these five to begin:

1. Open reduction, internal fixation of a fracture (ORIF)
2. Arthroscopic knee surgery–meniscus repair

3. Arthroscopic knee surgery–ACL reconstruction
4. Arthroscopic shoulder surgery–Bankart procedure
5. Removal of hardware

So you have contracted for case rates of $1800 for each of these cases, because you feel that there is some margin in doing them at that price, or because that was what the payer offered in its contract rate proposal as a percentage of Medicare rates, and you had no other interest in, time, software, or skill to model it differently.

The typical ORIF takes about 90 minutes of OR time with a slow surgeon. The typical knee surgery 90 minutes, shoulder 90 minutes, and removal of hardware 45 to 60 minutes. As far as equipment and supplies, the first four usually open up a major ortho pack, two gowns, three pairs of gloves, assorted suture, tapes, and dressings. The removal of hardware is generally a minor pack at best.

Anesthesia is usually monitored anesthesia care (MAC) or local or nerve block, and sometimes general anesthesia. If meperidine HCl and promethazine are used as anesthetics, there is considerable "barf time" and increased post-anesthesia care unit (PACU) nursing care budgeted in recovery, as opposed to a quicker recovery with propofol (but in patients allergic to eggs, we do what we have to). I find it amusing that surgeons who own their own surgical suites rarely know the cost of each minute of OR and PACU time and think they are saving money using less expensive drugs for anesthesia instead of maximizing throughput on the space and staffing resources they have with quicker, more costly drugs that recover the patient faster and more compassionately, but that is part of case cost too.

One other element that is part of the case cost is the instrumentation selection and all other supplies that are opened and tossed (they essentially are "pitched" onto the back table) onto the surgical field, back table, and Mayo stand. These instruments must be counted, sterilized, unpacked prior to the case, tossed if consumable, and resterilized, packed, and prepared for the next case. Therefore, in order to do multiple cases strung together one after another, you have to either have duplicate sets of instruments or schedule the cases accordingly, so that you have time to process the equipment between cases. That all has a cost implication and a quality implication too! (Longer anesthesia time and extended surgery time, etc.)

My experience in surgery tells me that many surgical preference cards for the surgeons are likely out of date and have not been updated recently to reflect what they really want or need for the case. Therefore, many things will be tossed onto the surgical field that take time and effort and staff to count; things that have been supplanted by newer things still remain. The Charge Description Master (CDM) has not been completely updated to reflect pricing for the new things, nor to retire the no-longer-used things. It probably also means that the costs attributed to the typical case have not been remodeled recently, and until these things are updated, the case cost remodeling will not occur.

All this is fine and dandy, but it is still based on that hypothetical "typical" case. Comes now the aberrance. A hemophiliac male patient is scheduled for surgery. Much more case management is needed; biological supplies such as expensive Factor K will be required. Pre- and postoperatively he will require additional care and monitoring to ensure hemostasis. He may end up in ICU. Let us take it a step further and assume it was the ORIF case, and in addition to the surgery and the comorbid condition, he experiences a nonunion of the fracture, requiring additional returns to the OR for additional surgeries. In one of these he becomes septic and infected; a true Murphy's Law case.

> *Issue 1*: Should this case have even been considered a case rate case? *or* should the contract have contained exceptions by example, condition, or some other indicia to trigger a different reimbursement methodology? Should any of these other subsequent triggering events or that of a malignant hyperthermia or other condition that might be encountered during surgery have given rise to an abandonment of the case rate methodology and a move to a different methodology?
>
> *Issue 2*: How detailed does the contract read? Does it even address this potential situation? Who gets to decide the final financial outcome? Based on what data or standards? Where are they published? Can they be unilaterally changed? Is the contract "mute" to this? Is the answer on the Web site in some obscure documents that may have never been reviewed? Have they been virtually referenced by the plan in the contract, but nobody ever checked to see of the documents really existed and what was contained in them? Assuming they were published, can the documents' established policies and coverage limitations be unilaterally amended at the sole and absolute discretion of the plan without any notice of the amendment to the provider? And if you took the case to dispute resolution, the arbiter can only decide the case based on what the Agreement states to begin with. So if you spend the money to file the dispute, but you cannot prove that something is wrong going solely by what is stated in the contract, can you win? (You probably do not have a snowball's chance.)
>
> *Issue 3*: How will the payer treat the treatment failure of the post-op infection? And the cost of the associated polypharmacy and likely intravenous therapy that will be required to treat it? Who pays that bill? How will you score on quality points, and will this injure your report with the little gold stars on the plan's Web site? What about any metrics being followed for pay-for-performance bonuses? Will this injure your position? How will

this messy outcome be addressed on a weighted scale or balanced score-card? Who has the discretion to score the outcome? Can you appeal the scoring methodology and statistical relevance?

Issue 4: Price transparency. You quoted this hemophiliac a price to come to your hospital. He planned to use his limited, banked, underfunded HSA and employer-contributed HRA funds to cover the front-end-loaded high deductible, which at your hospital and by your staff physician was pro-jected to come out less costly to him with a seemingly lower projected total price than the competitor up the street that was also "in network." After all, he was not planning on breaking his femur! Since he is not buying a car here, there is no list of options on the semiprivate or private room win-dow that faces the nurses' station from which to choose if he wants it or not. The fact is, he signed the consent form and stuff happens! Now there is a significant difference in price. Oh, but wait! Even though his funding mechanism is a CDHP, it is an "all-products" contract, so he is only fac-ing the maximum payout that the contract states is payable for the HMO and PPO folks. So who cares! His bill is $1800; it says so in the contract! Cool! And guess what? He has $1700 of it in the HSA fund. But now, he is angry. There was a less than stellar outcome. He has missed work, and he has had doctor visits, and he hurts, and the law says he does not have to choose to use his HSA fund money to pay *YOU!* He can keep it, bank it, roll it over to next year, or just choose to be a slow pay. What is worse is that your contract forbids you from asking for estimated patient financial responsibility up front, so not only do you have this runaway case expense, but you now have no money. Nada, zip, zero! The plan will not pay you, because the amount is within the high-deductible range, so they do not have to.

The moral of the story: Case rate contracts are extremely complex and should never be entered into without firm modeling, strategy, a plan for implemen-tation, and specific limitations and exclusions in addition to well-defined beginnings and endings of an episode of care. In addition, you need to determine so many of the things I brought up in the issues above, includ-ing payment and coverage policies, adverse outcome review and appeal rights, quality grades and publicity, pay for performance scoring methods and bonus calculations, and separate CDHP contracts. Oh, and then there is the clinical aspect of case rates; are the surgeon's preference cards cur-rent? Is the instrumentation reduced to only what is necessary? Have you eliminated all waste from the case? Is the CDM current? Is the case mod-eled appropriately for costs, and is there any other process improvement potential? I am asked to consult to hospitals all the time in this case cost strategic development. What is amazing to me is that those who ask for the assistance to structure such a program are far outnumbered by others who have signed these case rate agreements without any more preparation than accepting Medicare ASC Rates and moving to the next line item. If you are in the latter group, I implore you to at least examine a world where the homework is done.

Now let's chat about maternity rates. Most maternity case rates are based on DRG 374, normal newborn. First, I find it humorous that the average Medicare beneficiary is over 65, so that a Medicare DRG for any newborn born to a mother over the age of 65 could be classified as "normal." To quote Joan Rivers, "Can we tawk?" In the last 30 contracts I reviewed for clients, not once has there been mention of a different rate for vaginal births in comparison to Cesarean section births. One involves lots of pushing, breathing heavy, panting, sweating, and cursing, and threats of never ... well you get the picture. The other typically involves an epidural injection, knives, assistants at surgery, retractors, scissors, tapes, sponges, an OR, an OB pack, instrument tray, and nursery space for one normal, healthy baby.

Why is it that more than 95% of the contract proposals for maternal-child case rates that I reviewed in my entire career as a contract analyst and managed care expert never anticipate or mention rates for multiple births, stillborn babies, cases where the mother dies, or cases where the baby is tied to the father's plan as primary in accordance with the "birthday rule"? Is it that the plan forgot? Or is it that they never intended to pay for more than one normal newborn baby regardless of the outcome of the case or the number of babies delivered? And why do hospitals allow those contracts to be signed as proposed?

In conclusion to my discussion of case rates, I have included an example (see Table 10.3) of how I prepare the layout for case rate contract negotiations by procedure. It is not exhaustive, by any means, but it is significantly more detailed than the typical contract proposals I have seen for case rate negotiations.

One last consideration is with regards to hardware and implants and high-cost drugs. The old way to negotiate these was to agree to produce an invoice for each item. The new way is to assert in the contract that the price charged is reflective of not more than x% markup and allow up to two or three spot audits per year if the payer chooses to verify and audit that the rate charged is not more than the percentage markup asserted.

As I review contracts, my take on the situation is that the majority of hospital contract analysts, for the most part, have not developed a written set of contracting policies or business rules, and a written contracting strategy with a checklist of those things that cause modeling woes for the business office and reimbursement problems for the finance team. As such, the process becomes reactive, as opposed to responsive and proactive, and each contract is addressed with the

Table 10.3 Sample Case Rate Contract Attachment Form

CPT CODE:	29877	
Description:	Knee surgery–arthroscopy	
Includes:	Surgeon's history and physical	
Surgery		
90 days follow-up care: limited to evaluation and management services		
Surgical assistant, if requested		
Anesthesiologist		
Intraoperative X-ray and fluoroscopy, if required		
Intraoperative gross and anatomical pathologist review, as required		
Preoperative testing		
Limited to:	Finger-stick glucometry, HCG pregnancy test, if indicated, spin hematocrit, urinalysis, EKG	
NOTE: All other lab testing and pathology at Colorado WCRV Fee Schedule.		
Facility charges for routine procedure		
Recovery room		
Repricing from individual bills to case rate		
Disbursement to individual providers and MSO		
Excludes:	*Any hardware or implants	Fee: Invoice cost + 20% handling fee (however, this may be expressed in a myriad of ways that does not require the provider to tender an invoice)
*Facility overnight	Fee: $XXX	
*Any lab tests or follow-up X-ray or pathology services not included above		
*Emergency transfer fees by ambulance, as required		
*Physical therapy and DME fees, if any		
*Transition to inpatient status for any reason shall exclude this case from eligibility under this case rate program and revert the case back to traditional workers' compensation scheduled rates and reimbursement conditions		
Price:	$xxxx	

Source: HealthPro Consulting, Inc. (www.Mariatodd.com.)

time permitted to rush through the deal without method or data. The requisite forethought and preparation is not evident.

Managed care reimbursement takes lots of modeling capability to slowly and deliberately model the rate so that the surprises are reduced and the risk is managed. A fallback provision must be negotiated for when the system does not pay out as anticipated, and both parties need to have formulae that are stated within the terms of the agreement and its attachments, so that some third-party arbiter or mediator can get to the essence of the original understanding between the parties in the event of a dispute, without having to come up with a solution that was not part of the original understanding at the time it was signed. Unfortunately, most negotiators do not understand the terms of the contracts that they sign and therefore do not sweat the details as they should. Most also do not understand the mechanics of dispute resolution and, when a dispute arises, fail to use the prescribed remedies stated in the contract and simply quit. My apologies to all readers who have been through this and have the degree from Hard Knocks University. The vast majority of those who are unprepared for case rate and other alternatives to simple percent-of-charges reimbursement, by their very tolerance and execution of poor contract proposals, make it difficult for the rest of us to negotiate better contracts, as we are considered "troublemakers," squeaky wheels, and "difficult." I take pride in it; do you?

Chapter 11

Strategic Planning for Renewals and New Contracts: Understanding the Changing Competitive Environment

In health care, it is necessary for a contracted reimbursement strategy to remain increasingly flexible because of the many factors that influence change in the industry, including but not limited to:

- Insurance company market consolidation and dwindling HMO enrollments.
- Employer abandonment of traditional managed care health insurance coverage for employees and adoption of high-deductible policies.
- Increasingly prudent buyers who "shop" the cost of care and have the freedom to cross traditional geographic catchment areas, due to both the elimination of in-network "tethers" and the freedom to pay for travel to access care across the street or across the world out of both health reimbursement arrangements (HRAs) and health service agreement (HSAs) and other consumer driven savings accounts.
- Newly legislated changes to Medicare and Medicaid from government-direct reimbursement to that of reimbursement by a subcontracted

insurer that assumes risk of the cost of claims and needs to satisfy Wall Street simultaneously.

■ Globalization of health care that introduces competitors in previously insignificant markets, who compete on both price and accredited quality, and piques the interest of multinational employers with domestic and expatriate employees.

■ The advent of health plans' willingness to contract with those global health care sources for both medical services and supply of identical high-cost drugs and implants instead of permitting sourcing and markup through traditional domestic sources.

The strength of a contracted reimbursement strategy is determined not by an initial move, but rather by how well it anticipates and addresses the moves of competitors and shifts in customer (payers, employers, and individual consumers) demands over shorter and shorter timelines. I could be wrong, but I truly believe this alone is the greatest factor that has stymied most health care leaders and their contracting managers to commit to a well-developed, comprehensive written contracted reimbursement strategy and establishment of contracting business rules by which contracts are evaluated, negotiated, and/or rejected. As the rapidity of change increases, health care organizations must develop fluid and flexible reimbursement strategies that recognize and deal with this market dynamism in the development of their contracting strategies. In broad analysis of the clients I have worked with, together with more than 3500 respondents polled between 2006 and 2007 in my classes taught through the Healthcare Financial Management Association, my privately branded seminars, and other professional associations, only 3% to 7% respond affirmatively that they have a written contracting strategy, indicating that health care managers and executives have not kept pace to formulate and implement competitive strategies, but are simply reacting and not responding to the market.

Most providers' contracts are a patchwork quilt of terms and conditions, which make it impossible to truly manage or establish standardized business processes in revenue management departments. The staff is unable to assume that the organization's contracts would not contain the plethora of impracticable and unconscionable terms and conditions. If a well-developed contracting strategy and set of business rules were developed, communicated, and implemented to them, they would be correct to assume that the organization's business rules would never permit such terms to be accepted in contracts. The implementation of the strategy and business rules could arguably increase the efficiency and effectiveness of the revenue management department to draw out increased margin to the bottom line because of the standardization of process and approach. Lacking such standardization and adherence to strategy and business rules, the typical reimbursement contracts seen across the country require increasingly specialized, high-cost, and high-maintenance staff sensitive to the nuances of each contract in order to realize the compensation promised in the vague and ambiguous documents that are offered by most contracted reimbursement payer sources. What is worse is that, when I have dialogues with payers and ask why they do not wish to pay for the revenue management messes they create with these standard contracts, the resounding echo is "It's a cost of doing business." I really think their sentence is incomplete, as the more responsible and articulate response would be, "It's a cost of doing business *with us.*"

The organization's strategic success depends on how effective it is in addressing changes in the competitive environment from new drugs and technology and clinical interventions, newly introduced regulations, and consumer demands. For hospitals in particular, the added wild card of medical staff behavior and support is another significant element in assessing and managing the competitive environment. The impact of the strategy is determined by both the initial action of the organization and by the interaction of the strategy with competitors, customers, and others. The ripple effect of the strategy is characterized by how the market reacts to the strategy and then reflects back on the originating source. The complexity of the multiple waves of the strategy and the reactions to them shapes the ongoing refinements to the strategies, or the total abandonment of the strategy in favor of a distinctly different approach. The typical SWOT analysis (strengths, weaknesses, opportunities, and threats) is more complex and multidimensional in contracted health care reimbursement due to the ever-changing sources of monies available to pay for health care services.

Global health care sourcing and medical technology change, as well as new drugs in the market, also add to changes in the competitive environment. Markets are becoming increasingly complex as health plans open empanelment to foreign providers as "in-network" choices to increasingly prudent employers and consumers. In many instances, these networks offer pricing advantages that eclipse any steerage provisions in existing contracts that in the past created barriers to entry in what I refer to as the "provider directory" limited catchment area. With the advent of providers empanelled in Mexico, Thailand, and other countries, those glory days of steerage incentives as barriers to entry are null and void, in most cases. One must accept that every move of a competitor is to be met with a rapid and strategic countermove, and at best the advantage is only temporary.

Customers, whether health plans, employers, or individual patients, make their choices based on what they perceive each provider has to offer when compared to other available choices. As a hospital or physician group or other health care industry provider, there are several minimum requirements to be met in order to compete in the playing field. Among those requirements are accreditations and certifications, documentation of "assured" quality, possession of specific credentials, professional liability insurance, a clean history of regulatory compliance, continued compliance, and the training and development of revenue management staff to deal with the industry changes including coding, compliance, claims management, and reimbursement integrity benchmarking and its performance improvement, just to mention a few. These initial and ongoing burdens provide no significant advantage over rivals, but their continued maintenance and monitoring creates substantial ongoing business expense, which must be covered by the contracted reimbursement in order to remain alive as a business. (This is one reason why there is such interest by physicians to investigate direct practice or concierge care opportunities, because many of these overhead threshold expenses to enter the contracted reimbursement playing field are eliminated.) Therefore, that commitment to its maintenance is a small piece of the strategy that cannot be overlooked, because one cannot play without them. In short, the deciding factor is not how good the product or service being offered is, but how good a value it is relative to the competitor's offering. Those minimum standards referenced above are the "so what" aspect of all this. Everyone has them, so what makes you more special than your competitor—in the mind of the consumer? Can you express that differentiation in terms which the consumer can understand and use as the basis of comparison?

What is needed by American health care providers, in my humble but educated opinion, is to distill the complexities of the American health care reimbursement system, in recognition of its many diverse revenue sources, into a practicable, measurable, and manageable coherent strategic plan that serves as a framework to find and exploit new temporary sources of advantage, profit from sustainable advantages, and create sound barriers to entry for competitors. To the many diverse readers of this book, I do not envy you this task, but let us see if we can get you started with its formulation.

Begin at the Beginning: Define the Task

The key challenges for a well-developed strategy include:

1. Recognition of advantages in the changing competitive arena
2. Anticipating your competitors' actions
3. Developing the strategy
4. Evaluating alternative strategies

To develop an effective strategic plan, the leadership of the organization and its managers must understand the playing field and sources of competitive advantage, anticipate the moves of competitors, understand their advantages and leverage, and test proof of concept. This requires an accurate assessment of risk and rewards, the ability to communicate assumptions to others involved in the process, an assessment of both financial and operational sustainability (never negotiate what you cannot administrate!), and metrics to perform further refinements and responses to the ripples in the feedback loop.

Who Are Your Competitors?

To be a true competitor, each organization that competes with yours has to be selling to the same set of customers or market segment and serving many of the same functions. If they are not, or they focus on a distinctly different market segment, their actions may not affect your sales or profitability. How will you define the boundaries and the structure(s) of the competitive arenas? Are there single cases or multiple market segments? Where does the pool of available customers come from? What are the activities in the value chain?

Once you have identified the set of competitors, define in specific terms the advantage, if any, that you have over your competitors. Avoid oversimplifications that can result in fatal flaws from being blindsided by subtle changes to the competitive arena that result in serious consequences if overlooked. Take out a legal pad and do that now. Your foremost goal will be to sustain that advantage.

As the health care industry and its players become increasingly dynamic, the boundaries that define niche become overlapped and are less discernable. It is more difficult to identify your competitors or anticipate their moves. Next, on your pad, write down the identified sources of your advantage(s). Jot down any thoughts on how you assume they will change over time. Will they be changed by public policy, globalization, regulation, access to capital, consumer behavior and awareness, or technology? Who will the disruptors be and how will they disrupt?

Take a moment to consider any presently unserved or underserved market opportunities, changes in technology, pricing, and supply chain that could broaden the array of perceived substitutes, and the potential of entrants from adjacent markets that could influence market definitions. How will you identify them and deal with them? It is crucial that you recognize patterns of substitution, both from the demand side, to account for the ways customers meet their needs or have the needs addressed for them (as in closed panels of providers in an HMO setting), and the supply side, to include all competitors in the market with the capabilities to serve their needs. This is where one must take consumer behavior into consideration and assess the need to create affinities, loyalties, and self-selection of your brand and to determine if the customer is of the ilk to hop on a flight for a foreign land to save 80% on price for an acceptable substitution.

Properly defined markets are established by distinct discontinuities in the buyers' needs or benefits sought, and the degree of acceptable substitution of the product or service alternatives for satisfying those needs. Take a moment to jot down how the payers and other customers see your organization and the services you provide. Are you selling what they want to purchase, the way they wish to purchase it? Do you have enough to sell? If you sell too much to them, will you have enough inventory or capacity to sell to others who may wish to buy? What happens if they abandon their shopping cart without concluding the transaction? What happens if they switch to another supplier? How will you deal with the excess capacity or inventory that you previously sold to them? What will it take to win them back as a customer? Besides watching the customer's actions, (which may be too little, too late) you may need to inquire directly through the use of feedback or focus groups prior to making potentially incorrect assumptions upon which you stake your strategy and your business viability.

Now draw a vertical line down the middle of your paper. How will your competitor answer these same questions from their perspective?

Now let us give thought to your true competitors' actions and responses to any action prompted by your exploitation of this advantage. How will they move to respond or react to your move? How will they interpret what you have done and why you are doing it? Do what you can to guesstimate the mind of your competitor, and try to visualize their biases and experience that will affect their interpretation and decisions to respond or react to your move. Can you guesstimate how they will see the payoff? Is the payoff of significance or consequence to them or simply not on their radar? Have they discounted your actions to the extent of a fatal flaw? How quickly and effectively will they be able to respond to neutralize the advantage?

Keep in mind that both organizations' intellectual capital and experience will strongly color how the competitive intelligence and payoff relative value are calculated. The heuristics that influence each of the rivals are largely dependent on experience, predilection to entrepreneurial risk taking, and assumed or actual leverage. Sometimes a strategy is to simply shadow the leader. What happens if they take that tact with you and shadow your pricing by 5% or 10%? Is that enough to warrant the customer to shift purchasing behavior? How will your organization measure and evaluate your rivals' actions and reactions? Think of the metrics you will choose to monitor and how you will monitor them.

Forces That Influence Leverage and Competition

Five main forces influence both leverage and competition for your negotiations of contracted reimbursements:

1. Customer bargaining power
2. Threat of new entrants to the market
3. Direct rivalry among competitors on specific services or service lines
4. Pressure from acceptable substitutes
5. Bargaining power of suppliers

Strong bargaining power of payers and employers and threats from your competitors' substitutes will limit your ability to compete on price and value.

The intensity of competition between hospitals and physicians and other providers can drive down prices and raise costs of meeting the competition with new products, technology, drugs, service coverage, and promotion to win new business. These forces will be directly impacted by three other forces: government intervention, expensive technological change, and market growth or decline. The intersection of these eight forces, among others, can cause well-developed strategies to be short-lived or completely tossed out the window at a moment's notice. Reminder: our foremost goal is sustained competitive advantage.

Competition is most intense when there are only a few equally balanced competitors, or when numerous small players serve the same market and try to make moves that they hope their competition will not notice. Sometimes, payers and employers play this card to keep the competition intensified. Other times, competitors create the heat all by themselves. When competition is divided among a few companies with domination by one competitor that has at least 50% more advantage of market share or profit or sales volume than the competitor in the second position, the competition is more subdued. Generally, the followers position themselves in the shadow of the leader. This generally happens if the leader's costs are substantially lower than everyone else's. One case example that comes to mind is a medical group in a particularly heated market. The leader is a radiologist that has arrangements to be a beta test site with new technology in multiple locations in the marketplace. As such his arrangement includes access to cutting-edge technology with little or no capital equipment expense. His cost to produce cutting-edge technology is lower, and he cost-shares the expense of his marketing and promotion with the various technology suppliers to show off the fact that he has the ability to do the diagnostics with the latest and greatest—that the others in the marketplace do not. I cannot use the word other "competitors," because without the same technology the others have stumbled on at least one barrier to entry that is insurmountable. They do not have the cash to buy the same technology, the supplier does not have to sell it to them or cut them a similar deal as a beta site, and without it they are not true competitors. As such, this radiologist can compete at a much lower price point and higher sales volume than anyone in the area.

Next I examine his business model through the eyes of a patient—easy ingress and egress at a freestanding facility instead of the confusion and requirement to follow the yellow lines through the outpatient department of a large hospital Patients love not having to navigate large facilities if the smaller provider has what they need.

Decorative appointments and modern furnishings exude a perception of quality and modernity in all styles, including décor. Since patients cannot appreciate technical quality, their definition of perceived quality is what they base their purchase decision on, together with the fact that if they stay "in network" they get the best benefit level on their plan coverage. With his business model, he can afford to take everyone's low reimbursement, because his supply costs are far less than any competitor, thereby creating another barrier to entry. Is this sustainable? It has been for the 8 years that I have been aware of his practice. How long will it continue? As long as his suppliers continue to participate in this business model and not permit others to enter. Is it anticompetitive? Well, the feds assess the effect of the competition on the marketplace not between the competitors, so probably not. Customers can shop anywhere where they can get their price met. There are lots of radiologists, but many of them have failed to supply to the market what the customer wants or needs to buy. Therefore, one could say as I did, that they are not true competitors, just "other" radiologists. That actually gives him an advantage. Ponder for a moment, before reading ahead, how that can be applied to situations in which your organization competes. Who are your competitors? What are their advantages? How do they compare with your own? The ability to understand and evaluate how true competitors react to one another is critical to the development of a successful strategy. Much also depends on the heuristics and perceptions of the strategists and the data and leverage available.

One last concept we need to visit is that of exit barriers. Are you remaining in bad contracts as a participant in a market even when profitability is nonexistent or miserable? Why? If you exit, how will it affect the strategy of your competitors and the balance of competition in the market? In polling my audiences and clients, one thing is perfectly clear. Most providers have no exit strategy for poorly performing contracted reimbursement, and most do not have any established declination metrics to sound an alarm that it is time to employ the nonexistent exit strategy.

Step-by-Step Formulation of Your Competitive Strategy

Once you have taken into account the playing field and your understanding of true competitors, the next step is to design your contracted reimbursement strategy. In this phase, you must consider the need to develop a response rather than react to the move of competitors and market redirection and shifts. For example, instead of meeting a price cut by a payer, you might seek to increase volume of sales or increase service lines where others do not compete.

Better yet, preemption may, in some cases, be a better strategy. In other words, sometimes the best defensive move is a strong offense. To do this often requires insight into where your competitor will move next, or a crystal ball, or just plain luck. While some moves are fairly predictable, others can blindside you. Therefore, it is probably not wise to develop your entire strategy with just one approach, because preemption often requires a significant resource commitment that might produce an uncertain or unwanted result.

As in the old-fashioned SWOT analysis, options and opportunities must be evaluated. When developing a contracting strategy, you might be better served by narrowing options rather than expanding them; in other words, fewer but better contracts instead of poorer reimbursement by more payers. Can a commitment to tighter business rules yield an improved competitive position?

Is it right to just say "no" from time to time?

Since we are discussing competition in this chapter, I think it would be prudent to include qualified legal counsel in your development of a strategy to remain compliant in the area of antitrust. Rather than develop first and then submit for legal review, include the legal minds in the development process from the onset. Simply manage the relationship with them by formulating good questions and eliciting good guidance, rather than asking them to decide for you without understanding the nature of operational and managerial implications involved when revenue management and competitive strategy intersect. Most health lawyers do not have professional training in hospital and health services administration at the graduate or undergraduate level and have never walked a mile in those moccasins. The ones who have this are inherently successful and have a sustained competitive advantage among their fellow professionals, because their suggestions are practicable rather than just lawyerly. By the way, their names are in my contact manager if you want them!

Let us break down this formulation into different segments with questions to ponder for each.

Response to Competitor Actions

1. Should you react? If so, how aggressively? What is your rationale for this stance? Could you ignore the stance? Accommodate it? Abandon it? Retaliate?

2. What should be the relative magnitude of your response compared to the reaction? Should you meet or match their move or outdo them? Why? If you match them, will the customer deem there is no perceivable competitive advantage? If you outdo them, will you impede the competitor's chance of success? For how long?
3. How quickly should you respond? Would a more appropriate approach be to "wait and observe?" Or is a more immediate response necessary? Is a commitment of resource to a preemptive strike more appropriate? What indicators do you have that give one choice more weight than the other?
4. Where do you want to fight this battle? In the market that was attacked? Or in some other battlefield where they do not see you coming? What about a more neutral ground, if applicable? Perhaps a choice to step aside and let them have the business. Why did you make this choice?
5. Which weapon will you choose to fight the battle? Price, reputation, promotion, perceived quality, differentiation, repositioning, new product development? Something else? Why is that the right weapon of choice? Is there a need for multiple weapons used simultaneously? Which ones? How will they be employed?

It will be necessary to carefully explore the possible reactions and responses to competitors' moves to elect the best overall strategy. Rather than take action on the basis of gut and intuition, you will likely move toward a sustainable strategy instead of one that is short-lived and costly to rectify.

Next, we will look at preemption. While a reactive move tries to stop, impede, divert, or limit damage and exposure to further loss after the competitor's move is initiated, preemption deals with offensive attack or movement in a different direction. With preemption, you attack the other's intention to attack. You are taking control of the chessboard by owning squares that limit the opponent's choices and access to key positions. You impede their growth and limit or stop their progression before they have had a chance to act.

Preemptive Response Questions

First, determine where the market is headed or where it might head. Next, identify potential strategies for getting there first or creating a blockade. Then begin to assess feasibility and consistency with the current overall business strategy if there is one, and whether they are likely to affect your competitor's response and position in the market. While easily said, it is not easily done, and errors will likely prove more costly than will yield serendipitous outcomes. They could easily be career-limiting errors if one is not careful and acts like a maverick.

Consider these questions:

1. Can you lock up capacity?
2. Are you able to own and lock up markets?
3. Can you lock up customer preference?
4. Can you block your competitor's intended actions?

In developing a preemptive strategy, you may save time and costly errors by calling upon a small number of outside experts for brainstorming sessions. I have had the pleasure of working with several "dream teams," many of whom I have assembled for clients in order to bring the intellectual capital together in a conference room over an intense two-day brainstorming retreat with organizational leadership, legal counsel, board members, and industry experts. These sessions have taken me to Capitol Hill, Jackson Hole, and other retreats, and hospital cafeterias alike. Often these sessions involve a relatively small number of participants (usually fewer than 10), who are encouraged to come up with new approaches and solutions, as opposed to being constrained by the way the organization has done things in the past. At first, the wildest ideas possible are laid out without reservation, criticism, or judgment. It is always easier to trim down than it is to add more ideas to the mix. By calling upon experts with national experience, you bring to the table an insight into the applicability and lessons learned. Just select carefully, so that you are not entrusting your future to a consultant with little experience and a "one-size-fits-all" approach to your situation. Also consider that the most active consultant in your market may also work for your competitor and may have a conflict of interest in their advice to you. Consider that, in all likelihood, they would place themselves in a difficult position if they fought as aggressively or made creative solutions such that their position elsewhere in the community is jeopardized, especially if the revenue they generate from your project is far less than that which they generate from your competitor.

There are many facets to preemptive options that one should consider:

Market Segmentation

1. Existing customers
2. New customers
3. Former customers
4. Prospects

These should be evaluated in three formats: payers, employers, and individual patients seeking your services.

Pricing

1. Discount off charges
2. Package or bundled pricing
3. Fee schedules
4. DRGs and case rates
5. Capitation
6. New pricing formulae

Promotion

1. Frequent buyer programs
2. Special affinity ventures with employers
3. Steerage
4. Endorsements by clients
5. Endorsements by media
6. Endorsements by payers (e.g., gold star ratings on Web sites)

Products and Services

1. New services
2. Expansion of existing service lines
3. New generation products
4. Cutting-edge technologies

Distribution and Logistics

1. Exclusive deals
2. Loading the channels
3. Strategic partnerships and alliances
4. Mergers and acquisitions

Positioning

1. Technical quality
2. Perceived quality
3. Premium and branding
4. Cost savings and sensitivities
5. Value added

Create a preemptive worksheet that includes four, five, or six vertical columns.

Competitor's Move:		Criteria for Evaluation			
Strategy	Consistent with our existing objectives and strategy?	Is it feasible and practicable?	Effect on the competitor?	What will it cost us to implement?	Time frame
1					
2					
3					
4					

Rather than evaluate each column on its own merits, do not be afraid to examine the competitive effect of the criteria overall. Just because an approach is inconsistent with current strategic goals and objectives does not mean it should be abandoned. Perhaps the current strategy and objectives should be reexamined? Likewise, if it has consistency but is not feasible or costs too much to endeavor, it may not be the right choice either. Create a similar worksheet for each preemptive move you will consider, rather than mixing the moves over one sheet. Paper is cheap. Sort your thoughts into distinct chunks at this point.

How long will the competitive advantage last with this preemptive strike? Consider the magnitudes of impacts of each choice by positioning options in a grid, where the vertical axis depicts the duration of the impact, whether permanent (high) or short-term (low), and the horizontal axis depicts the magnitude of impact from minimum (left) to maximum (right). At a high degree of permanence and maximum impact, your competitor will likely be stopped dead in their tracks. While that permanent maximum impact is ideal, it may not always be possible, and other outcomes should be planned for to provide viable alternative outcomes.

Remember, the stakes are high with preemption and involve a considerable element of the ability to predict the future with considerable risk and cost for mistakes. Still, even with the risk potential, one should not dismiss preemption as part of the planning for a competitive strategy. Just be prudent about your ability to take on risk, and have a backup plan in case it shows signs of failure.

Signaling to Your Competition

How you signal to your competitors will have an impact on their behavior.

Signals come in two main forms, including announcements and actions. There are signals that can be used to discourage attack, other signals used to block entry or dissuade excess capacity in the absence of certificate of need regulations and considerations, and signals used to discipline bad actors and uncooperative behavior among rivals. The latter often happens in pricing initiatives where a leader signals a price increase and a competitor breaks ranks to drop prices or keep them steady.

Signals can also set a code of conduct and be used to segment the market or to gain acceptance of de facto position that will ensure peaceful coexistence in a marketplace. These require careful legal analysis to ensure that the hands-off message to the market will not be viewed as collusive to artificially manipulate price and competition among a select few competitors. That would be a bad thing.

Signals can also be used to send up trial messages to test market response. Finally, there is always the bluff. An organization can often confuse customers and competitors by signaling an action without any intention of following through. I have seen this all too often with hospital administrators and the interactions with their medical staff members, especially when they want to plant misinformation. Unfortunately, this approach often leads to credibility issues, and soon the administrator is rendered ineffective and is replaced. In contracting, this might be the case when the hospital is considering a relationship with a particular payer and they "leak" the information to a select few on the medical staff known to be blabbermouths.

The docs pass the message on in the operating room (OR) and the cafeteria, and soon each physician is empanelled with the plan. If the hospital chooses not to complete the transaction, the doctors have no place else to admit patients unless they go to the facility down the road, where they may or may not have privileges. Soon, doctors begin to plan their day with the cases strung together in block time in the OR or begin to direct admissions to one hospital over the other so that it is more convenient and less time-consuming to make rounds.

The ripple effect is with the patients who may have choice, because the payer with which they have their coverage has contracts with both hospitals; therefore, the limited market segment that is forced down the road is sleeping in the same semiprivate room as the patient that could have been in the bluff hospital generating revenues. The bluff backfires and can facilitate demise when not used appropriately. It is not usually sustainable as a competitive approach.

Signals are interpreted in three main ways: aggression, clarity, and consequences, as well as how committed and consistent the sender is with the message. It can also be affected by the similarity of the sender and receiver, because the outcome is highly dependent on the interpretation of the signal.

Take the time to develop explanations and rationale of why a move was initiated, and how it will likely play out, with all the intended "what if" qualifiers and limitations. Reserve the right to change tack if indicated because of new information, data, or circumstances.

It is important that a strategist spend time and resource to understand the reason behind a competitor's move. If the signal makes no sense, it should not be dismissed out of hand. It may be that the strategist is missing some key information or is inexperienced in this particular evaluation.

Keep your eyes moving and your ears open. Do not dismiss what is happening in the periphery, lest you be blindsided by it. Part of the SWOT analysis includes threats. Take heed of all signals and impute weighted values to all of them, large or small.

It is crucial to avoid overreaction. Keep in mind that bias and heuristics may be in play on both sides. Inexperienced strategists may be reacting to ghosts and shadows. Test and prove concepts and interpretations whenever feasible.

Consider your risks. If too much information is revealed or too little information released, taking the wrong action could be counterproductive and cause serious setbacks. A signal that causes allegations of unfair competition or deceptive trade practices could be construed as collusive and could trigger serious legal consequences and antitrust allegations.

Never underestimate your opponent. It is imprudent to assume that competitors will react to signals as expected and act accordingly. Keep in mind that you do not know all the situations ongoing at the rivals' camp that may contribute to their interpretation and reaction and produce an unanticipated result.

Developing Alternative Strategies

Your mom told you to never put all your eggs in one basket. She was right. Now you are all grown up. It is time to come up with different options, each of which may produce intended results based on application, planning, feasibility, and best overall fit.

You will need to build a "big picture" view of your strategy, one that can permit you to see multiple competitive dynamics over time and across several futures, especially in light of what is happening in the health care reimbursement arena.

You might build one view to analyze a market-based approach. The preferred method for this analysis is the conjoint technique, a market research tool that captures perceptions in the market from payers, employers and the general public that might self-select your services without payer or employer influence, or benefit design incentives.

Another view can feature strategic assets, whereby the view includes industry characteristics, your service line capabilities, unique talents and notorieties within your medical staff, and some "what-if" scenarios. This view might include some new service bundle packaging, such as executive health, medical tourism, and new technology offerings that set you apart from your competitors. Keep in mind that these assets and capabilities will change over time, with the departure or retirement of a physician that was integral to one of the packages, or because of politics within the medical staff and management, and with developments in technology applications, just to name a few. The magic here is to try to determine what will be considered a valuable asset in the future.

Your strategic plan should enable you to run competitive simulations to proof concepts and assist both the developers of the plan and those who will be charged to implement it in feeling more comfortable that it is the right decision and a sound plan. These simulations can incorporate the above two methods and other approaches to test out the plan before investing serious time and money to implement them. Since strategy is not the domain of management or the contracting team alone, in order to get the most out of the strategic plan and associated business rules, you must have emotional buy-in from all members of the leadership and board members, revenue management staff that will live with the effects of the strategy from day to day, the physicians, and contracting team members.

Simulations enable those involved in executing the strategy to gain experience before meeting with the marketplace. It is like a practice match for a chess competition. It involves lots of formal logic; if "P" then "Q," if not "P, then "R," and so on. The more at risk, the more important the simulation will be. A study that I reviewed more than 20 years ago while still an undergraduate involved positioning of M&Ms, and the introduction of peanut M&Ms. It seems the strategists thought that the introduction of the peanut variety would add market share. Instead, the introduction of the peanut variety segmented the existing plain M&Ms market share, and a poor outcome was experienced. How could Mars have done that rollout differently? How does that translate to contracted reimbursement? Will your method and strategy simply cause segmentation and shift within the existing market share for no net gain? How can you test that to avoid a segmentation outcome and arrive at the intended gain you are shooting for?

Do not forget to use your contract management software for modeling simulation of reimbursement rates and forecasting. You should be able to ask for customized reports that can provide trend lines that can analyze historical rate changes over the last 5 years, as well as forecasting what the numbers will look like given a change in technology, surgical and treatment approach, and differences in the book of business held by a payer from various employers, over certain zip codes, and with select diagnoses and procedures.

Finally, decide how you will handle uncertainty. Put in place some key performance indicators and a few initial values that will serve as alarms that call your attention to problems or assurances that things are going as planned. Once you have your plan and business rules developed, consider how you will convey the information about what has been decided to those who will be charged to execute it. Ensure that they understand the strategy so that they do not undermine it, and ask for a written nondisclosure agreement with severe penalties for leaks and inappropriate dissemination. Like Coca-Cola and Kentucky Fried Chicken, you may wish to consider not giving everyone the entire recipe and releasing only those pieces of information necessary to do a task on a need-to-know basis.

Chapter 12

Developing Business Rules for Better Contracts

As part of a contracting strategy, it is a best practice for the leadership of the organization contracting with a health plan to develop a set of business rules or contracting policies to help frame up the parameters by which the contracts will be evaluated and negotiated.

Every variation in operation and maintenance of a contract diminishes revenue and profitability. It is like a factory that has to change tooling and die casting for each and every product instead of standardizing to one preferred model and selling lots of them. In the same way, contracts that require variation in pricing, modeling, terms and conditions of participation, notice requirement deviations, and the like each cost more per unit to evaluate, implement, and maintain than they would if there were one "best" to conform to.

In a perfect world where a provider had all the leverage in the world, it is highly unlikely that the provider would be able to achieve the one "best" standard contract, especially when each payer has different roles, customers, interests, and products to sell, each with their own benefit package, actuarial underwriting projections, and premium loads. Still, a movement to standardized contracting policy can reduce the expense and improve the inefficiency of having so many variables to contend with.

Rather than go on and on with explanations of what it takes to make up contracting polices, I would prefer to offer examples of the contracting policies that I have developed and implemented over the years for clients and for the entities with which I have worked in the past. These contracting policies are in effect in a variety of contracts throughout the country, so they are not in the least bit theoretical and are most practicable.

First, an initial contracting policy should include the acquisition of information produced for due diligence review of the payer. For this, I use the following questionnaire and request return not less than 2 weeks prior to an initial meeting to discuss the contract.

In preparation for contracting with a new payer or an existing payer where a change has taken place over the last year in strategy or ownership, or where the relationship is new to the physician or practice manager, this questionnaire (or parts of it) may be helpful to gain a better comfort level by the physician and/or practice manager before blindly proceeding into a business agreement.

This is a standard of practice for me, and I make sure I do it for commercial, Medicaid, and Medicare Advantage payers, in addition to Employee Retirement Income Security Act (ERISA) direct-to-employer contracts. In each case, the document is tweaked only slightly to fit the payer type.

In cases where you have an all-products contract, you may need to separate out the document into separate questionnaires or redundant questionnaires for the different lines of business they bring to the deal.

Precontracting Due Diligence

The cover letter generally includes the following text:

In preparation for our meeting scheduled for _____, please prepare two copies of the following information and bring it with you to our meeting. (Alternate: provide 2 weeks prior to the meeting to give you a chance to review the materials and verify their accuracy.)

A. Contact Information
   Name
   Title
   Address
   City, State, Zip
   Phone
   Fax
   E-mail
B. Organization Management
   1. Please attach an organizational history and ownership summary.
   2. Please attach an organizational chart including job titles.
   3. Please attach a description of senior management and their credentials.
   4. Please attach the CV of the Chief Medical Officer or Medical Director

C. Insurance
   Please attach copies of the following declaration sheets:
   1. Officers and directors coverage
   2. E&O or Liability insurance
   3. State Certificate of Authority from the Department of Insurance in all counties in the service regions in which the plan operates
   4. Insolvency Protection for Inpatient Claims, if any
D. Excess Loss—Reinsurance
   1. Please attach proof of present reinsurance policy, if any.
   2. Which reinsurance carrier will underwrite your excess loss coverage?
   3. What is the threshold for the reinsurance?
   4. In other states, what is the percentage of claims that go to reinsurance?
   5. Please provide claims info (below) for reinsurance claims history separate from your information.
E. Certifications and Accreditations
   1. NCQA, URAC, or other certifications
   2. JCAHO Accreditation
   3. Other Certification or Accreditation
F. Contracting
   1. Is your organization seeking providers for other lines of business in addition to this program on the same contract? If so, please elaborate.
   2. Is your organization willing to sign a single-program contract for HMO, PPO, or CDHPs only?
   3. (Include only if applicable): Is your company willing to sign a PHO or IPA contract? If not, please explain.
   4. Enclose a sample contract including all documents that are referred to in the contract and amendments.
   8. Please discuss proposed payment methodology/ies and formulae for physician services, physician-supplied drugs and supplies (i.e., discount formula, fee schedules, capitation, etc.).
G. Claims Management
   Please provide a description of your claims management and other health care information systems, including the claims payment system, and required Web-based claims verification, filing, and EFT/ACH payment mechanisms. (Attach a separate sheet, if necessary.)
H. Detailed Claims Payment Experience
   If you have experience in [State] or in other states where the payer has a managed care product, please provide recent statistical data, including:
   1. Number of claims processed per month.
   2. Accuracy rate.
   3. Performance standards for claims processing personnel.

4. Claims processors' performance compared to standards.
5. Average claims turn-around time.
6. Retrospectively denied days percent for lack of medical necessity.
7. Number of days payer will be able to readjudicate (reconsider) claims after payment.
8. Please provide historical payment to claims denial ratio (from Medicare Advantage, Medicaid, and commercial HMO products, if applicable). If none in [State], please provide data from other states where you presently conduct business.
9. Describe policy regarding retroactive charge back. Provide detailed retroactive review data on other managed care programs.
   a. Ratio of reconsidered claims to claims paid.
   b. Ratio of reconsidered claims that provider was allowed to refund without offset.

I. Sales/Marketing
   1. Please provide a brief summary of your marketing plan, including copies of sales/marketing collateral materials for our area.
   2. Please provide a sample or "mock-up" of what the member ID cards will look like for the patients enrolled with your plan.
   3. Please describe by example how our staff and physicians will discern payer information on the Identification Card (i.e., logo and/or name of plan, name of member, ID #, PCP, customer service number, claims address, etc.).
   Listing of past and present clients
   4. Describe how often your listing of providers is updated and distributed and how often new copies are published and distributed (i.e., Hard copy provider directory and/or Internet directory? Updated and distributed monthly, quarterly, yearly?).

J. Provider Relations
   1. Please describe the education program you will use to prepare hospital, physicians, and ancillary providers for your product(s). How frequently will training sessions be held to keep our staff informed of changes?
   2. Please provide a list of hospitals/physicians in the [local] region that have already executed a contract with you.
   3. Please provide a listing of completed or expected exclusive specialist agreements in either this region and other states (i.e., exclusive agreement with one specialty type/practice/physician network).
   4. Please provide a listing of completed or expected exclusive ancillary contracts in both this region and other states which will affect our participation and reimbursement (i.e., exclusive agreements for

laboratory, testing facilities, specialty pharmacies, or pharmacy benefit managers).

5. Please provide a copy of the provider operations manual, including policies and procedures.
6. Please provide a description of how provider issues/complaints are handled.
7. Please provide copy of the outcomes of the organization's last two provider satisfaction surveys.
8. Please describe the method providers use to determine enrollee eligibility.
9. Please describe what happens if eligibility is given by payer in error.
10. Please describe the method of determining which PHO providers will be on panel.

K. Clinical/Utilization Management/Case Management

1. Please attach a description of the utilization management policies and procedures (including referral, precertification, and prenotification requirements). Are there any guidelines such as InterQual or M&R currently implemented or under consideration? Please describe the standards and/or any published or self-developed guidelines used to develop utilization management/case management protocols.
2. Please attach a description of the nurses involved in case management, including their specialties and number of hours they work per month for the organization. Are they full-time regular employees or contracted independently?
3. Describe the access our physicians will have to the plan's medical director. Is the medical director licensed as a physician in [State]?
4. Will your organization be willing to participate in quarterly review/joint operations meetings with practice to address issues at our facility?
   a. Will the medical director, case manager, claims director, and director of medical management agree to attend?
   b. Is your organization willing to include quality, utilization, outcomes, problems, claims payment, and denial issues as agenda items for such meetings?

L. Member Services

Description of member services policies and procedures (please attach).

1. Please describe the educational program you will use to prepare enrollees for the HMO product.
2. Please describe any programs used to educate enrollees regarding ER usage, wellness, and disease management.

M. Financial

1. Please attach an audited balance sheet for the most recent fiscal quarter and year.

2. Please attach the last four quarterly audited income statements and the last two audited annual income statements.

N. Miscellaneous

1. What has your company done that is innovative in the managed care market?

2. What has your company done that is innovative demonstrating provider collaboration in managed care?

3. What sets you apart from the other payers?

4. Why should we choose to execute an agreement with your company over the other offers we have received?

5. Have you conducted any pay-for-performance programs in other states? If so, please describe.

6. Do you anticipate a pay-for-performance program in [state]? If so, please describe.

7. List of references both physicians and hospitals from other states.

Undoubtedly, the experiences you have encountered over the years will lend themselves to even more questions, but the above model questionnaire should get your creative juices flowing. Please note that most of the facts and figures requested are routinely produced for periodic reports to the state and federal authorities, and none are considered "proprietary," just in case you encounter reticence in the plan providing you with the requested data and materials.

Also, please note that for preferred provider organizations, this questionnaire would likely be impossible to answer in a state where the PPO is unregulated and nothing more than a marketing vehicle to negotiate discounts between payers and providers, for which the PPO middleman derives a networking deal-making fee. The information would have to be obtained from the individual payers that access your discount through the PPO brand name label.

Next, let us look at some sample contracting policies that I routinely attempt to preserve with clients and contracts for organizations for whom I contract as the actual negotiator. Again, the organization's leadership should determine which policies it would like to emphasize and which ones may not be of issue to the organization. I would prefer to give you more and have you eliminate some of mine or trade a few out with your own, rather than to have you try to come up with some from scratch. An old Chinese proverb attributed to an unknown author says, "Give a boy a fish, he eats for today; teach a boy to fish and he eats for a lifetime." I am a firm believer in showing the student what a fish looks like, rather than trying to describe it and let the student test the waters without ever having seen the fish. So here goes:

Model Contracting Policy for Hospitals

1. The offering party must be currently qualified, and in good standing, to do business in the State of Arkansas.
2. The offering party must have a current and valid Arkansas Certificate of Authority from the Department of Insurance in all counties in the Service Regions in which the offering party operates. (Alternate: List specific counties that the hospital considers its Service Region)
3. The offering party must sign Hospital's mutual confidentiality agreement prior to discussions.
4. Hospital prefers to contract with a plan that is already NCQA or URAC accredited, and has had at least three (3) years favorable experience in managing Medicare Advantage populations in other states and can supply valid current references of providers attesting to same.
5. Hospital prefers to contract with at least (#) Payers who have been awarded contracts to cover individuals this [Service Region], as Hospital currently services Beneficiaries from these areas.
6. All participating providers of Hospital's Active and Courtesy Medical Staff shall be included in the contract unless reasonable documented quality concerns exist with regard to a specific provider. Such concerns, if any, shall be noted to Hospital's Executive Board, in writing, prior to the onset of negotiations of any Participation Agreement. (*Especially prudent if a PHO exists!*)
7. The offering party shall provide Hospital with a copy of its Physician and Hospital Selection and Retention Policies and Procedures to be included as a part of the Provider Agreement.
8. In accordance with Hospital Policy, hospital-based providers must retain the right to opt out of the agreement if they so desire.
9. The offering party shall share with Hospital its methodology and algorithm for auto assignment of enrollees without a Historical Provider Relationship to a PCP prior to the conclusion of negotiations of the Provider Agreement, if applicable. (A serious concern if capitation is anticipated!)
10. In the event that any enrollee chooses to disenroll in accordance with 42 CFR § 438.56(d)(2), citing reasons including, but not limited to, poor quality of care, lack of access to services covered under the Contract, or lack of providers experienced in dealing with the enrollee's health care needs, Plan shall notify Hospital or Physician within 3 business days from the time it receives such notice. Hospital or Physician member provider shall have the opportunity for due process before any action may be taken against provider.

11. Plan shall provide enough copies of [Commercial, Medicaid, ERISA, Medicare Advantage, etc.] Summary Plan Description to Hospital for distribution of one retention copy for each Participating Provider to keep for reference and for the convenience of the enrollee at the providers' location.

12. Plan shall provide Web-based claims verification, claims filing, and Electronic Fund Transfer (EFT) of all payments to all providers. Timely payment shall be made to providers via EFT within a stated negotiated time frame. Plan shall clearly define to the satisfaction of Hospital and hospital-based physicians, a written definition of a "Clean or Complete Claim," which shall be attached to the provider agreement as an Exhibit.

13. Failure of or a delay in giving notice or furnishing written notice of claim to the insurer does not absolutely and under all circumstances bar a recovery on the claim. Failure to submit claims with the negotiated time frame shall not invalidate nor reduce any claim if it was not reasonably possible to give proof within such time, provided such proof is furnished as soon as reasonably possible and in no event, except in the absence of legal capacity, later than 18 months from the time proof is otherwise required. Plan and Hospital shall establish timely filing limits and timely payment standards to which both parties shall use their respective best efforts to adhere. Hospital PHO network providers shall be permitted to file claims for all services rendered for a period of 18 months after the provider receives notice that the patient has received eligibility process or period of retroactive eligibility.

14. The parties shall negotiate a time limit of not more than 120 days after which payments cannot be readjudicated or refunds to the offering party requested for any reason other than fraud or abuse. Refund requests shall only be upheld when mutually agreed that the reason for the refund is valid and appropriate. Any request for refund or readjudication by the offering party shall be accompanied by any and all relevant source documentation indicating the rationale of the decision to facilitate Hospital's consideration and/or agreement to such request.

15. In the event of a mutually agreed refund due to the offering party, provider shall have a negotiated time limit to submit the offering party a check, in order to facilitate an audit trail. There shall be no right of offset against future claims paid.

16. For services that the offering party deems retroactively to be considered noncovered or for any benefit reductions, Plan shall provide sufficient documentation to support the request, including a copy of the offering party rules and terms, the date the error was detected and by whom, and proof that the patient is aware and agrees with the action taken on the policy.

Any necessary recuperation of funds after the claim has been closed shall be a private matter between the enrollee and the Plan.

17. If an enrollee demonstrates abusive or threatening behavior as defined by the CMS or the State of [name] Department of Health, or if the enrollee demonstrates a pattern of disruptive or abusive behavior that could be construed as noncompliant and is not caused by a presenting illness, Hospital or Physician may choose to end the provider–patient relationship by giving the usual written 30 day notice of intention to terminate care, without first having to request permission from the Plan.

18. Plan shall provide payment for Emergency Services when furnished by a qualified provider, regardless of whether that provider is in the Plan network. These services shall not be subject to prior authorization requirements. The offering party shall be required to pay for all Emergency Services that are Medically Necessary until the enrollee is stabilized. The offering party shall also pay for any screening examination services conducted to determine whether an Emergency Medical Condition exists. Medical Necessity shall be solely determined by the attending physician. Plan may make coverage determinations deemed valid by the plan.

19. The Plan shall not refuse to cover an Emergency Service based on the emergency provider, hospital, or fiscal agent's failure to notify the enrollee's PCP, or the Plan's for screening and treatment within Emergency Medical Treatment and Labor Act (EMTALA) required time frames.

20. The Plan shall be responsible for providing Poststabilization care services 24 hours a day, 7 days a week, both inpatient and outpatient, related to an Emergency Medical Condition, that are provided after a enrollee is stabilized in order to maintain the stabilized condition, or, pursuant to 42 CFR § 438.114(e), to improve or resolve the enrollee's condition. Prior authorization is assumed granted unless denied or direction of the enrollee's care is initiated by the Plan within a reasonable period of time after the offering party receives the prior authorization request. Plan must approve or deny coverage of post-stabilization care as requested by a treating physician, dentist, or other provider within the time appropriate to the circumstances relating to the delivery of the services and the condition of the patient, but in no case to exceed one hour.

21. For Coding and Bundling interpretations, Plan shall acknowledge and adhere to Official Coding Guidelines and official coding advice as approved by the four cooperating parties (American Hospital Association, American Health Information Management Association, Center for Medicare and Medicaid Services, and National Center for Health Statistics) responsible for administering the ICD-9-CM coding system. *Coding Clinic for ICD-9-CM* is the official publication for the ICD-9-CM coding guidelines and

advice as designated by the four cooperating parties. Any deviation from the above shall be included as an attachment to the agreement. At such time that ICD-10 is implemented in the United States, this policy shall be assumed to be updated concurrently.

22. The Plan shall acknowledge and adhere to Current Procedural Terminology (CPT-4) coding principles and guidelines as developed by the American Medical Association. *CPT Assistant* Newsletter is the official publication for the CPT-4 coding guidelines and advice as designated by the American Medical Association.

23. Should the Plan (or its pharmacy benefit manager (PBM), as applicable) develop a formulary, then that list and its updates, if any, shall be provided to Hospital and/or provider network prior to completion of negotiation of and made a part of the provider Agreement as an Exhibit. Changes to same will be addressed through the Notice and Amendment provisions of the finalized Contract.

24. Providers may rely on telephone or electronic verification of eligibility. Plan shall provide a confirmation or other tracking number to keep with the record in the event eligibility is at issue with regards to claims payment.

25. Plan shall establish a Joint Operating Committee (JOC) to review relevant performance measures, quality, and utilization. Together with Hospital, Plan shall establish target benchmarks for utilization of certain services related to disease management and overall utilization assessment. Not less than monthly, Plan shall provide Hospital with relevant feedback to the mutual satisfaction of both Hospital and Plan, including monthly quality and utilization detail reports for ambulatory encounters, inpatient days, ED Visits for specific diagnoses, pharmacy utilization, generic equivalent compliance by specialists and primary care physicians, and other quality indicators or matters similar in nature.

26. Plan shall develop a way to extrapolate Encounter Data from CMS-1500 and UB-04 claim formats whenever possible and shall avoid manual Encounter Data logs or other manual entry if possible.

27. Plan shall provide timely and accurate claims and encounter data feedback to Hospital for all enrollees assigned to Hospital or PHO Network providers and shall certify all data pursuant to 42 CFR § 438.606. The data that must be certified include, but are not limited to, enrollment information, Encounter Data, and other information required by the State and contained in Contracts, proposals, and related documents. A copy of the same data submitted to the state shall satisfy this requirement.

28. It is a proven fact that managing medical conditions and disease in a more comprehensive and coordinated manner can reap tremendous

clinical benefits for patients and cost savings for health plans and providers. Implementing new care programs requires the development and adoption of case-tested pathways, protocols, and guidelines. To this end, Hospital and its Medical Staff have developed and continue to develop many of these case-tested pathways, protocols, and guidelines for the purpose of this and other participation agreements.

29. Hospital is aware that many Commercial, ERISA, and Medicare Advantage contract awards include bonus amounts or other substantial operating funds in addition to funds available to pay claims for Enhanced Services required under their contract. These bonuses are often tied to Special Needs Populations (SNPs), Disease Management, and quality issues that require participation, support, and adherence by the provider network in order for the offering party to reach established goals and objectives of the bonus program set forth by such state or federal programs. Hospital hereby states a desire to participate in such activities and to develop a bonus structure in addition to the claims payment amounts paid by the plan in furtherance of these financial performance and/or quality goals and objectives as is mentioned above. The parties agree that any such incentives shall be in compliance with the federal managed care Incentive Arrangement requirements pursuant to 42 CFR § 438.6 and any other state or federal regulations.

30. The plan shall use its best efforts to adhere to the following standards with regards to communications between provider and Plan: At a minimum, the standards shall require that 99% of calls are answered by the fourth ring, the call abandonment rate is 5% or less, and the average hold time is 2 minutes or less.

31. If Plan is at risk for cost of enrollee claims, without backup reinsurance, Plan shall provide information regarding reinsurance demonstrating that the Plan can and shall at all times maintain net equity (assets minus liability) equal to at least 1 month's CMS payments under this Contract, the dollar amount of which shall be disclosed in compliance with this requirement. In addition, the offering party shall maintain a current ratio (current assets/current liabilities) of greater than or equal to 1.0.

As stated previously, the organization's leadership should take a proactive and participative role in structuring the contracting policy for those who are charged with the analysis and negotiation of the deals being offered to the providers. An added bonus to the creation and adherence to these policies will be that the leadership will be able to evaluate the performance of both the contracts and the contractors by pairing the outcome of contracts metrics tied to Key Performance Indicators (KPIs), the development and utilization of Payer

Report Cards, and benchmarking day-to-day business costs associated with the contracts negotiated along with how they fared against established policies that were developed in the best interest of the provider.

Chapter 13

Negotiation Techniques, Tactics, and Strategies

This chapter focuses on the art of persuasion, a subject which includes much controversy as to which negotiation techniques, tactics, and strategies are considered best. What I am *not* going to do in this chapter is teach negotiation. There are many books already written by many experts far more knowledgeable than me to teach the art of negotiation. A chapter on the topic from me would do both professional discourtesy and disrespect to my author colleagues and to those wonderful resources and would be remiss in the treatment of such an important topic. What I will attempt to do in this chapter instead is address how I have used the skills that I have learned from the many resources both written and taught to me by mentors, and lots of coursework at "Hard Knocks University" in order to persuade, not manipulate, others, many of which include primarily health plans serving as my opponent at a negotiation table.

Here are a few observations: First, most health care administrators (and contract negotiators) have never taken a formal course in negotiation. My assessment comes from direct inquiry at the hundreds of seminars I have taught to more than 50,000 attendees of my signature seminars on managed care contract analysis over the course of more than 18 years. Second, most health plan contract negotiators are untrained and unskilled in the art of negotiation, nor do they have any refined techniques in negotiation, and the majority of plans would like to keep them that way. This conclusion comes from having to negotiate with many of them on behalf of clients, and also having worked for health plans as a contract negotiator. Third, most hospital administrators, physicians, practice administrators, and those who are charged with the responsibility for carrying out the negotiations are under the mistaken impression that the health plan folks have lots of data at their disposal and polished negotiation skills, and that they are no match for the health plans' soldiers, tactics, and strategies, and therefore have little to no leverage. This conclusion comes from direct inquiry of hundreds of clients and thousands of seminar attendees, and makes me want to scream and throw tantrums!

Open up *Barrett's Quotations* or any other readily available quotation source, either in print or on the Internet, and read the sage wisdom of anyone who has been quoted on the powers of positive attitudes, defeatist attitudes, and leverage! I do not need to include any of them in this chapter. You have already heard them, but why are so few taking those quotes and philosophies to heart?

With all the years in the industry and teaching, observing, and negotiating contracts for clients and for employers, I could never understand why the negotiation skills set is so poorly developed, let alone why there is so little emphasis (or interest) in mastery of both persuasion and strategic development. Then, last week while presenting to one of many state association meetings of hospital and health care executives, the answer came to me as I was on the stage presenting a 90-minute session on "Payer Report Card Development and Preparation for Renegotiation." I surveyed the audience using audience response technology, and when I asked the first question, "What size hospital do you represent?" more than 34% of the respondents came from hospitals with more than 300 beds. A follow-up question of: "Do you have a written contracting strategy and a set of business rules by which to guide your contract analysts and negotiators?" yielded a 2% positive response. A third question, "Do you feel that your contracting position is strategic or reactive?" received a response of 49% strategic and 51% reactive. As George Carlin says in one of his skits, "There are some things that just make you go 'Hmm.'" Had I not been the experienced presenter that I am, the distraction of this epiphany could have derailed my entire program. I both love and hate equally those "Aha!" moments, especially when they hit me on the stage, and I cannot stop to write things down. I will bet my publisher hates them too, but does not know it, since the end result that she sees is a delayed manuscript, while I again sort out the approach for this one of the most difficult chapters to write in this book. Difficult because, in this chapter, I must practice what I preach; I must convince and persuade you to buy into my philosophies enough to turn the page, and why you should adopt them and take a suggested action.

A few more observations if you will kindly indulge me:

Observation 1: Most health care providers and administrators are not happy with their contracted reimbursement agreements. (I did not need a Ph.D. to make that deduction.)

Observation 2: Few of those providers and administrators have likely ever written down specifically why they are unhappy with those agreements. They have likely never written down what makes them happy with the contracts that they do express satisfaction with.

Observation 3: Fewer have likely expressed in written form what they want and do not want specifically, if they could identify and wordsmith the perfect contract. I have heard the proposed, "I send them the bill, and they pay it correctly and timely"; we all have. The problem is, we would need, at a very minimum, to define correctly and timely. And therein lies the challenge. How does the hospital administrator persuade the health plan that the bill is correct and accurate, such that a claim—which is filed for services that are assumed to be "covered expenses" under a contract for such financial exposures as may be experienced by the patient or insured—should be paid using investor-entitled monies to satisfy the claim to the satisfaction of both the claimant and its authorized assignee of benefits (the hospital), and for which the hospital, in anticipation of receiving steered business volume directed to itself because of a preagreed discount price that is less than the billed amount and payable under certain conditions and situations, has agreed to participate in this arrangement? Did you follow that? Read it again. The challenge is in the myriad of definitions that must be laid down and mutually agreed to by the parties.

Observation 4: Most medical providers do not have a clue how much it costs to render care on a line-item basis, let alone the cost to manage contracted reimbursement. Heck, it is safe to say that most providers and their administrators do not even have a handle on exactly what contracted business they have and where all the executed contracts are kept, when they are next renewed, and exactly how much is payable under each! So, if they do not know what they have, it is almost certain they are not managing it, and if they are not managing it, they most certainly do not have a clue what it costs to do so. Therefore, when someone tells me a contract is or is not profitable, I just have to challenge them on that notion. Forgive me, but this is soooo frustrating!

So I must ask: "First, how can one feel that their contracting position is strategic without a strategy established?" Were those who responded that they are in a strategic mode kidding themselves? Or do they not have a clue what contracting strategy is all about and lack the understanding of how it can be used to persuade, strengthen their position, increase leverage, increase revenues, decrease costs, and increase margins and efficiency?

Second, if they did understand, would they continue putting off the development of a contracting strategy and a set of business rules? Would they bother to commit to a contracting process improvement that required some investment into modeling tools, data set development, skills set development, and commitment to proof of concept? And would that lead them to a mind-set of empowerment and the courage of their convictions to say "No" when it was appropriate to do so? Would they go so far as to determine forensically if there are real dollars or real losses in the checks they deposit in the bank from the various health plans for the services rendered under contracted reimbursement arrangements?

What a revolution could occur in contracting if just 15% did! Who wants to be first to get their own way and become happier and more satisfied with their contracted reimbursements? If you did not raise your hand, throw this book in the recycle bin. You do not need to read the rest of it. The rest of you, follow me.

In order to get our way and persuade others that our way is best, we need to first define what is "our way." For many years, Burger King's slogan was "Have it your way." When I drove up to the little squawk box in the drive-through lane, I had "my way" down to the very last detail. I wanted a Whopper, with cheese, cut in half, extra mayo, no onions, and a diet Coke. I no longer eat fast food, but I have the same routine at Starbucks. I know exactly what my way is for coffee, and so does every other coffee pilgrim in the line in front of me and behind me. We make our way there every morning, dutifully, and we are prepared when it is our turn to tell them exactly what we want. We do this quickly, because we also do not want to offend the other pilgrims with unnecessary delay because we see ourselves as considerate, civilized people, and we want to persuade others that we are that way. If I go to a steak house, I have a plan for what I want and what I do not want. I want my steak medium rare, depending on the cut; I know how I want my side dishes; I know which brand of Scotch I want, and I will tell you exactly how I want it served. (Johnny Walker Blue, neat.) If they do not have Johnny Walker Blue, I have a backup strategy for how I want my unblended Scotch, in rank order by brand and age. Barring that, I will resort to bottled water and not drink what I do not like. I simply do not settle for what is unacceptable.

Funny, I do that with contracts too. I know exactly what I want, what I do not want. I have specified what I will accept if they will not give me my first preference, and when to walk away. It is all on a checklist and committed to by the client before I sit at the table.

It is no surprise that I am successful at that negotiation table, because I am committed to those chosen preferences and deal breakers that have been confirmed and committed to in writing by the client and any board of trustees of the hospital. I can be very persuasive, because I can defend the strategy by which they were conceived, and I am committed to the business rules that support the strategy.

As such, that level of commitment shows through in how I present my arguments, defend my data, offer what alternatives are acceptable, and know when to push my chair back away from the table and leave. The commitment to the strategy and business rules or contracting policy shows in my confident demeanor, my style of dress, the accessories I carry, how I command my space at the table, my use of props, and the techniques employed to carry out the act of negotiating, including caucus technique, use of time, data, and market intelligence. It shows in the precise vocabulary I choose to use in discussions, and the subliminal messages I send through the use of color psychology, cultural sensitivities, the use of humor I carefully employ during the meeting, and my social grace as hostess as I make my "guests" comfortable and relaxed during the meeting on my turf with my own home field advantage. Is any of the above something that cannot be learned? Hardly! Yet everything is purposeful, and each and every subliminal message I plant as well as those messages sent on the surface exude that I am successful, I am correct, I am confident, and it all contributes to my power of persuasion. What it does not support is any impression that would bring about an accusation of being manipulative, dishonest, lacking integrity, unprepared, or uninformed. In order for me to be convincing, I must first convince myself that I am not those things; I do have to convince myself that I am doing right by my client, maintaining my integrity, upholding the rules of compliance as far as antitrust, Sarbanes-Oxley, fraud and abuse regulations, among others, and that the client has agreed that the strategies and rules are good for the organization and that, if not upheld, the agreement is worthless and should not be pursued. To do this takes hours of due diligence, preparation, and homework long before the first meeting to discuss the merits of the "proposed" or "draft" agreement (I do not use the word "contract" until it is fully executed and signed, because it is not a contract until that point). With all my years doing this, I still never permit myself to become overconfident, and I never permit myself to negotiate from a position that is unprepared. So why do those with less experience, less practice, less preparation, no written strategy or business rules, no commitment from the leadership, and no exit strategy or defined deal breakers have the audacity to think they can do it as well, if not better, without that planning, preparation, and the commitment that leads to such persuasiveness without those tools, techniques, tactics, and strategies? That is simply insane! And to do it repeatedly and expect a different outcome defies all logic. You will never be happy with the contracted reimbursement agreements you have executed (notice that I did not say "negotiated") until the preparation, training, and due diligence is done, whether undertaken in-house or outsourced to someone who can. And if your level of commitment and belief in yourself and your objectives are not strong enough to evoke and emote your passion, then others will never be convinced or persuaded that your way is best, for them and for you.

So how do we get to that level of preparation so that we are ready for negotiation?

Understand the organizations out there that are offering the proposals and draft agreements:

1. What do they want? Why do they want it?
2. What do they not want? Why do they not want those things?
3. Who are their stakeholders? What is at stake for them?
4. What regulations must they uphold? What consequences do they face if they do not uphold them?
5. What is in their wallets? How much can they afford? What happens if they go over budget? Are they insured for their excess losses? Self-insured or externally indemnified? Is their budget actuarially realistic, or have they decided to make do with an insufficient premium, which might cause them to deny or delay claims or face insolvency?
6. What accountability do they face in the marketplace? What are the consequences of not meeting or exceeding that accountability?
7. Why should they want to do business with you?
8. What should they want to buy from you? How much of it should they buy?
9. Should they assume that you cannot fill their every need? If so, who else should they buy from, and for what contingencies should they plan? How should they buy from others? What will it cost them in time and effort and maintenance to keep up with so many vendors?
10. How do they define quality? Is it consistent with how they should define quality? How do they reward quality as they define it? How do they penalize the lack thereof, if the quality perceived or measured does not meet their standards?
11. Before they are entitled to a discount or any other consideration from you, what level of business volume, revenue, or profitability should they be able to steer your way in a quantifiable, objective, and proven way? What if they fall short? What if they fall short only once? Repeatedly? Or variably per quarter, per anum, per whatever period you wish to stipulate?
12. How have they acted in the past? With you? With others? What would you like to see changed or improved? Why?
13. What if they choose not to change or improve? Can you live with continued bad or unsatisfactory behavior? For how long? How much will it cost you to endure the continued behavior as compared to other payers? At what point is it time to declare it untenable?
14. How many times have they caused you unnecessary expense which only eroded any contribution margin?

Chapter 14

Contract Law Basics

Managed care participation, like practically every other business activity, involves a contract. The contract is essential to free enterprise in our economic system. Each party in the contract is legally obligated to observe the terms of the agreement and the rights of others created and protected by those contracts.

A contract is a binding agreement. In the Uniform Commercial Code (UCC), a contract is defined as a "total legal obligation that results from the parties' agreement as affected by [the Code] and any other applicable rules of law."* By one definition, a contract is a promise or set of promises, the performance of which the law in some way recognizes as a duty, and the breach of which the law gives a remedy for. Contracts arise out of agreements; hence, a contract is often defined as an agreement that creates an obligation.

The essential elements of a contract include (1) an agreement between competent parties based upon genuine assent of the parties and (2) supported by consideration (money) and made for a lawful objective in the form required by the law. The parties to a contract include the promisor, or *obligor,* and the promisee, or *obligee.* A party to a contract may be an individual, a partnership, a corporation, or a government. A party to a contract may be an agent acting on behalf of another person. There may be one or more persons on each side of the contract. In some cases, there may be three-sided contracts, such as a managed care agreement between provider, payer, and patient. In addition to the original parties to the contract, other persons may have rights or duties with respect to it.

---

* The Uniform Commercial Code UCC §1-201(11).

A contract arises when an agreement is reached. The offeror makes an offer, and the offeree accepts. If either is lacking, there is no contract. Each contract includes specific information, including but not limited to (1) the date, (2) the name and address of each party, (3) the promise or consideration of the seller, (4) the promise or consideration of the buyer, and (5) the signatures of the two parties.

Working arrangements between two parties are sometimes not regarded as contracts, because it is not the intention of the parties to enter into a binding agreement that could be interpreted as nonperformance if the two parties are not satisfied with the outcome. When a working arrangement is part of a clearly contractual relationship, the transaction remains a binding agreement, because the purpose of a working arrangement is merely to provide flexibility to a contract. Are all parties to the contract clearly identified by name? Sometimes a contract only identifies the Preferred Provider Organization (PPO) or Third-Party Administrator (TPA), not the payers. Before a provider enters into a contract with a managed care entity, the provider needs to assure predictability of patients and revenue. The provider needs to obtain the following information:

- Who owns the entity and what type of management/administration does it have? Is the contracting entity the actual risk holder or payer, or is it a shell corporation or a rental or consignment network? The party identified in the contract will be the entity legally responsible for the managed care entity's financial undertakings. The provider must review the financial stability and the management expertise of the legal organization identified in the contract.
- Who are the other providers under the contract with the entity?
- What is the entity's volume of enrollees? How are they marketing to new enrollees?
- What obligations would be imposed upon you as a contracting provider? Are you able and willing to comply with them? Must the physician accept all patients referred to him or her?
- Must the hospital accept all patients for all procedures requested, even if it conflicts with religious missions?

In theory, if there is an increase in patient volume and the provider costs are fixed, the increase in volume more than compensates for the discount on services. But, if the managed care patient takes the place of a full-charge cash or indemnity patient because of limited capacity, the economics shift.

Providers must also review whether the agreement requires providers to provide care for a certain number of patients, or if it requires the provider to be available to all patients who visit the provider. The provider should have the right to notify the managed care entity that he or she no longer has the capacity to accept new patients. Otherwise, the provider risks loss of practice control.

Incorporation of Exhibits or Attachments

Many contracts contemplate future events or benefits. In the course of negotiation or discussion leading up to a contract, one party may show the other party various charts, tables, and statistical projections into the future to show the actual dollar value of the particular transaction to the other party. It is a question of intent to what extent such a matter is merely illustrative and to what extent it is part of the contract. This is why it is necessary to have all exhibits and attachments incorporated into the contract so that, in the event of default, there can be a proven breach of contract and liability can be imposed accordingly.

Sometimes, the contract will expressly refer to and incorporate the terms and conditions of the other writing or statement. In this case, it is necessary to have the words *"a copy of which is attached hereto and made a part of this contract."*

Specified Services

A detailed list of the services required is necessary, especially under capitation systems where the provider agrees to perform services for an up-front fee. Otherwise, the provider takes the risk that the managed care entity can determine what services should be provided in its sole discretion.

Standards of Care

Providers must avoid provisions that require them to provide services under a different standard of care than otherwise required by state law. Many times, contracts require providers to provide care "of the highest quality." In a malpractice context, if a physician agrees to provide care "of the highest quality," a higher standard of care than required by state law will be imposed upon the provider.

Exclusion of Other Statements

In the opposite of incorporation, the contract may declare that there is nothing outside of the contract. This means that, in the offerror's eyes, there was never anything offered or promised or that any prior agreement was merely a preliminary step that is finally canceled out or erased when the contract in its final form is stated in writing.

Contract of Record

A contract of record arises when one acknowledges before a proper court the obligation to pay a certain sum unless a specified thing is not done. Some of these obligations may be known as recognizance. When an agreement is made with an administrative agency such as the Federal Trade Commission (FTC) that the entity will cease and desist engaging in a particular business practice that the FTC has found unlawful, the business is bound by its agreement and cannot disregard it afterwards.

Express or Implied Contracts

Simple contracts may be classified in terms of the way they are created as express or implied contracts. An *express contract* is one where the parties have made oral or written declarations of their intentions and the terms of the agreement. An *implied contract* is one where the evidence of the agreement is shown by acts and the conduct of the parties. An example of an implied contract would be where one party orders a meal in a restaurant, eats the meal, and then honors the bill for the meal and pays it. In terms of effect, there is no difference between an implied contract and an express contract. The difference relates solely to the manner of proving the existence of a contract.

Quasi-Contracts

Under certain circumstances, the law imposes an obligation to pay for a benefit received as though a contract had actually been made. This will be done in a few situations in order to attain an equitable or just result. When a health care provider delivers services with the expectation of being paid for emergency services, it may be implied that the patient receiving the services would be unjustly enriched if the services delivered their expected outcome but the patient did not pay for them. In order to distinguish this from a true contract, which is based on the agreement of both parties, the obligation is called a *quasi-contract.*

While the objective of the quasi-contract is to do justice, one must not jump to conclusions that a quasi-contract will arise every time there is an injustice. For example, no quasi-contractual agreement arises when a provider merely confers upon the payer a benefit that the payer was already entitled to.

A quasi-contractual obligation would not exist if performance of a contract proves more difficult or more expensive than expected, as in the case of adverse selection. It would also not entitle a party to extra compensation when there was no misrepresentation as to the conditions that would be encountered or the events that would occur, and particularly when the party complaining is experienced with the particular type of contract and the problems that are likely to be encountered. Does the term *full-risk* contract remind you of this situation?

Another case where a quasi-contract would not exist is in the event of disappointed expectations. If a person wrongly concludes that there is a binding contract and proceeds to make a purchase on that assumption, there is no right to recover for the loss sustained when the other person refuses thereafter to enter into a contract that is binding. A third example where there is no quasi-contract is in the case of contracts involving third parties. When a person has a binding contract with a third party, only that person is required to pay for performance made under the contract. Even though the performance has conferred a benefit upon the defendant, the person cannot sue the defendant for quasi-contract when the third party fails to make payment under the contract. For example, in private indemnity insurance circumstances, a physician who does not accept assignment of insurance benefits from a patient but bills the insurance company as a courtesy cannot sue the insurance company if it fails to pay.

One of the most important sections of contract law that you must understand is the agreement. An agreement is formed when an offer is accepted. Offers are conditional promises upon an act, a forbearance, or a return promise that is given in exchange for the promise or its performance.

To constitute an offer, the managed care payer or case manager must intend to create a legal obligation or appear to intend to do so. It is not necessary for him or her to expressly state that he or she is making a contract. When there is neither intention nor the appearance of intention to make a binding agreement, there is no contract. It makes no difference whether the provider takes any action on the apparent offer.

Definiteness

An offer, and the resulting contract, must be definite and certain. If an offer is indefinite or vague, or if an essential provision is lacking, no contract arises from an attempt to accept it. The problem arises because the court cannot ascertain the intentions of both parties.

An offer and the resulting contract, which by themselves may appear "too indefinite," may be made definite by referencing another writing (or exhibit or attachment), such as a fee schedule, table of inclusions in case rate contracts, or capitation inclusion listings, utilization management program details, quality assurance program details, formularies, sanction policies, and the like. An agreement may also be made definite by reference to the prior dealings of the parties and to trade practices. This might include "rollover contract terms and conditions."

Although an offer must be definite and certain, not all of its terms need to be expressed, because some omitted terms may be implied by law, and other omissions are often skillful omissions intended to mislead a careless or ignorant reviewer. For example, a contract must be for a lawful purpose. In the language of the contract, it states that the hospital or physician or other providers must abide by and comply with all terms and conditions of applicable state and federal laws and regulations. In addition, the provider must comply with and abide by the health plan's utilization and quality management policies and procedures, coverage policies, formulary selections, etc. Likewise, one would think that the plan has the same requirements incumbent upon it or will be held accountable for any breach of this policy. So, when the plan does not comply with state statute on timely payment, or ignores its own published policies and procedures for utilization or quality or coverage, for example, is it in breach of the contract for breaking the law or the policy? Not at all! The contract terms did no specify that. When the payer refuses to pay the statutorily established medical records copy fee, are they in breach of the contract? Not necessarily.

This is why it is so important to have a contracting checklist, written strategy, and business rules implemented. Attorneys can help eliminate these ignorant or careless assumptions, even if they are unskilled in the business of health care; they can follow what it is we want and ensure that our expectations are what is enforceable in the contract. Attorneys may not have gone to health administration school, but we can help them pair up what they learned in law school with what we know as far as the operational difficulties of the contract to make a better, more practicable *and* enforceable contract for us.

Terms may also be implied by conduct. There may also be an agreement known as a *divisible,* which consists of two or more parts and calls for corresponding performances by each part by the parties. Such may be the case in home health and durable medical equipment (DME) contracts. The purchaser agrees to purchase different articles at different prices at the same time. When the contract contains a number of provisions or performances to be rendered, the question arises as to whether the parties intended merely a group of separate, divisible contracts, or whether the agreement was for a package deal so that complete performance by each party is essential to delivery. The same is true of situations where we allow breach of contract to go on repetitively for an

indefinite time. The other side may argue that we never took issue before, so why the change in position all of a sudden? One defense back at that could be recent enlightenment—you took a class, read a book, sought professional guidance, and realized that there was an action that you could take instead of continuing to just accept unfair business practices and continued poor conduct.

If the term of an agreement that is too vague is not important, it may sometimes be ignored. If the balance of the agreement is definite, there can be a binding contract. Consider unspecified basic terms in the contract where no example is given—terms like adequate, reasonable, material, sufficient, timely, prompt, appropriate, fair, among others. Often without any other explanation or clarification elsewhere, say in an attachment or exhibit or formula in the contract language, the resolver of the dispute, usually an arbiter, would look to the author of the contract. This should make you take heed and sweat the details of additional clarification and creating a memorandum that is annexed to the contract as an exhibit or attachment, so that these vague terms do not come back to haunt you in the future.

The law has come to recognize certain situations where business necessity makes it desirable to have some form of a contract, yet the situation makes it impossible to make the terms and conditions definite in advance. There are three common situations in which this can occur.

Cost-plus contracts are valid as against the contention that (1) the amount to be paid is not definite when the contract is made. Futures contracts or *output contracts* are valid against the contention that the contract was not binding and was illusory because there was no obligation on the part of the buyer to purchase any quantity from the seller. A contract to supply medical goods as necessary is likewise binding as against the objection that it is (2) too indefinite and does not state a price. An entity may desire to be assured that the services of a given person, ordinarily a specialist or professional, (3) will be available when needed. It is thus becoming valid to make a contract with the professional to supply such services as in the professional's opinion will be required, although this is indefinite and would appear to give the professional the choice of doing nothing. Under such contracts, the duty to act in good faith supplies the protection found in most contracts in the usual rules as to certainty and definiteness.

Contracts with no specific time limits are valid. The law meets the objection that there is a lack of definiteness by interpreting the contract as being subject to termination at the election of either party. An agreement is not too indefinite to enforce because it does not state the exact price to be paid, but states that the price shall be prevailing market terms or the "usual reasonable and customary" marketplace allowance.

A contract may contain preemptive rights when the payer gives the provider first right of refusal or privilege to engage in a certain activity.

Termination of an Offer

An offer gives the provider power to bind the payer by contract. This power does not last forever, though, and the law specifies that under certain conditions the power ends or is terminated. Offers may be terminated in a number of ways: counteroffer, revocation of the offer by the offeree, lapse of time, death or disability of either party, illegality, and rejection. For example, in specialty capitation it would be wise to negotiate terms to an agreement that in the event not enough covered lives sign up with a particular plan, a specialty provider might reserve the right to rescind their agreement to accept risk if there is not enough critical mass to reasonably expect to manage the risk transferred through the contract.

Duress Issues

Economic pressures on a contracting party may be so great that it will be held to constitute duress. Economic duress occurs when the victim will be threatened with irreparable loss for which adequate recovery could not be obtained by suing the wrongdoer. Usually, a threat of economic loss or the pressure caused by economic conditions does not constitute duress, which makes a contract voidable. The fact also that a payer drove a hard bargain does not give rise to the defense of economic duress, or that the provider gave in too easily because the contract was too complex, the time to review it was insufficient, or that the provider "assumed" one thing or another but has no documentation demonstrating a clarification was sought.

Mistake, fraud, undue influence, and duress may make the agreement voidable or, in some instances, void. If this happens, the following remedies are available: recision, liquidated damages, or reformation. Do not permit yourself to make assumptions that these options are readily available and easy to come by on a poorly negotiated contract. That preceding sentence is a legal mouthful and will cost tens of thousands to prove and correct.

Interpretation of Contracts

The terms of managed care contracts and agreements should be clearly stated, and all important terms should be defined and included as recitals. If they are not, the parties may construe different meanings. The author of the offer always retains the privilege of interpreting the offer. When such differences cannot be resolved satisfactorily by the parties and the issues are brought forth to an arbitrator or court, certain principles of construction and interpretation are applied.

A contract is to be enforced according to its terms. It is the binding intention of the parties that must prevail. A word will not be given its literal meaning when it is clear that the parties did not intend such a meaning. For example, "and" may be substituted for "or," and "may" for "shall" when the parties' intentions are clear.

Unspecified Terms of an Agreement

Managed care agreements require providers to participate in utilization review and quality assurance activities and abide by the terms, conditions, and operating policies. Providers should not blindly agree to participate in such programs. The agreement must specifically reference and incorporate the specific utilization review and quality assurance programs so that the programs cannot be changed without notification or approval from the provider, by U.S. mail, prepaid, certified, return receipt requested. Providers should make sure that these programs are consistent with the quality of care rendered in their practice and that they do not unduly interfere with the provider's practice of medicine.

Must the provider abide by unspecified "medical policies?" Who establishes these policies? Where can they be obtained in writing?

Tip: Beware of phrases such as these:

■ A utilization review program *shall be established* to review the medical necessity of covered health services furnished to enrollees. ...
■ Such program will be established by the PPO, in its sole and absolute discretion.
■ Provider shall comply with and, subject to provider's rights of appeal, shall be bound by such utilization review program. ...

When a contract is partly printed or typewritten, and the written part conflicts with the typewritten part, the written part prevails over the typewritten part. If there is an ambiguity, it is interpreted more strictly against the drafting party. Thus, printed forms of a contract, such as insurance policies, which are supplied by one party to the transaction, are interpreted against the supplier and in favor of the other party when two interpretations are reasonably possible. If the contract is clear and unambiguous, it will be enforced to its terms even though this benefits the party who drafted the contract. The rule that an ambiguous contract is interpreted against the drafter is not applied when the other party knew what the drafter intended.

Assignments

The parties to a contract have both rights and duties. This is so in managed care agreements as well. An assignment of rights is a transfer of rights. The party making the assignment is the assignor, and the party to whom the assignment is made is the assignee. An assignee may generally sue directly on the contract, rather than suing in the name of the assignor. An assignment may take any form, written or spoken, to show that intention to transfer or assign will be given the effect of an assignment.

In managed care agreements, there should be mutuality as to the ability or privilege to assign the benefits of performance under a contract, provided that both parties agree to obtain the written consent of the other party before doing so. This is especially important when contemplating the future sale of a business or additions such as mergers or new providers coming under the same corporation as the assignor.

As we observe the insurance industry cope with changes in underwriting, consumer driven health plan (CDHP) shifts in membership, and reduced premium outcry, we will notice fewer and fewer companies surviving and more mergers and acquisitions. Assignment paragraphs will play a major role in the calculation of the ongoing business value for a health plan as the merging plans carry out due diligence to determine what they get as a package deal with the purchase. If you have contracts with both merging plans, which fee schedule and contract terms and conditions will survive? You may wish to consider requiring that both contracts cease and a new contract is evaluated with the new entity after you assess the position in the marketplace, its enrollment, and how you wish to facilitate the market transition, as your participation may well be pivotal in the marketplace. You may also find that to do so walks the risk of being eliminated from both plans and the new combined entity, so relationship both with the plan and with the community may be vital to an ongoing relationship with the new player. It is all a matter of business strategy and should never be decided under pressure or at a time of volatility in the marketplace.

Delegation of Duties

In certain instances in managed care agreements, it may be necessary to execute a contract that requires duties that you cannot personally perform. The service may be lab testing or radiologic or psych or skilled nursing facility or rehab services that you may not be able to render personally for whatever reason: no equipment, restrictive covenants on leases, services that you normally outsource, cross-coverage, and so on. You will be required to make or buy those services, delegate their duties, and perhaps maintain ostensible liability on their performance.

In the case of integrated delivery systems such as independent practice association (IPAs), physician–hospital organization (PHO) single-signature contracts, management services organization (MSO) contracts, and the like, a contracting party may obtain someone else to do the work. This also arises when health plans hire companies that do claims and bill audits or in the case of Health Insurance Portability and Accountability Act of 1996 (HIPAA) Business Associate Addenda. When the performance is standardized and nonpersonal, so that it is not material who performs, the law will permit the delegation of performance of the contract. In such cases, however, the contracting party remains liable for the default, if any, of the person doing the work just as though the contracting party had performed or attempted to perform the job, unless the agreement states otherwise. One who is entitled to receive performance under the contract may agree to release the person who is bound to perform and to permit another person to render the required performance. When this occurs, it is not merely a question of assignment of liability under the contract, but is really one of abandoning the old contract and substituting in its place a new contract. This change of contracts is called a *novation.*

Discharge of Contract

When two parties enter into a binding agreement, performance, mutual consent, impossibility of performance, operation of law, or material breach may discharge a contract. Please do not assume that this too is a fallback for a poorly negotiated contract, as it is easier said than done. A contract is usually discharged by the performance of the terms of the agreement. In most cases, both parties perform their duties and promises, and if the contract ceases to exist it is thereby discharged.

If performance of the contract on or within the exact time specified is vital, it is said that "time is of the essence." Time is of the essence when the contract relates to property that is perishable or that is fluctuating rapidly in value. An express statement in the contract that time is of the essence is not controlling. When it is obvious that time is not important, the courts may set such a statement aside. Time may be essential, for example, when a contract for discharge planning or start-up of outpatient therapy is required within 24 hours of the initiation to dispatch services. This may be more commonplace in outpatient ancillary and behavioral health agreements. When the time for performance is not indicated, it will be assumed that the performance called for in the contract will be rendered within a reasonable amount of time.

A contract may be discharged by the operation of one or more of its clauses, such as bankruptcy terms, mutual consent and notification to the other, material breach without remedy, waiver of responsibility by one party to another, substitution, novation, accord and satisfaction, release, temporary impossibility due to weather or weather clauses, impossibility due to materials not available anymore, death or disability or change of law, economic or commercial frustration, or discharge by operation of law such as alteration, destruction of the contract, merger, bankruptcy, statute of limitations, contractual limitations, renunciation, or incapacitating self. We will examine a few of these that are more germane to managed care contracts.

A discharge by agreement may be terminated by the operation of one of its provisions or by a subsequent agreement. Often we see this in the "rollover" clause, where the contract automatically renews with the mutual consent of both parties. When a contract provides for a continuing performance but is nonspecific as to how long the contract is good, it is terminable by either party, with the same consequences as though it had expressly authorized termination upon notice.

A contract is discharged by waiver when one party fails to demand performance by the other party or to object when the other party fails to demand performance according to contract terms.

The parties may also decide that the contract is not the one they want. They may mutually consent to replace it with another contract. If they do, the original contract is said to be discharged by substitution.

Impossibility of performance refers to external or extrinsic conditions as contracted with the obligor's personal inability to perform them. Thus, the fact that a debtor does not have money to pay and cannot pay a debt does not present a case of impossibility. The fact that it will prove more costly to provide a service than originally contemplated or that the obligor has voluntarily gone out of business does not constitute impossibility that excuses performance. No distinction is made in this connection between acts of nature, people, or governments.

Bankruptcy

In the event of bankruptcy, most debtors either voluntarily enter into federal bankruptcy court or are compelled to do so by their creditors. In HMO situations, the administrative oversight body such as the department of insurance or, in California, the department of corporations, may, after an audit of the cash assets set aside for claims incurred but not reported (IBNR), require that an HMO declare itself bankrupt if the state does not feel the HMO has enough cash set aside in reserve to pay its claims. In bankruptcy court, a trustee takes the assets that a debtor has and distributes them as far as they will go. Insurance companies also have reinsurance policies that may well add value to the debtor's property or net value. Once the trustee distributes the property as far as it will go, the court grants the creditor a discharge in bankruptcy if it concludes that the debtor has acted honestly and has not attempted to defraud its creditors.

Even though all creditors have not been paid in full, the discharge in bankruptcy is a bar to subsequent enforcement of ordinary contract claims against the debtor. The cause of action or contract claim is not destroyed, but a bankruptcy discharge bars a proceeding to enforce it. As the obligation is not extinguished, the debtor may waive the defense of discharge in bankruptcy by promising later to pay the debt. Such a waiver is governed by state law. In a few states, the waiver must be written.

What are the physician's obligations if the plan goes bankrupt? Is there a provision of the contract requiring notification of filing for protection under bankruptcy laws? Does the contract allow for post-termination retroactive denials/recovery of previously paid payments to the physician? For how long? Does the contract provide for timely payment of pretermination services within a reasonable (45 days) time frame?

> **Tip:** Ask for notification of any petition for bankruptcy protection by U.S. mail, certified, return receipt requested, within 72 hours of the submission of the appeal for protection under bankruptcy.

Breach of Contract

There is a breach of contract whenever one of the parties fails to perform the contract. A contract is discharged by breach if, when the breaching party breaks the contract, the other party accepts the breach. A breach does not result in the discharge of a contract if the term broken is not sufficiently important. (So define sufficiently!) When there is a failure to perform under a contract, the agreement is not terminated, but the defaulting party may be liable for liquidated damages.

There are several remedies for breach of contract, one or more of which may be available to the injured party. The injured party may bring action for damages, rescind the contract, bring suit to obtain specific performance, or commence a proceeding to obtain relief from an administrative agency of the government.

In a claim for damages, the injured party is under duty to mitigate the damages if reasonably possible. In other words, the injured party is required to take measures to generally stop any performance under the contract in order to avoid running up a larger bill. Here, recovery is limited to direct loss, not consequential loss. If there is nothing that the injured party can do to reduce damages, there is, by definition, no duty to mitigate damages.

Liquidated Damages

The parties may stipulate in their contract that a certain amount shall be paid in case of a default. Such an amount will be enforced if the amount is not excessive, and if the contract is of such a nature that it would be difficult to establish the actual damages. When a liquidated damages clause is held valid, the injured party cannot collect more than the amount specified by the clause. If the liquidated damages clause calls for payment of a sum that is clearly unreasonably large and unrelated to the possible actual damages that may be sustained, the clause will be held void as penalty.

Liquidated damage clauses require a sum of money to be paid by one party to the other party if he or she breaches a term in the agreement. The fact that this has happened in the past has led payers to insert liquidated damages clauses in managed care agreements. In the event that a provider might use this influence or make disparaging remarks about a plan that causes patients to choose another plan, the payor might reserve the right to sue for liquidated damages to recover business losses as a remedy.

In a court challenge with Humana and a Florida physician, Humana filed an action against the physician for failure to pay $700 (ancient history!) per patient that remained after the physician's termination of the agreement. The courts found that the physician was not held responsible for this sum of money for several reasons: the patients were not the property of the insurance company; the clause interfered with the patient/physician relationship; and the patients had the right to see whomever they chose as a provider of health care services.

A Checklist for Managed Care Agreements

Now that we have examined the basic concepts in contract law, let us apply them to some of the most popular terms of the managed care agreements seen in both PPO and HMO contracts, as well as IPA, PHO, and MSO contracts of late.

A. Does anyone or any organization, other than physicians, control deter- minations of medical necessity or quality of care? Is the plan entertaining NCQA accreditation or reaccreditation?
B. Does the provider indemnify the managed care entity against liability? If so, does the provider's professional liability policy cover such contract liability? Will the managed care indemnify the provider in case of liability on the behalf of the managed care entity?

Hold-harmless agreements require a provider to reimburse a managed care entity for any costs, expenses, and liabilities incurred by the managed care entity because of action by the provider. These provisions jeopardize the coverage of a provider's professional liability insurance coverage. These provisions are known as liabilities assumed by contract. If a provider agrees to this type of arrangement, he or she often does so without the benefit of reimbursement from his or her professional liability policy and must often pay for these expenses himself or herself.

Change wording that requires you to indemnify the managed care payer to language that reflects responsibility by each party for own their own acts. The following is an example of the preferred language.

Responsibility for Own Acts

Each party will be responsible for its own acts or omissions and any and all claims, liabilities, injuries, suits, and demands and expenses of all kinds which may result or arise out of any alleged malfeasance or neglect caused or alleged to be caused by that party, its employees, or representatives in the performance or omission of any act or responsibility of that party under this Agreement. In the event that a claim is made against both par- ties, it is the intent of both parties to cooperate in the defense of said claim and to cause their insurers to do likewise. However, both parties shall have the right to take any and all actions they believe necessary to protect their interest.

C. Does the contract permit unilateral changes in terms and conditions of the contract without the prior notice to the provider or without the prior consent of the provider?

If the contract states that the provider will be bound by articles of incor- poration, bylaws, or other documents of the managed care entity, has the provider perused such documents? Is there a contractual provision for the providers to be advised of modification of such documents? Is the provider bound by such modifications?

Does the contract make reference to peer review or a utilization review program? Has the provider obtained and perused the program documents? Might they conflict with the provider's own published by The Joint Commission or the Accreditation Association for Ambulatory Health Care also known as AAAHC or other accreditation documents? Are the procedures of these programs subject to unilateral change without prior notice to the provider or without the prior consent of the provider?

The following is sample wording to beware of: "The payer shall provide to the provider any changes in policy regarding payment, withholds, or fee reductions within 30 days of implementation of said changes."

Allow them to make changes, but reserve the right to notification at least 60 days in excess of the "bailout" time provided in the "termination without cause" clause prior to your responsibility to the change, and request that notification be provided by U.S. mail, postage prepaid, certified, return receipt requested, or by hand delivery.

D. Are limitations on referrals realistic? How are they granted? What level of intrusiveness in the decision making of the provider may be encountered for routine preventive services such as mammography and gynecological exams? Who must the provider refer to? What physicians, hospitals, pharmacies, and ancillary services are available to patients? Is the referring provider satisfied with the quality of the panel of referral specialists, ancillaries, and hospitals? How are out-of-network services handled? Are there negative financial sanctions for out-of-network referrals? What services have limited or noncoverage that may require the use of out-of-plan providers due to unavailability?

E. What are the requirements for prior authorization for nursing home and home health initiation of care and hospital inpatient admissions? Is the mechanism reasonably available when needed?

F. Does the contract provision on medical records comport with state law? Is there a reimbursement mechanism to cover direct costs associated with photocopying medical records when requested by the insurance carrier?

G. For what co-payments, if any, are patients responsible? Can the amount of co-payment be unilaterally changed or eliminated under the contract? Will the managed care entity support the provider in endeavors to collect co-payments unpaid by the patient? Can the provider discharge a patient for not cooperating with co-payment policies on a habitual basis? If a co-payment is eliminated from a particular service encounter, what recovery mechanism is built into the contract to allow the provider to recuperate the fully negotiated amount for services rendered?

H. Is there a contractual time limit for the submission and payment of such claims? Is there any perfunctory leniency to do recovery of "lost" claims at least one occasion per year, per provider? Is there a provision for additional time to submit claims in the event of key staff loss or equipment failure, upon advance notice to the managed care entity? Is there a contractual time penalty, such as some defined rate of interest, for delay in the receipt of payment?

I. What is the exact definition of a "clean claim?" How long does it take for the managed care entity to pay clean claims? Who can attest to these date ranges? Is there any statutory requirement on timeliness of payment for clean claims?

J. Is the contracting organization subject to statutory licensing requirements? Has it complied? As an HMO, there are reserve amounts that must be maintained to sustain risk. Have they provided the figures to verify these reserves? What is their "medical loss ratio?"

Medical loss ratio is the equivalent of costs of goods and services. It equals the cost of delivering health care, with the rest going to administrative costs and profits. In general, it is best to shy away from entities that have less than an 80% medical loss ratio, because they are in effect taking more than their fair share of the monies available.

K. How are disputes resolved? Does the provider have any meaningful right to participate in his or her own defense?

The grievance procedure should be spelled out specifically. Each step of the process should be outlined so that the provider may know all of the remedies available before giving up the grievance and making a business decision as to whether to go forth with the contract or "opt out."

L. Will the provider have some readily available method to identify patients under a contractual relationship? Does the contract require that the provider call and verify patient identification prior to each consultation or service other than emergencies? Do they permit standing referrals for services that are anticipated to be repeat frequency? How recent are the updates maintained on federal Consolidated Omnibus Budget Reconciliation Act (COBRA) participants?

M. What obligation does the provider assume if physicians covering for the contracting physician see his or her patients? Does the contract require the physician to be available on a 24-hour basis? Does the contract require a "contracted" physician to arrange for another contracted physician to cover during absences and vacations? What about hospitalists? Must the physician guarantee/warranty performance or indemnify the carrier for any professional liability issues arising from the treatment of patients by the covering physician? Must the participating physician cover payments

> **Tip:** When these guarantee or warranty words appear, counteroffer the negotiated phrase with words such as "encourage."

in excess of the fee schedule for the treatment of patients by a nonparticipating covering physician?

N. Does the contract obligate the physician to perform any services after the contract is terminated? Is there a provision to receive 100% of billed charges for post-termination services delivered to patients who wish to continue with the physician?

Even without a contractual provision, providers have an ethical, continuing duty not to abandon their patients. Managed care contracts typically require the continued care and treatment of assigned members who are under the provider's care until the member is reassigned to another provider.

Reimbursement should continue at the provider's usual and customary charge rather than at the discounted rate. There should be provisions providing that the managed care entity cannot assign new patients to the provider and that the entity will reassign outpatients as quickly as possible.

O. What are the provisions for retroactive denials of payments?

P. What is the term and termination policy? How much time is required to give notice of termination without cause? Does this window of time match all prenotification for unilateral changes in the contract, with an additional window of time to make business decisions relative to those unilateral changes?

Q. What is the renewal system? Is the renewal of the contract covered under an "evergreen" or "rollover" clause? If so, what is time frame to request renegotiation of terms prior to automatic renewal of the contract? Are there provisions for increases in the negotiated fee schedule that keep reimbursement current with market conditions with these automatic renewal clauses?

R. What are the definitions of material breach of the contract? Are there remedies available and a limited time frame to implement remedies by either party, in the event of a material breach?

S. Does the contract require the physician to inform the patient whether the physician's services are covered or noncovered under the patient's health plan? Are there special waiver forms required to prove such notification was given? Can the same format as the Medicare noncovered services form be used?

T. Are there "most-favored nations" clauses in the contract?

Most-favored nations clauses provide that the rate of reimbursement negotiated by the managed care entity will be the lowest rate offered to any other managed care entity by the provider during the term of the agreement. If the provider offers a lower rate, the original managed care entity is entitled to the lower rate. Often, the agreement will further stipulate that the original entity must be notified of the lower rate at such time as it has been negotiated with the new entity. Whether any adjustment is retroactive is usually subject to negotiation. These clauses should be avoided.

U. Check the boilerplate clauses, such as entire agreement and assignability clauses.

Entire agreement clauses mean that any verbal representations or other marketing materials do not become part of the agreement. Therefore, promises made in recruiting that are not specifically mentioned as an addendum or attachment in the agreement and incorporated into the agreement as referenced do not become part of the agreement. This also implies that the signer read and understood all materials (including any referenced and contained on the plan's Web site) referenced in the contract before signing. Such documents as the provider relation's manuals, utilization management, quality assurance policies, bylaws, and so on are part of this consideration.

Are assignment clauses mutually beneficial? A provider should ensure that the contract is not assignable to a third party. Otherwise, the managed care entity may assign the contract to another organization with less financial or managed resources or an entirely different patient base.

V. Liability issues may arise by signing a managed care agreement. Make sure that you are aware of any assumed or created liabilities.

1. *Ostensible Agency Liability.* Realize that you may be held accountable for the actions of those providers you refer patients to.

2. *Respondeat-Superior Liability.* Realize that you may be held accountable for utilization management decisions if you deny care or discontinue care because the carrier states they will not pay for more care, visits, and so on. The provider carries the ultimate decision-making responsibility on clinical issues.

3. *Vicarious Liability.* Realize that in an IPA or a PHO, due diligence is required for credentialing and recredentialing members.

W. Let words be your cue that there may be some unstated, unclear, or unfinished policies in development that you are agreeing to uphold sight unseen. Am, is, are, was, were, be, being, been, do, does, did, have, had, has, shall, will, should, would, could, may, might, must, can. These words suggest a state of being. The text may imply that the policy is unspecified or indefinite at the time of signing. Seek to clarify. For example:

Unspecified terms. You will see wording such as this from time to time: "A withhold of fifteen percent (15%) *shall be taken from* all payments subject to provisions as allowed in the Manual. *At such as time as it* shall be *deemed necessary,* withholds shall increase or be decreased and the provider notified within sixty (60) days of the increase or decrease." Ask for the withhold policy and a methodology for determination of the necessity to increase or decrease withholds.

Policies and procedures undefined. "Provider *shall be bound by* and abide by all policies and procedures as set forth in the Manual."

Ask for disclosure on all policies and procedures you must be bound by and list them as exhibits to the contract. Then add the language into the contract.

Identify language suggestive of hidden incremental direct costs. For example, "The Provider shall abide by all terms and conditions of participation as is specified in the Manual with regards to Utilization Management, Quality Improvement, Denials and Appeals, Claims Submission, Preauthorization Procedures, Timely Filing, Staffing, and Compliance with waiting time and appointment policies."

Peruse that manual! Identify things that will have to be done differently to accommodate performance obligations on the contract.

As always, it is wise to seek out competent health law attorneys to evaluate a contract before signing a managed care agreement. This chapter is provided to make you more able to do some prenegotiation and review before incurring charges for such evaluation and to make the attorney review more meaningful to you as a provider.

Chapter 15

Evaluating a Managed Care Agreement— Step-by-Step

A Checklist to Guide You

The purpose of this contracting checklist is to enable you to have a tool that you can use to undertake an organized and focused evaluation of managed care agreements with payers.

Most physicians and managers and many hospital contractors and chief financial officers (CFOs) or chief executive officers (CEOs) have never had formal training in contract analysis, but worse yet, may have never done any critical analysis to understand what the contract says. Often intimidated by the language and ambiguity, they simply turned to the fee schedule page, determined if the amount described as payment for their services was adequate, signed, and hoped for the best.

Unlike some hospital administrators, physicians frequently verbalize frustration with their apparent lack of leverage to negotiate contracts. What they fail to acknowledge is that they have the right to:

☐ Ask lots of questions of clarification and obtain written responses to those inquiries.

☐ Obtain additional documentation and data.
☐ Request and review current policies and procedures.
☐ Possess enough information to model each and every fee for every service they offer.

Every provider has the right to be treated with courtesy and respect instead of summarily dismissed with answers that do not explain why something is written in a certain way, or required of them in the contract. For example, when a physician, practice administrator, or contracting manager asks the provider relations representative for clarifications, they should always ask open-ended questions in writing, by e-mail, or in regular written correspondence, rather than questions that can be easily answered with a "yes" or "no" response. Many inexperienced provider relations representatives will not be prepared to answer the questions in the checklist for which no answer exists in the contract without some research and guidance from their supervisors. As a best practice, the responses obtained from the plan should be reduced to writing so that the provider has notes from his/her research and due diligence to produce in the event of a future dispute on the same point. Upon execution, the responses should be incorporated into the contract and attached as one of the exhibits or attachments so that it is made a part of the Entire Agreement.

Often, the Entire Agreement reads as follows:

> *This Agreement together with all Program Attachments, Fee Schedules, Exhibits, Provider Manuals, Memorandums, and other writings attached hereto and incorporated herein by reference as exhibits contains all the terms and conditions agreed upon by the parties, and supersedes all other agreements, express or implied, verbal or written, regarding the subject matter.*

As you can see, without incorporating the document containing the clarifications as an attachment or exhibit, the provider will have made the effort to obtain and review the information, but will not be able to rely upon those explanations, responses, or additional data, because the agreement in its vague and ambiguous form will supersede the clarification. Without proper incorporation into the contract, the clarifications and additional data would simply be reduced to hearsay, just as if the responses had been answered over the phone or in casual conversation.

I cannot stress enough the importance of a healthy respect for the Entire Agreement paragraph while reviewing the checklist in order to understand the importance of obtaining the additional information in a manner in which you can rely upon your research and evaluation efforts.

Particular attention should be paid to the clarification and provision of coverage policies and fee schedules that are in effect at the time the contract is executed. The reliance upon coverage policies, coding and rebundling policies and procedures, and medical necessity definitions may only be made if incorporated as they are at the time of contract execution as specific exhibits or attachments. Failing to ensure this incorporation or annexation may result in tacit approval to changes that are made by the plan from time to time. Only your attorney will know for sure by the way it is expressed in the contract. You can and should do the homework so that the attorney may more effectively assist you. Inquiries should be made and responses attached so that the provider is prepared in the event of future denials. Simply obtaining these data and clarifications for review without attachment and incorporation into the executed contract is the most frustrating "Gotcha!" in denials management. When I teach denials management courses, I teach providers to obtain and review the information. Without doing the due diligence and specific attachment of those polices and reliances to the contract, many providers fail to complete the process of negotiation. Without specific inclusion into the contract, they cannot rely upon that which they read and accepted as policy. If the policy is not attached and incorporated into the Entire Agreement, no reliance is assumed, and therefore, ad hoc changes to the policies at the unilateral whim of the plan can be made without the burden of adherence to the notice and amendment provisions of the contract.

Providers are entitled to these data and clarifications whether they have leverage or not. Attaching these as exhibits or attachments to the final executed contract is a matter of negotiation, and is for the provider or their contracting expert to push for. That attachment and incorporation is the part that is going to require leverage, and all providers may not be able to achieve the desired end result.

In the end, one has to ask rhetorically, "Should I sign a contract with a payer that will not stand behind its clarifications, policies and procedures, and data that they have supplied to me in reliance of how my fees will be calculated and against which my claims adjudicated?" That is a business decision that each provider must make on his/her own.

Preliminary Questions

List five points that summarize why you want this contract as part of your reimbursement strategy. (*Distill your rationale for executing this contract. You will have another opportunity to reassess your priorities post-review at the conclusion of the checklist.*)

1.

2.

3.

4.

5.

List your five major concerns with your managed care contracts. (*Do not be afraid to reveal your overall concerns in this section of the checklist. The epiphany will come post-review at the completion of the checklist. The exercise will enable you to measure their awareness of new areas of concern that relate to reimbursement and more upon completion of the contract review.*)

1.

2.

3.

4.

5.

Complete Contract

Do you have the complete contract and all attachments and exhibits necessary for review? (*Remember, the Entire Agreement provision may or may not assume that all of the parts of the contract may be relied upon. Read it carefully; it may require modification.*)

- ☐ Identification of the parties
- ☐ Recitals
- ☐ Definitions
- ☐ Obligations of the provider
- ☐ Obligations of the health plan
- ☐ Medical records policies and procedures
- ☐ Billing, coding, documentation and claim submission procedures
- ☐ Complete fee schedule(s) detailing fees for their specific services
- ☐ Utilization management attachments and exhibits
- ☐ Quality management attachments and exhibits
- ☐ Term and termination provisions
- ☐ Denials and appeals procedures
- ☐ List of participating providers
- ☐ Provider manual
- ☐ List of affiliated payers and plan types
- ☐ Coverage determination policies
- ☐ Sample copies of identification cards from significant employer groups in my market
- ☐ Contact information for key support individuals and medical director

Identification of the Parties

(Who will owe you money? Do they really want another contract with this payer? If they already have access to patients, why do you want it? In the event that there is more than one access point, which fee schedule, policies, and procedures will prevail?)

1. Name of the Plan: _____

2. Are they a Subsidiary/Affiliate of another plan? _____

3. Do we already have a relationship with them through another contract?

   ☐ Yes   ☐ No

4. If yes, through which contract do they presently access our services?

   _____

5. Which major employers in our area offer this health plan?

   ☐ _____ # Employees _____

   ☐ _____ # Employees _____

   ☐ _____ # Employees _____

   ☐ _____ # Employees _____

   ☐ _____ # Employees _____

6. Can I be reimbursed for all service lines that I offer?

   _____

7. Are any services I routinely offer reserved exclusively for certain providers in the network? If yes, which ones? _____

   _____

(Are there any services upon which the bulk of your income is derived that are not included in the contract? Has another provider or hospital contracted for the exclusive right to perform and be reimbursed for special services lines you offer? If not, are they interested in negotiating for that position?)

Fact-Finding
Term and Termination

Contract Effective Date:

_____

Contract Termination Date:

_____

Notice of termination window for Termination Without Cause: _____ Days

Termination is permitted by   ☐ Plan Only   ☐ Either Party

Reason(s) for Termination:
☐ Without Cause ☐ With Cause ☐ Material Breach

Material Breach Remedy Opportunity: _____ Days

Correspondence

To whom shall bills be addressed?

_____

Billing address:

_____

Corporate address:

_____

Contact List

Provider Relations Contact

Name: _____

Phone: _____

Fax: _____

E-mail: _____

Mobile: _____

Medical Director

Name: _____

Phone: _____

Fax: _____

E-mail: _____

Secretary: _____

Claims Manager

Name: _____

Phone: _____

Fax: _____

E-mail: _____

Secretary: _____

Prior Authorization Contact

Name: _____

Phone: _____

Fax: _____

E-mail: _____

Electronic Billing Contact

Name: _____

Phone: _____

Fax: _____

E-mail: _____

Precertification/Eligibility Contact

Name: _____

Phone: _____

Fax: _____

E-mail: _____

Secretary: _____

Notice Recipient

Name: _____

Phone: _____

Fax: _____

E-mail: _____

Type of Plans Covered by the Contract

- ☐ HMO
- ☐ PPO
- ☐ ERISA self-insured employer
- ☐ Workers' compensation
- ☐ Motor vehicle/no fault
- ☐ Medicare Advantage
- ☐ Medicaid managed care
- ☐ TriCare
- ☐ Discount card arrangement (self-pay)
- ☐ Consumer driven health plan
- ☐ Continuous discount arranger/silent PPO arrangement

List some of the names of plans that may access services under this contract:

Utilization Management Program

(While the fee schedule may detail how much money will be paid, careful attention to detail in the utilization management program details will provide insight as to "if" the money will ever be paid and under which circumstances the plan has a legitimate reason not to pay. Tacit agreement to these policies and program documents without review and clarification is the reason that many denials are upheld against the claim.)

1. Are **all** utilization/coverage policies attached to the contract as Exhibits?

   ☐ Yes   ☐ No

2. Will each payer under the contract follow one standard coverage policy?

   ☐ Yes   ☐ No

   (It is important to inquire whether or not these coverage policies will be standardized across all plans including the ERISA payers, or just the contracting payers' own policies for their own plans, and not the network lessees.)

3. Are stated coverage policies adequate to address the needs of my patients?

   ☐ Yes   ☐ No

   (Smaller local health plans may actually welcome assistance with the coverage policy development in certain subspecialties. You should ask if you can be of assistance if those policies are not yet developed. If invited to meaningfully participate, you would be in a very influential position, especially in the case of new and exclusive technologies.)

   If not, what is understated or missing? _____

   _____

4. Who determines medical necessity?

   ☐ Attending Physician   ☐ Health Plan

   (Often this right is reserved for the plan and stated as such in the contract. If this is the case, attempt to negotiate that all services deemed not medically necessary are labeled "noncovered," instead of "nonallowed." This may mitigate perfunctory write-offs, because nonallowed services are rarely, if ever, permitted to be transferred to patient responsibility.)

5. Are services deemed not medically necessary subject to appeal?

   ☐ Yes   ☐ No

6. Must we write off services deemed by the plan as "noncovered" or "not medically necessary," or can they be billed to the patient?

   ☐ Mandatory write-off

   ☐ Patient responsibility

   ☐ Patient responsibility, but only after advising the patient in writing similar to a Medicare ABN

   Cite relevant contract provisions that support this position:

   _____

   Is this cited elsewhere in the provider manual, attachments, or policies and procedures?

   ☐ Yes   ☐ No

   If yes, note where it is mentioned: _____

   _____

   (*About medical necessity: If the plan agrees that it has vetted the credentials of the physician and has determined that the physician has the requisite training and education to make all decisions related to patient care and must exercise independent, professional medical judgment as an independent contractor with respect to all such matters, then why should the plan be permitted to interfere with the physician's professional independent medical judgment with regard to treatment or utilization issues? Consider negotiating that any payment or absence of payment for services should not constitute an opinion or affirmation by plan that the services or procedures recommended or rendered by the physician are, are not, were, or were not medically appropriate, but only that the service or procedure was not a covered service.*)

7. Under what circumstances can denied claims be presented for external review by regulatory authorities? _____

   _____

If applicable, who pays for the proceedings? _____

_____

(*If a claim is submitted for external review, the plan is often responsible to pay the cost of the entire proceeding, whether they win or lose. The external review mechanism is there for the benefit of the insured. While the physician may assist in the preparation of the case with the patient, the physician may not initiate the proceedings in most states. The physician's staff may assist the patient with completion of all the necessary paperwork, which is usually a single-page questionnaire available on the state insurance commissioner's Web site. This does not apply to ERISA plan members. For ERISA plan members, refer to your notes from the Denver managed care training on ERISA authorized representatives, a process that the physician can initiate in order to assist with an appeal and possibly overturn a denial.*)

8. How long are we permitted to reopen a claim for appeal of a denial?

_____

(*At a minimum, this time frame should be no less than the time frame the plan has to ask for a refund or recalculate the benefit on a claim. As a best practice, the window of opportunity for an appeal of a denial or short-paid claim should be not less than 2 years from the date the claim was paid or denied.*)

9. Which peer in my specialty makes final decisions of medical necessity or clinical appropriateness regarding my claims if a claim is questioned?

_____

(*When determining who will make decisions about medical necessity, if the health plan hires the services of a local or outside specialist as an expert, the provider should be able to request, receive, and review that expert's CV as well as any opinions rendered regarding treatment rendered. If the provider perceives a conflict of interest or an inadequacy as to the expert's training or experience with the provider, the issue should be raised and any understandings negotiated as documented in the contract or a memorandum referenced in the contract as part of the Entire Agreement.*)

10. Am I permitted to review and challenge expert opinions or committee decisions of denied claims?

    ☐ Yes   ☐ No

    If not, why? _____

    _____

11. Are any employer groups accessing services under this contract that do not cover physician-administered injectable drug therapy for their employees?

    ☐ Yes   ☐ No

    If yes, which ones?

    _____

Authorizations

(In many instances, the contract will mention the preauthorization requirement for specialty services, diagnostic testing, and treatment, in addition to preauthorization for evaluation and management services. The procedures may often be detailed in the provider manual or on a Web site.

One would be wise to obtain a retention copy of what was on the manual or Web site the day the contract was executed, so that any updates are required to go through the notice and amendment process as part of the Entire Agreement. This could be a "cut and paste" from the Web to a paper document, or burned to a CD and labeled as an exhibit or attachment as a digitized document. The main point is to record what was in effect at the time the contract was executed so that no new requirements are added to the responsibilities of the physician and staff as a surprise and a new reason for a denial to be upheld.)

1. Are prior authorizations required?

   ☐ Yes   ☐ No

   If yes, what is the process to obtain authorizations? _____

   _____

2. When is authorization required?

   ☐ Initial referral

   ☐ Each service or procedure

   ☐ Other: _____

   _____ (Specify)

3. Will a written authorization number be issued to office?

   ☐ Yes   ☐ No

4. Are we required to submit written authorization with claim?

   ☐ Yes   ☐ No

5. Is supporting documentation required?

   ☐ Yes   ☐ No

6. Describe supporting documentation: _____

_____

7. How long are prior authorizations valid? _____

_____

8. Will the plan occasionally cooperate to provide retroactive referrals under extenuating circumstances?

    ☐ Yes   ☐ No

    If not, why? _____

    _____

9. Describe a sample authorization number (i.e. alpha/numeric): _____

    _____

10. Does prior authorization guarantee payment?

    ☐ Yes   ☐ No

    If not, why? _____

    _____

    (If we think in the context of the Entire Agreement, unless the contract states "prior authorization guarantees payment," then all prior authorizations are outside the Entire Agreement, because they happen after the contract is executed and are not an exhibit or an attachment.)

11. Are preauthorizations able to be issued online?

    ☐ Yes   ☐ No

    Average processing time: _____ Average turnaround time: _____

Billing and Reimbursement

1. What is the timely filing limit to file claims when the payer is primary?

---

2. What is the timely filing limit to file claims when the payer is secondary?

---

3. When this payer is secondary, what is the maximum reimbursement amount I can receive when combined with the payment from the primary payer?

   ☐ The maximum allowable amount payable under this contract

   ☐ The maximum allowable amount payable under the primary contract

   ☐ 100% of my billed charges

   Cite the relevant contract provisions that support or explain this:

(Often the coordination of benefits (COB) reimbursement provisions in a contract do not match the state administrative code. In fact, most plans add restrictions to the contract that enable the plan to avoid additional payment for services that they have assumed the insurance risk of claims payment. They do this by requiring the provider to discount their fees to less than 100% of billed charges when that payer is not primary, rather than transferring the risk of additional cost to the patient—a practice that might be construed as racketeering (if they collected premium from the patient and gave nothing in exchange and then transferred financial responsibility to the patient).

This is a matter where the provider should obtain counsel or comparison of the contract language with any applicable regulatory requirements from their attorney, consultant, or medical society before proceeding. The cost of the consultation may be far outweighed by the ability to collect additional reimbursement to which they may otherwise be entitled through proper negotiation of this situation.)

4. What is the penalty for filing claims beyond the timely filing limit?

(The penalty for late filing should never be 100% if the plan cannot prove prejudice. Many states have enacted laws and/or regulations that require a showing of prejudice to the insurer to deny benefits for late notice. Prejudice would be interpreted as the inability to verify that the claim was really the responsibility of that payer and not another party. Often, the provider unknowingly accepts a 100% penalty on late-filed claims by negotiation, thereby excusing the plan from responsibility of risk for payment of late-billed claims. This is a matter where the provider should obtain professional counsel or comparison of the contract language with any applicable regulatory requirements from their attorney, consultant, or medical society or other professional association attorney before proceeding.)

5. Where in the contract is a clean or complete claim defined? _____

_____

6. What is the prompt payment time limit? _____

_____

7. What is the penalty if the claim is paid late? _____

_____

(While the health plan may not initially offer to pay a penalty or sustain any consequence, providers should look for some deterrent for poor performance in this area either in statute, administrative code, or by negotiation if there is nothing to address this by regulation. If there is law or regulation to address this, the provider should be careful to reiterate it in the contract, and not to unknowingly forego this protection by negotiating away contract provisions to the contrary.)

8. Are ERISA self-funded employers required to follow the same timely payment contract provisions?

☐ Yes   ☐ No

If not, why? _____

_____

(Many states have enacted laws to define a clean or complete claim and timely payment rules. Providers often unknowingly allow for a departure from state requirements, enabling the plan to negotiate extensions or liberties not elsewhere provided and excusing the plan or its affiliates from upholding the laws and regulations. Again, this is a matter where the provider should obtain professional counsel or comparison of the contract language with any applicable regulatory requirements from their attorney, consultant, or medical society or other professional association attorney before proceeding.)

9. Is the fee schedule attached?

   ☐ Yes   ☐ No

   (A word about representative or sample fee schedules:
   Because of the Entire Agreement provision, any abbreviated listing of fees in the fee schedule means that only those fees detailed in the abbreviated list are a part of the contract, and that reimbursement for all other unlisted fees is subject to the changes that the plan may establish or change from time to time in its sole and absolute discretion.)

10. Is the fee for each service for which we routinely bill able to be financially modeled?

    ☐ Yes   ☐ No

    Does the fee schedule list a fee for every service rendered for which we routinely bill by specific Current Procedural Terminology (CPT) and Healthcare Common Procedure Coding System (HCPCS) code?

    ☐ Yes   ☐ No

    If not, which ones are missing? _____

    _____

    (Modeling: The contract should provide enough detail so that a fee can be calculated for every CPT or HCPCS code submitted by the physician, including those codes that have variances because of modifier use. The only codes that should not be able to be modeled would be those codes for which a fee must be determined "by report." Generally, those codes end in XXX99. For those codes, the physician might be wise to negotiate a formula into the contract for unlisted procedures or codes at a straight discount percentage from billed charges.)

11. Is there a formula stated in the contract to calculate fees not stated in the fee schedule?

☐ Yes   ☐ No

If yes, what is that formula? _____

_____

12. Does the fee schedule specifically address reimbursement for unavoidable injectable drug wastage?

☐ Yes   ☐ No

(Physicians or office manager should attach a superbill, charge slip, or a computer printout of their charges and enter the allowable amounts under each contract for each service, drug, or supply. Note any that cannot be accurately modeled for reimbursement with the information provided in the contract. Only procedures ending in 99 (by report) should pose modeling difficulty. All other fees, including those codes that are routinely submitted with modifiers, should be modeled and the worksheet attached as an exhibit to specify actual reimbursement expected under the contract.)

13. Does the contract stipulate that Medicare billing and interpretation rules for bundling and coding will apply?

☐ Yes   ☐ No

If not, what rules will apply? _____

_____

Cite the relevant section of the contract where this is specified: _____

_____

(Most providers, including experienced hospital contractors, mistakenly assume that all health plans follow Medicare guidelines and coding and bundling rules when calculating payments. This is not the case unless the contract or some other document tied to the Entire Agreement states this as an understanding within the agreement. Physicians should always ask for written clarification if the coding and billing standards follow Medicare regulations exactly, or if not, which deviations will apply.)

14. Can the plan unilaterally change billing and interpretation rules for bundling and coding unilaterally and arbitrarily without a formal amendment to the contract in accordance with the notice and amendment provisions of the contract?

☐ Yes   ☐ No

If yes, how will I receive notice of such changes to policy? _____

_____

(*Providers often fail to request clarification on this important privilege of interpretation. If the provider does not obtain and attach coverage, billing, bundling, and other relevant rules as exhibits or attachments to the contract, they are not considered part of the Entire Agreement, and interpretation would be subject to the pleasure and convenience of the plan without the requirement of a formal amendment or notification to the provider other than an incidental mention on an* explanation of benefits *(EOB) as a denial or reduction in payment. Obtain documentation for everything that relates to your revenue, and request that your attorney determine if the clarification and documentation will be enforceable if a dispute arises as incorporated.*)

15. Can the plan(s) delete or revise drug and other coverage decisions policies without providing us with advance written notice prior to the effective date of the change?

☐ Yes   ☐ No

If yes, how will I receive notice of such deletions or revisions to policy?

_____

(*The plan may be able to revise coverage policies, but there are many state-required notifications that the plan will give the employer, insured, or other authorized representative. Require clarification on this point, and negotiate a method for inclusion on updates to relevant policies for their specific services. In the case of ERISA plan participants, the physician will have no right to receive these notifications without possession of an Authorized Representative designation from the patient, parent, or guardian.*)

16. What is the procedure to follow if a claim is paid at less than the contractually stated amount? _____

_____

(This procedure is often overlooked or mishandled by most billing managers. They continue to resubmit the claims to the same department that paid the claim incorrectly in the first place. A claim paid at less than the agreed-upon amount may represent a breach of contract—especially if it is paid inaccurately on a repeated basis. Those claims should be submitted to the notice recipient with a letter requesting that full payment be made and the breach corrected within the amount of time specified in the remedy section and the root cause of the error be corrected.)

17. Does the payer require sourcing of drugs, implants, or supplies through an exclusive provider?

    ☐ Yes   ☐ No

    (If the contract or provider manual does not specify this, the provider should ask for written clarification as to the plan reimbursement policy for physician- or hospital-supplied drugs or supplies for which a pass-through reimbursement is anticipated. If there is none, that clarification should be attached to the contract as a formal understanding, so that any change in policy in the future cannot be imposed upon the provider without a formal contract amendment and notification.)

18. If the payer requests copies of medical records, will they pay the state statutory copy fee, if any?

    a. If yes, how much is that fee? _____

    b. How should we bill for it? _____

    c. When should we expect payment for copies of records? _____

Capitation

   ☐ N/A

19. Will any of our reimbursement be in the form of capitation?

    ☐ Yes   ☐ No

    If yes, for which services? _____

    _____

20. Is capitated reimbursement in the plans for any of your product lines in the near future?

    ☐ Yes   ☐ No

21. What is the minimum number of patients that will be assigned to us before a capitated reimbursement method takes effect? _____

22. What is the threshold dollar amount of claims paid to all providers (if any) that would transition a patient to stop loss status from the capitated risk pool? _____

    (*Capitation is not dead! It is thriving in certain markets and returning to others. In the event that provider fee reimbursement changes to capitation, answers to these questions should be obtained and evaluated by an experienced actuary before the physician agrees to capitation reimbursement for any services.*)

Quality Management

Clinical Quality Issues

1. Must we participate in and comply with the health plans' quality management and peer review programs?

   ☐ Yes   ☐ No

   If yes, briefly cite sections where details of these programs are found:

   _____

2. What will happen if we do not agree with a particular aspect or element of the quality management or peer review program? Can we object without being found in breach of contract?

   ☐ Yes   ☐ No

   If yes, cite section:_____

3. If the plan requires the use of a designated source for drugs acquisition, interpretations of lab and diagnostic testing, etc., can you review the quality or handling standards that address these matters with the plan to ensure your satisfaction with standards set for safety and product integrity?

   ☐ Yes   ☐ No   ☐ N/A

   If undisclosed and unavailable, can you ethically agree to comply?

   ☐ Yes   ☐ No

4. Can you request and receive the designated sources' standards for drugs and supplies to ensure your satisfaction with standards set for safety and product integrity?

☐ Yes   ☐ No   ☐ N/A

If undisclosed and unavailable, can you ethically agree to comply?

☐ Yes   ☐ No

The physician or hospital medical staff or chief medical officer can and should obtain and review these policies and procedures.

5. Is there a provider grievance mechanism?

☐ Yes   ☐ No

If yes, can you meaningfully participate?

☐ Yes   ☐ No

If yes, cite section of the contract where details of this program are found:

_____

Credentialing

6. Can we begin treating patients as a participating provider before all credentialing activities are complete?

☐ Yes   ☐ No

7. Is specialty board certification required for empanelment with this plan?

☐ Yes   ☐ No

Pay for Performance

8. Is there a pay-for-performance program established or slated for the near future?

☐ Yes   ☐ No

If yes, please describe: _____

_____

9. Will the plan incorporate episode treatment groups (ETGs) as part of their quality metrics?

☐ Yes   ☐ No

If yes, please describe: _____

_____

10. If yes, will there be an opportunity to earn bonuses for meeting certain quality metrics and benchmarks?

☐ Yes   ☐ No

If yes, please describe: _____

_____

11. Does the contract contain specifics as to how such bonuses or penalties will be calculated?

☐ Yes   ☐ No

If yes, cite section: _____

12. Does the contract contain specifics as to when the money shall be paid?
☐ Yes   ☐ No

If yes, cite section: _____

13. Does the contract contain specifics that enable use to determine exactly how much bonus or penalty is due?

☐ Yes   ☐ No

If yes, cite section: _____

14. Does the contract contain specifics that enable use to determine the penalty for late payment of any bonus or penalty?

☐ Yes   ☐ No

If yes, cite section: _____

Term, Termination, and Contract Renewals

Term of the Contract

1. The initial term of the contract begins on: _____

2. The length of the initial term of the contract is: _____

3. At the conclusion of the initial term of the contract, the contract:

   ☐ ends ☐ rolls over

   If applicable, the subsequent rollover terms, if any, are for what length of time?

   _____

   Cite relevant section of the contract: _____

4. If a rollover or evergreen feature is included, then upon the anniversary of the contract, what provision is in the contract for fee adjustment or escalation?

   _____

   Cite relevant section of the contract: _____

5. If automatic fee escalation does not take effect or is implemented late, what process is necessary to enforce the provision? _____

   _____

   Cite relevant section of the contract: _____

Termination of the Contract

6. In the event we wish to terminate the contract, may we do so without citing a cause?

   ☐ Yes ☐ No

   If yes, how much advance notice is required? _____

   Cite relevant section of the contract: _____

7. In the event the plan wishes to terminate the contract, may they do so without citing a cause?

   ☐ Yes   ☐ No

   If yes, how much advance notice is required?_____

   Cite relevant section of the contract: _____

8. In the event that the plan terminates the contract, who notifies the patient? _____

   Cite relevant section of the contract: _____

9. In the event that either party terminates the contract, how long must we honor the fee schedule? _____
   Cite relevant section of the contract: _____

10. In the event that the plan terminates the contract, who absorbs the cost of medical records copies for continuity of care? _____

    Cite relevant section of the contract: _____

11. Upon termination of the contract, how much time is allowed to close the books with any final auditing and finalize any outstanding payments? _____

    Cite relevant section of the contract: _____

12. In the event that a payer under the contract (who is not a signatory) habitually breaches the contract to the extent that we no longer wish to honor their status as a payer under this contract, are we permitted to terminate the individual payer without terminating the entire contract?

    ☐ Yes   ☐ No

    If yes, cite relevant section of the contract: _____

13. Are you permitted to discharge a patient for the usual and customary reasons without interference or first seeking permission from the plan?

    ☐ Yes   ☐ No

14. Which specific provisions, if any, survive the termination of the contract?

    _____

Assignment of the Contract

15. Is either of the signatories to the contract permitted to assign the contract to others without the express written consent of the other party?

   ☐ Yes ☐ No

16. Are there any mergers or acquisitions planned in the near future?

   ☐ Yes ☐ No

   If yes, and we have executed contracts with both entities, which contract and fee schedule will survive? _____

   Cite relevant section of the contract: _____

   (*While this will not be found in the contract, inquire and obtain a written response to the question. Careful attention should be paid to the "Assignment" paragraph, which may imply that the plan has the right to transfer or "assign" this contract to its successor in the event of a merger or acquisition, with or without the provider's express written consent, as the contract may specify. If a case like the example above arises, and the provider has contracts with both plans, the provider may wish to have some say as to which contract will remain in effect, and which coverage policies will be used to adjudicate claims.*)

17. If a new assignee expects discounted rates to be honored under this contract, how will we recognize their patients? _____

   _____

   (*While this will not be found in the contract, inquire and obtain a written response to the question. One best practice would be to require that the logo be present on the identification card presented by the patient in order for a discount to be applied. A few contracts throughout the country now specifically state this for the record.*)

18. How will we decipher cards and model rates if multiple logos are found on the identification card? _____

19. Does the plan include access by entities solely involved in brokering continuous discount arrangements without the requirement of adherence to other provisions of the contract?

□ Yes   □ No

If yes, can you limit or restrict their activities as they relate to your discount?

□ Yes   □ No

Miscellaneous Provisions

Notice

1. Is the plan required to provide notice of any contracting issues by certified mail, with return receipt requested?

□ Yes   □ No

Amendment

2. Is the plan able to unilaterally change the contract provisions, fee schedules, policy manuals, and provider manuals during the term of the contract without giving you written notice and obtaining your agreement to such changes in advance?

□ Yes   □ No

Entire Agreement

3. Does the contract and Entire Agreement provision include the base agreement together with all attachments, exhibits, fee schedules, published policies and procedures, provider manual, and other documents from which reliance and consideration is given at the time the contract is executed?

□ Yes   □ No

Cite where this is found in the contract: _____

4. Do you have a copy of each of these items for your files, either on a CD/ DVD or printed on paper?

□ Yes   □ No

If not, why not?_____

Dispute Resolution

5. If a dispute arises, what is the method of formal dispute resolution?

☐ Mediation

☐ Arbitration

☐ Litigation

6. If arbitration, which rules apply to the proceedings?

☐ American Arbitration Association

☐ American Health Lawyers Alternative Dispute Resolution Service

☐ Other

7. Under which state's governing law is the contract interpreted? _____

8. In which city and county is the dispute resolution conducted? _____

9. Is the dispute resolution final, conclusive, and binding?

☐ Yes   ☐ No

10. Who pays the dispute resolution fees and costs?

☐ Winner   ☐ Loser   ☐ Each pays ½

Organize Your Thoughts

List five points that summarize why you still want this contract as part of your reimbursement strategy:

1.

2.

3.

4.

5.

List your five major concerns with this contract:

1.

2.

3.

4.

5.

Next Steps

List follow-up actions, clarifications needed, and any change requests necessary in order to execute this contract:

☐

☐

☐

☐

☐

☐

☐

☐

☐

☐

☐

☐

☐

☐

☐

☐

☐

☐

What obstacles, if any, would I like to overcome in order to feel more comfortable with this contract?

- ☐
- ☐
- ☐
- ☐
- ☐
- ☐
- ☐
- ☐
- ☐
- ☐
- ☐
- ☐
- ☐
- ☐
- ☐
- ☐
- ☐
- ☐
- ☐

Notes:

Frequently Asked Questions

Q: **How flexible are the health plans when setting up contracts with providers?**

A: Often they are not very flexible with changes to existing language unless the contract does not address a specific point that has been promised. However, they will often provide additional information that may answer many of the questions in the checklist.

Q: **What recourse do providers have when dealing with denied claims?**

A: The contract, exhibits, and attachments, as well as the provider manual will often spell out options and limitations for denials and appeals.

Q: **Can contracts automatically roll over or renew without automatically increasing the fee schedule to current reimbursement rates?**

A: Yes. It is important to negotiate this point into your contract if you want some escalation formula tied to the automatic renewals. Otherwise, you should not expect any automatic increases.

Q: **Can you negotiate reimbursement on specific CPT codes?**

A: Yes. A best practice would be to be able to have an exact expectation of the reimbursement for every service you provide, whenever possible.

Q: **How do you negotiate prompt payment?**

A: First, check with your attorney or state medical association regarding any prompt payment laws that may be in effect in your state. Second, you may wish to consider negotiating a window for timely payment, in accordance with any existing state laws, together with a penalty for late payments.

Q: **Can different providers within the same practice have different contracts with different rates?**

A: It is possible, but often proves very difficult to administrate. Typically, they all seek to have the contract modified to one standard across all providers in the group.

Q: **Where can I get more information or assistance with negotiating managed care contracts?**

A: Attorneys with specific subject matter expertise and insight into the operational and financial aspects of the contract, not just the legalities, are a good resource. Additionally, a wide variety of consultants are available with operational and financial expertise, as well as knowledge of practice management and contracting trends in the marketplace. You may find good referral sources through professional associations that you or your practice administrator may belong to.

Q: How often should I review my managed care agreements?

A: At least annually if the contracts review annually. It is always a good practice to begin reviews of ongoing contracts not less than 4 months prior to the anniversary or renewal date.

Appendix: Insurance and Managed Care Glossary

A

AAPC: *See* Adjusted Average per Capita Cost

ABC: *See* Activity-Based Costing

Abuse: When used as a legal term in the business of health care, it normally refers to actions that do not involve intentional misrepresentations in billing but which, nevertheless, result in improper conduct. Consequences can result in civil liability and administrative sanctions. An example of abuse is the excessive use of medical supplies.

Access: The patient's ability to obtain medical care. The ease of access is determined by such components as the availability of medical services and their acceptability to the patient, the location of health care facilities, transportation, hours of operation, and cost of care. An individual's ability to obtain appropriate health care services. Barriers to access can be financial (insufficient monetary resources), geographic (distance to providers), organizational (lack of available providers), and sociological (e.g., discrimination, language barriers). Efforts to improve access often focus on providing/improving health coverage.

Accident and Health Insurance: Coverage for accidental injury, accidental death, and related health expenses. Benefits will pay for preventative services, medical expenses, and catastrophic care, with limits.

Accountable Health Partnership: An organization of doctors and hospitals that provides care for people organized into large groups of purchasers.

Accountable Health Plan (AHP): AHPs can be IDSs, MCOs, health networks, partnerships, or joint ventures between practitioners, providers, or payers that would assume responsibility for delivering medical care and managing the funds required to pay for the services rendered. Physicians and other providers would work for, contract with, or own these health plans. When an IDS or hospital group or IPA operates one or more health insurance benefit products, or a managed care organization acquires a large-scale medical delivery component, it qualifies as an accountable health system or accountable health plan.

Accreditation: The process by which an organization recognizes a provider, a program of study, or an institution as meeting predetermined standards. Two organizations that accredit managed care plans are the National Committee for Quality Assurance (NCQA) and the Joint Commission on Accreditation of Health Care Organizations (JCAHO). JCAHO also accredits hospitals and clinics. CARF accredits rehabilitation providers.

Accrete: The addition of new recipients to a health plan; a Medicare term.

Accrual: The amount of money that is set aside to cover expenses. The accrual is the plan's best estimate of what those expenses are and (for medical expenses) is based on a combination of data from the authorization system, the claims system, lag studies, and the plan's prior history.

ACR: *See* Adjusted Community Rate OR Adjusted Community Rating

Actively at Work: Describes insurer's policy requirement indicating that coverage will not go into effect until the employee's first day of work on or after the effective date of coverage. May also apply to dependents disabled on the effective date.

Activities of Daily Living (ADLs, ADL): An individual's daily habits such as bathing, dressing and eating. ADLs are often used as an assessment tool to determine an individual's ability to function at home, or in a less restricted environment of care.

Activity-Based Costing (ABC): Activity-based costing defines health care costs in terms of a health care organization's processes or activities. The costs are then associated with significant activities or events. It relies on the following three-step process: (1) activity mapping, which involves mapping activities in an illustrated sequence; (2) activity analysis, which involves defining and assigning a time value to activities; and (3) bill of activities, which involves generating a cost for each main activity.

Actuarial: Refers to the statistical calculations used to determine the managed care company's rates and premiums charged their customers based on projections of utilization and cost for a defined population.

Actuarial Soundness: The requirement that the development of capitation rates meets common actuarial principles and rules.

Actuary: In insurance, a person trained in statistics, accounting, and mathematics, who determines policy rates, reserves, and dividends by deciding what assumptions should be made with respect to each of the risk factors involved (such as the frequency of occurrence of the peril, the average benefit that will be payable, the rate of investment earnings, if any, expenses, and persistency rates), and who endeavors to secure as valid statistics as possible on which to base his assumptions. Professionally trained individual, usually with experience or education in insurance, who conducts statistical studies such as determining insurance policy rates, dividend reserves, and dividends and also conducts various other statistical studies. A capitated health provider would not accept or contract for capitated rates, or agree to a capitated contract without an actuarial determining the reasonableness of the rates.

Acute Care: A pattern of health care in which a patient is treated for an acute (immediate and severe) episode of illness, for the subsequent treatment of injuries related to an accident or other trauma, or during recovery from surgery. Specialized personnel using complex and sophisticated technical equipment and materials usually give acute care in a hospital. Unlike chronic care, acute care is often necessary for only a short time.

Adjudication: Processing claims according to contract.

Adjusted Admissions: Adjusted admissions are equivalent to the sum of inpatient admissions and an estimate of the volume of outpatient services. This is a measure of all patient care activity undertaken in a hospital, both inpatient and outpatient. This estimate is calculated by multiplying outpatient visits by the ratio of outpatient charges per visit to inpatient charges per admission.

Adjusted Average per Capita Cost (AAPCC): The basis for HMO or CMP reimbursement under Medicare risk contracts. The average monthly amount received per enrollee is currently calculated as 95% of the average costs to deliver medical care in the fee-for-service sector. CMS's best estimate of the amount of money care costs for Medicare recipients under fee-for-service Medicare in a given area. The AAPCC is made up of 122 different rate cells; 120 of them are factored for age, sex, Medicaid eligibility, institutional status, and whether a person has both Part A and Part B of Medicare. Actuarial projections of per capita Medicare spending for enrollees in fee-for-service Medicare. Separate AAPCCs are calculated—usually at the county level—for Part A services and Part B services for the aged, disabled, and people with end-stage renal disease (ESRD). Medicare pays risk plans by applying adjustment factors to 95% of the Part A and Part B AAPCCs. The adjustment factors reflect differences in Medicare per capita fee-for-service spending related to age, sex, institutional status, Medicaid status, and employment status.

A county-level estimate of the average cost incurred by Medicare for each beneficiary in the fee-for-service system. Adjustments are made so that the AAPCC represents the level of spending that would occur if each county contained the same mix of beneficiaries. Medicare pays health plans 95% of the AAPCC, adjusted for the characteristics of the enrollees in each plan.

Adjusted Community Rate (ACR): Health plans and insurance companies estimate their ACRs annually and adjust subsequent year supplemental benefits or premiums to return any excess Medicare revenue above the ACR to enrollees. These are the estimated payment rates that health plans with Medicare risk contracts would have received for their Medicare enrollees if paid their private market premiums, adjusted for differences in benefit packages and service use.

Adjusted Community Rating (ACR): ACR is a rating by community influenced by certain group demographics. Estimated payment rates that health plans with Medicare risk contracts would have received for their Medicare enrollees if paid their private market premiums, adjusted for differences in benefit packages and service use. Health plans estimate their ACRs annually and adjust subsequent year supplemental benefits or premiums to return any excess Medicare revenue above the ACR to enrollees.

Adjusted Drug Benefit List: A small number of medications often prescribed to long-term patients. Also called a drug maintenance list. A health plan, CMS or third-party administrator can modify it from time to time.

Adjusted Payment Rate (APR): The Medicare capitated payment to risk-contract HMOs. For a given health plan, the APR is determined by adjusting county-level AAPCCs to reflect the relative risks of the plan's enrollees.

Adjusted per Capita Cost (APCC): Medicare benefits estimation for a person in a given county using sex, age, institutional status, Medicaid disability, and end-stage renal disease status as a basis.

Adjuster: An individual employed by a property/casualty insurer to evaluate losses and settle policyholder claims. These adjusters differ from public adjusters, who negotiate with insurers on behalf of policyholders and receive a portion of a claims settlement. Independent adjusters are independent contractors who adjust claims for different insurance companies.

ADL: *See* Activities of Daily Living

Administrative Code Sets: Code sets that characterize a general business situation, rather than a medical condition or service. Under HIPAA, these are sometimes referred to as nonclinical or nonmedical code sets. Compare to medical code sets.

Administrative Costs: Costs related to utilization review, insurance marketing, medical underwriting, agents' commissions, premium collection, claims processing, insurer profit, quality assurance programs, and risk management. Administrative costs also refer to certain allowable costs on hospital CMS cost reports, usually considered overhead. Rules exist which disallow certain expenses, such as marketing. Costs not linked directly to the provision of medical care. Includes marketing, claims processing, billing, and medical record keeping, among others.

Administrative Services Only (ASO): A relationship between an insurance company or other management entity and a self-funded plan or group of providers in which the insurance company or management entity performs administrative services only, such as billing, practice management, marketing, etc. and does not assume any risk. The client bears the financial risk for the claims. Clients contracting for ASO can include health plans, hospitals, delivery networks, IPAs, etc. A provider system wishing to capitate might contract with a TPA for ASO for certain services which the provider group does not want to bring in house. This is a form of outsourcing. *See also* TPA.

Administrative Services Organization (ASO): A contract between an insurance company and a self-funded plan where the insurance company performs administrative services only, and the self-funded entity assumes all risk.

Administrative Simplification: Title II, Subtitle F, of HIPAA which authorizes HHS to (1) adopt standards for transactions and code sets that are used to exchange health data; (2) adopt standard identifiers for health plans, health care providers, employers, and individuals for use on standard transactions; and (3) adopt standards to protect the security and privacy of personally identifiable health information.

Admission Certification: Methods of assuring that only those patients who need hospital care are admitted. Certification can be granted before admission (preadmission) or shortly after (concurrent). Length of stay for the patient's diagnosed problem is usually assigned upon admission under a certification program.

Admissions per 1000: Number of patients admitted to a hospital or hospitals per 1000 health plan members. An indicator calculated by taking the total number of inpatient and/or outpatient admissions from a specific group (e.g., employer group, HMO population at risk) for a specific period of time (usually one year), dividing it by the average number of covered members in that group during the same period, and multiplying the result by 1000. This indicator can be calculated for behavioral health or any disease in the aggregate and by modality of treatment (inpatient, residential, and partial hospitalization, etc.).

Admitted Company: An insurance company licensed and authorized to do business in a particular state.

ADR: *See* Alternative Dispute Resolution

Adverse Event: An injury to a patient resulting from a medical intervention.

Adverse Selection: The problem of attracting members who are sicker than the general population, specifically, members who are sicker than was anticipated when developing the budget for medical costs. A tendency for utilization of health services in a population group to be higher than average or the tendency for a person who is in poor health to be enrolled in a health plan where he or she is below the average risk of the group. From an insurance perspective, adverse selection occurs when persons with poorer-than-average health status apply for, or continue, insurance coverage to a greater extent than do persons with average or better health expectations. Occurs when premium does not cover cost. Some populations, perhaps due to age or health status, have a great potential for high utilization. Some population parameter, such as age (for example, a much greater number of 65-year-olds or older to young population), that increases the potential for higher utilization and often increases costs above those covered by a payer's capitation rate. Among applicants for a given group or individual program, the tendency for those with an impaired health status, or who are prone to higher than average utilization of benefits, to be enrolled in disproportionate numbers and lower deductible plans.

AFDC: *See* Aid to Families with Dependent Children

Affiliated Provider: A health care provider or facility that is part of the HMO's network, usually having formal arrangements to provide services to the HMO member.

Affiliation: An agreement between two or more otherwise independent entities or individuals that defines how they will relate to one another. Agreements between hospitals may specify procedures for referring or transferring patients. Agreements between providers may include joint managed care contracting.

Affinity Sales: Selling insurance through groups such as professional and business associations.

Age-at-Issuance Rating: A method for establishing health insurance premiums whereby an insurer's premium is based on the age of individuals when they first purchased health insurance coverage. This is an older form of actuarial assessment.

Age-Attained Rating: Similar to the above, this method for establishing health insurance premiums whereby an insurer's premium is based on the current age of the beneficiary. Age-attained-rated premiums increase in price, as the purchasers grow older.

Age/Sex Factor: Underwriting measurement representing the medical risk costs of one population compared to another based on age and sex factors.

Age/Sex Rates (ASR): Also called table rates, they are given group products' set of rates where each grouping, by age and sex, has its own rates. Rates are used to calculate premiums for group billing and demographic changes are adjusted automatically in the group.

Agency Companies: Companies that market and sell products via independent agents.

Agency for Health Care Policy and Research (AHCPR): The agency of the Public Health Service responsible for enhancing the quality, appropriateness, and effectiveness of health care services.

Agent: Insurance is sold by two types of agents: independent agents, who are self-employed, represent several insurance companies, and are paid on commission, and exclusive or captive agents, who represent only one insurance company and are either salaried or work on commission. Insurance companies that use exclusive or captive agents are called direct writers.

Aggregate Margin: This is computed by subtracting the sum of expenses for all hospitals in the group from the sum of revenues and dividing by the sum of revenues. The aggregate margin compares revenues to expenses for a group of hospitals, rather than one single hospital.

Aggregate PPS Operating Margin/Aggregate Total Margin: This is computed by subtracting the sum of expenses for all hospitals in the group from the sum of revenues and dividing by the sum of revenues. A PPS operating margin or total margin compares revenue to expenses for a group of hospitals, rather than a single hospital.

Aggregate Stop Loss: The form of excess risk coverage that provides protection for the employer against accumulation of claims exceeding a certain level. This is protection against abnormal frequency of claims in total, rather than abnormal severity of a single claim.

AHCPR: *See* Agency for Health Care Policy and Research

AHP: *See* Accountable Health Plan

Aid to Families with Dependent Children (AFDC): The federal AFDC program provides cash welfare to (1) needy children who have been deprived of parental support and (2) certain others in the household of such children. States administer the AFDC program with funding from both the federal government and state. The Personal Responsibility and

Work Responsibility Act of 1996, enacted in August 1996, replaced AFDC with a new program called Temporary Assistance for Needy Families (TANF).

Alien Insurance Company: An insurance company incorporated under the laws of a foreign country, as opposed to a foreign insurance company that does business in states outside its own.

All-Inclusive Visit Rate: Aggregate costs for any one patient visit based upon annual operating costs divided by patient visits per year. This rate incorporates costs for all services at the visit.

Allowable Charge: The maximum charge for which a third party will reimburse a provider for a given service. An allowable charge is not necessarily the same as either a reasonable, customary, maximum, actual, or prevailing charge.

Allowable Costs: Covered expenses within a given health plan. Items or elements of an institution's costs, which are reimbursable under a payment formula. Both Medicare and Medicaid reimburse hospitals on the basis of only certain costs. Allowable costs may exclude, for example, luxury travel or marketing. CMS publishes an extensive list of rules governing these costs and provides software for determining costs. Normally the costs which are not reasonable expenditures, which are unnecessary, which are for the efficient delivery of health services to persons covered under the program in question are not reimbursed. The most common form of cost reimbursement is the "cost report" methodology used for DRG-exempt services, such as many outpatient hospital-based programs, long-term care and skilled nursing units, physical rehab, psychiatric and substance abuse inpatient programs. Some specialty hospitals receive all of their CMS reimbursement as cost-based reimbursement.

Allowed Amount: Maximum dollar amount assigned for a procedure based on various pricing mechanisms. Also known as a maximum allowable.

Allowed Charge: This is the amount Medicare approves for payment to a physician, but may not match the amount the physician gets paid by Medicare (due to co-pay or deductibles) and usually does not match what the physician charges patients. Medicare normally pays 80% of the approved charge, and the beneficiary pays the remaining 20%. The allowed charge for a nonparticipating physician is 95% of that for a participating physician. Nonparticipating physicians may bill beneficiaries for an additional amount above the allowed charge. The CMS intermediary in each state publishes these rates.

All Patient Diagnosis-Related Groups (APDRG): An enhancement of the original DRGs, designed to apply to a population broader than that of Medicare beneficiaries, who are predominately older individuals. The

APDRG set includes groupings for pediatric and maternity cases as well as of services for HIV-related conditions and other special cases.

All-Payer System: A system in which prices for health services and payment methods are the same, regardless of who is paying. For instance, in an all-payer system, federal or state government, a private insurer, a self-insured employer plan, an individual, or any other payer could pay the same rates. The uniform fee bars health care providers from shifting costs from one payer to another.

ALOS: *See* Average Length of Stay

Alternate Delivery Systems: Health services provided in other than an inpatient, acute-care hospital or private practice. A phrase used to describe all forms of health care delivery except traditional fee-for-service, private practice. The term includes HMOs, PPOs, IPAs, and other systems of providing health care. Examples within general health services include skilled and intermediary nursing facilities, hospice programs, and home health care. Alternate delivery systems are designed to provide needed services in a more cost-effective manner. Most of the services provided by community mental health centers fall into this category.

Alternative Dispute Resolution (ADR): Alternative to going to court to settle disputes. Methods include arbitration, where disputing parties agree to be bound to the decision of an independent third party, and mediation, where a third party tries to arrange a settlement between the two sides.

Alternative Markets: Mechanisms used to fund self-insurance. This includes captives, which are insurers owned by one or more noninsurers to provide owners with coverage. Risk-retention groups, formed by members of similar professions or businesses to obtain liability insurance, are also a form of self-insurance.

Ambulatory Care: Health services provided without the patient being admitted. Also called outpatient care. The services of ambulatory care centers, hospital outpatient departments, physicians' offices, and home health care services fall under this heading provided that the patient remains at the facility less than 24 hours. No overnight stay in a hospital is required.

Ancillary Services (Ancillary Charges): Supplemental services, including laboratory, radiology, physical therapy, and inhalation therapy that are provided in conjunction with medical or hospital care.

Anniversary Date: The beginning of an employer group's benefit year. The first day of effective coverage as contained in the policy group application and subsequent annual anniversaries of that date. An insured has the option to transfer from an indemnity plan (which may have maximum benefit levels) to an HMO.

Annual Statement: Summary of an insurer's or reinsurer's financial operations for a particular year, including a balance sheet. It is filed with the state insurance department of each jurisdiction in which the company is licensed to conduct business.

Anonymized Data: Previously identifiable data that have been deidentified and for which a code or other link no longer exists. A provider, third party, or investigator would not be able to link anonymized information back to a specific individual.

Anonymous Data: Under HIPAA, this refers to data that were collected without identifiers and that were never linked to an individual. Coded data are not anonymous.

ANSI (American National Standards Institute): A national organization founded to develop voluntary business standards in the United States.

Antitrust: A legal term encompassing a variety of efforts on the part of government to assure that sellers do not conspire to restrain trade or fix prices for their goods or services in the market.

Antitrust Laws: Laws that prohibit companies from working as a group to set prices, restrict supplies, or stop competition in the marketplace. The insurance industry is subject to state antitrust laws, but has a limited exemption from federal antitrust laws. This exemption, set out in the McCarran–Ferguson Act, permits insurers to jointly develop common insurance forms and share loss data to help them price policies.

Any Willing Provider: A requirement that a health plan contract for the delivery of health care services with any provider in the area who would like to provide such services to the plan's enrollees.

Any Willing Provider Laws: Laws that require managed care plans to contract with all health care providers that meet their terms and conditions.

APCC: *See* Adjusted per Capita Cost

APDRG: *See* All Patient Diagnosis-Related Groups

Application Integrators: Software that transparently provides application-to-application functionality, primarily through data conversion and transmission, while eliminating the need for custom programming. Also referred to as application integration gateway, application interface gateway, integration engine, and intelligent gateway. This type of software is key to developing networks of information systems, making client-specific information available in real time to all members of an IHDS.

Apportionment: The dividing of a loss proportionately among two or more insurers that cover the same loss.

Appropriateness: Appropriate health care is care for which the expected health benefit exceeds the expected negative consequences by a wide enough margin to justify treatment. This term is not to be confused with "usual and customary" or "approved" service. The extent to which a particular procedure, treatment, test, or service is clearly indicated, not excessive, adequate in quantity, and provided in the setting best suited to a patient's or member's needs.

Approval: A term used extensively in managed care that, to many, implies the primary process of "managing" managed care. Approval usually is used to describe treatments or procedures that have been certified by utilization review. Can also refer to the status of certain hospitals or doctors, as members of a plan. Can describe benefits or services, which will be covered under a plan. Generally, approval is either granted by the managed care organization (MCO), third-party administrator (TPA), or by the primary care physician (PCP), depending on the circumstances.

Approved Charge: Limits of expenses paid by Medicare in a given area of covered service. Charges approved by payment by private health plans. Items that are likely to be reimbursed by the insurance company.

Approved Health Care Facility, Hospital, or Program: A facility or program authorized to provide health services and allowed by a given health plan to provide services stipulated in contract.

APR: *See* Adjusted Payment Rate

Arbitration: Procedure in which an insurance company and the insured or a vendor agree to settle a claim dispute by accepting a decision made by a third party.

ASO: *See* Administrative Services Only OR Administrative Services Organization

Assignment of Benefits: Method used when a claimant directs that payment be made directly to the health care provider by the health plan.

Assisted Living: Broad range of residential care services, which does not include nursing services. Normally lower in cost than nursing homes.

ASR: *See* Age/Sex Rates

Attestation: The requirement that the attending physician certify, in writing, the accuracy and completion of the clinical information used for DRG assignment.

Audit of Provider Treatment or Charges: A qualitative or quantitative review of services rendered or proposed by a health provider. The review can be carried out in a number of ways: a comparison of patient records and claim form information, a patient questionnaire, a review of hospital and practitioner records, or a pre- or posttreatment clinical examination of a patient. Some audits may involve fee verification. Something we had better get used to being subjected to since this is usually first type or "first generation" managed care approach.

Authorization: Any document designating any permission. The HIPAA Privacy Rule requires authorization or waiver of authorization for the use or disclosure of identifiable health information for research (among other activities). The authorization must indicate if the health information used or disclosed is existing information and/or new information that will be created. The authorization form may be combined with the informed consent form, so that a patient need sign only one form. An authorization must include the following specific elements: a description of what information will be used and disclosed and for what purposes; a description of any information that will not be disclosed, if applicable; a list of who will disclose the information and to whom it will be disclosed; an expiration date for the disclosure; a statement that the authorization can be revoked; a statement that disclosed information may be redisclosed and no longer protected; a statement that if the individual does not provide an authorization, s/he may not be able to receive the intended treatment; the subject's signature and date.

Autoassignment or Auto Assignment: A term used with Medicaid mandatory managed care enrollment plans. Medicaid recipients who do not specify their choice for a contracted plan within a specified time frame are assigned to a plan by the state.

Auto-Enrollment: The automatic assignment of a person to a health insurance plan, typically done under Medicaid plans.

Auto Insurance Policy: There are basically six different types of coverages. Some may be required by law. Others are optional. They are:

1. Bodily injury liability, for injuries the policyholder causes to someone else
2. Medical payments or personal injury protection (PIP) for treatment of injuries to the driver and passengers of the policyholder's car
3. Property damage liability, for damage the policyholder causes to someone else's property
4. Collision, for damage to the policyholder's car from a collision
5. Comprehensive, for damage to the policyholder's car not involving a collision with another car (including damage from fire, explosions, earthquakes, floods, and riots), and theft
6. Uninsured motorists coverage, for costs resulting from an accident involving a hit-and-run driver or a driver who does not have insurance

Average Length of Stay (ALOS): Refers to the average length of stay per inpatient hospital visit. Figure is typically calculated for both commercial and Medicare patient populations.

Average Wholesale Price (AWP): Commonly used in pharmacy contracting, the AWP is generally determined through reference to a common source of information. Average cost of a nondiscounted item to a pharmacy provider by wholesale providers. Drug manufacturers commonly publish suggested wholesale prices.

Avoidable Hospital Condition: Medical diagnosis for which hospitalization could have been avoided if ambulatory care had been provided in a timely and efficient manner.

AWP: *See* Average Wholesale Price

B

Balance Billing: The practice of billing a patient for the fee amount remaining after insurer payment and co-payment have been made. Under Medicare, the excess amount cannot be more than 15% above the approved charge.

Base Capitation: Specified amount per person per month to cover health care cost, usually excluding pharmacy and administrative costs as well as optional coverages such as mental health/substance abuse services.

Base Year Costs: In Medicare, the amount a hospital actually spent to render care in a previous time period. Depending on the hospital's Medicare cost reporting period, the base year was the fiscal year ending on or after September 30, 1982 and before September 30, 1983 for hospitals in operation at that time. Recent legislation has made dramatic changes in cost reporting opportunities for health care providers, limiting these reimbursements.

Bed Days: Number of inpatient hospital days per 1000 health plan members for a specified period, usually annual.

Behavioral Health, Behavioral Health Care: An umbrella term that includes mental health, psychiatric, marriage and family counseling, addictions treatment, and substance abuse. Services are provided by a myriad of providers, including social workers, counselors, psychiatrists, psychologists, neurologists, and even family practice physicians. Many states have "parity" laws that attempt to require that behavioral health insurance coverage be provided "on par" to physical health coverage.

Behavioral Offset: This is the change in the number and type of services that is projected to occur in response to a change in fees. A 50% behavioral offset suggests that 50% of the savings from fee reductions will be offset by increased volume and intensity of services.

Benchmark: A goal to be attained. These goals are chosen by comparisons with other providers, by consulting statistical reports available, or are drawn from the best practices within the organization or industry. Benchmarks are used in quality improvement programs to encourage improvement of care, efficiencies, or services. Benchmarks are also used for length-of-stay comparisons, costs, utilization review, risk management, and financial analysis. The benchmarking process identifies the best performance in the industry (health care or nonhealth care) for a particular process or outcome, determines how that performance is achieved, and applies the lessons learned to improve performance.

Beneficiary (*Also* Eligible; Enrollee; Member): Individual who is either using or eligible to use insurance benefits, including health insurance benefits, under an insurance contract. Any person eligible as either a subscriber or a dependent for a managed care service in accordance with a contract. An individual who receives benefits from or is covered by an insurance policy or other health care financing program.

Beneficiary Liability: The amount beneficiaries must pay providers for Medicare-covered services. Liabilities include co-payments, deductibles, and balance billing amounts. CMS has very strict rules about health providers billing patients for their liabilities. Cost-based facilities are not allowed to charge nonpayment by beneficiaries to bad debt unless a clear history of collection activity is recorded.

Benefit Limitations: Any provision, other than an exclusion, which restricts coverage in the evidence of coverage, regardless of medical necessity. Limitations are often expressed in terms of dollar amounts, length of stay, diagnosis, or treatment descriptions.

Benefit Package: Aggregate services specifically defined by an insurance policy or HMO that can be provided to patients. The services a payer offers to a group or individual. The package will specify cost, limitation on the amounts of services, and annual or lifetime spending limits.

Benefit Payment Schedule: A list of the amounts an insurance plan will pay for covered health care services.

Benefits: Benefits are specific areas of plan coverages (outpatient visits, hospitalization, and so forth) that make up the range of medical services that a payer markets to its subscribers. Also, a contractual agreement, specified in an evidence of coverage, determining covered services provided by insurers to members.

Billed Claims: Fees submitted by a health care provider for services rendered to a covered person. Fees billed and fees paid are rarely synonymous.

Biometric Identifier: Identifying information based on a physical characteristic, such as a fingerprint. Confidentiality laws and HIPAA privacy rules refer to biometric identifiers.

Bioterrorism or Biological Warfare: The unlawful use, wartime use, or threatened use of microorganisms or toxins to produce death or disease in humans. Often viewed as the preferred choice of warfare of less powerful groups of people in attempt to wage war or protect themselves from more powerful groups or nations. However, biological agents could be used by individuals or by powerful nations as well.

Block Grant: Federal funds made to a state for the delivery of a specific group of related services, such as drug abuse–related services.

Board Certified (Boarded, Diplomate): Describes a physician who has passed a written and oral examination given by a medical specialty board and who has been certified as a specialist in that area.

Board Eligible: Describes a physician who is eligible to take the specialty board examination by virtue of being graduated from an approved medical school, completing a specific type and length of training, and practicing for a specified amount of time. Some HMOs and other health facilities accept board eligibility as equivalent to board certification, significant in that many managed care companies restrict referrals to physicians without certification.

Bodily Injury Liability Coverage: Portion of an automobile insurance policy that covers injuries the policyholder causes to someone else.

Bonus Payment: An additional amount paid by Medicare for services provided by physicians in health professional shortage areas. Currently, the bonus payment is 10% of Medicare's share of allowed charges. This is not to be confused with other payments to hospitals, such as the disproportionate share payment or the settlement made to facilities at the end of a cost report year.

Book of Business: Total amount of insurance on an insurer's books at a particular point in time.

Broker: One who represents an insured in solicitation, negotiation, or procurement of contracts of insurance, and who may render services incidental to those functions. By law, the broker may also be an agent of the insurer for certain purposes such as delivery of the policy or collection of the premium.

Bundled Payment: A single comprehensive payment for a group of related services. Bundled payments have become the norm in recent years, and CMS and other payers investigate unbundled services closely. Unbundling service charges has been a common form of fraud as defined by CMS.

Business Associate: Under HIPAA rules, this term refers to an outside person/entity that performs a service on behalf of the health care provider (including a researcher) or the health care institution, during which individually identifiable health information is created, used, or disclosed. For example, Web hosting or data storage companies will be business associates if they receive protected health information. In addition, third parties that handle billing for a research study, or recruitment and screening, will also be business associates. Certain exceptions apply.

C

Cafeteria Plan: Arrangements under which employees may choose their own benefit structure. Sometimes these are varying benefit plans or add-ons provided through the same insurer or third-party administrator; other times this refers to the offering of different plans or HMOs provided by different managed care or insurance companies.

Capacity: The supply of insurance available to meet demand. Capacity depends on the industry's financial ability to accept risk. For an individual insurer, the maximum amount of risk it can underwrite based on its financial condition. The adequacy of an insurer's capital relative to its exposure to loss is an important measure of solvency.

Capital: Shareholder's equity (for publicly traded insurance companies) and retained earnings (for mutual insurance companies). There is no general measure of capital adequacy for property/casualty insurers. Capital adequacy is linked to the riskiness of an insurer's business. A company underwriting medical device manufacturers needs a larger cushion of capital than a company writing Main Street business, for example.

Capital Cost Report: Similar to the above review, but normally produced retrospectively rather than prospectively.

Capital Costs: Capital costs usually involve equipment and physical plant costs, not consumable supplies. Included in these costs can be interest, leases, rentals, taxes, and insurance on physical assets like plant and equipment. Capital costs are usually reimbursed to cost-based facilities through submission of these costs on annual cost reports to the CMS intermediaries. Depreciation schedules apply.

Capital Expenditure Review: A review of proposed capital expenditures of hospitals or providers to determine the need for, and appropriateness of, the proposed expenditures. The review is usually done by a designated regulatory agency and has a sanction attached that prevents or discourages unneeded expenditures. Often this is related to CMS or Medicare and the willingness of the federal government to provide allowances for capital costs.

Capitation (Cap, Capped, Capitate): Specified amount paid periodically to health provider for a group of specified health services, regardless of quantity rendered. Amounts are determined by assessing a payment "per covered life" or per member. The method of payment in which the provider is paid a fixed amount for each person served no matter what the actual number or nature of services delivered. The cost of providing an individual with a specific set of services over a set period of time, usually a month or a year. A payment system whereby managed care plans pay health care providers a fixed amount to care for a patient over a given period. Providers are not reimbursed for services that exceed the allotted amount. The rate may be fixed for all members, or it can be adjusted for the age and gender of the member, based on actuarial projections of medical utilization.

Carrier: An insurer; an underwriter of risk that finances health care. Also refers to any organization that underwrites or administers life, health, or other insurance programs. When an employer has a "self-insured" plan, the carrier (such as Aetna or Blue Cross) may not serve as carrier in this case, but may serve only as "third-party administrator."

Carve-In: A generic term that refers to any of a continuum of joint efforts between clinicians and service providers; also used specifically to refer to health care delivery and financing arrangements in which all covered benefits, such as behavioral and general health care, are administered and funded by an integrated system.

Carve-Out: Practice of excluding specific services from a managed care organization's capitated rate. In some instances, the same provider will still provide the service, but they will be reimbursed on a fee-for-service basis. In other instances, carved out services will be provided by an entirely different provider. A payer strategy in which a payer separates ("carves out") a portion of the benefit and hires an MCO to provide these benefits. A health care delivery and financing arrangement in which certain specific health care services that are covered benefits (for example, behavioral health care) are administered and funded separately from general health care services. The carve out is typically done through separate contracting or subcontracting for services to the special population. Common carve outs include such services as psychiatric, rehab, chemical dependency, and ambulatory services. Increasingly, oncology and cardiac services are being carved out. This permits the payer to create a separate health benefits package and assume greater control of their costs. Many HMOs and insurance companies adopt this strategy because they do not have in-house expertise related to the service "carved out." A "carve-out" is typically a service provided within a standard benefit package but delivered exclusively by a designated provider or group. This process may or may not seem transparent to the subscriber, but it often means that separate utilization review (UR) and precertification entities are involved as well as different payers and providers. Carve-outs are *also called* subcontractors, subcaptivators, or junior capitation contracts.

Case Management: A system of coordinating medical services to treat a patient, improve care, and reduce cost.

Case Manager: A nurse, doctor, or social worker who works with patients, providers, and insurers to coordinate all services deemed necessary to provide the patient with a plan of medically necessary and appropriate health care.

Case Mix: The mix of patients treated within a particular institutional setting, such as the hospital. Patient classification systems like DRGs can be used to measure hospital case mix. (*See also* DRGs and Case-Mix Index). Measurement reflecting servicing needs, uses of hospital capabilities, and the general rate of hospital admissions. The types of inpatients a hospital or post acute facility treats. The more complex the patients' needs, the greater the amount spent for patient care. Case mix is generally established by estimating the relative frequency of various types of patients seen by the provider in question during a given time period and may be measured by factors such as diagnosis, severity of illness, utilization of services, and provider characteristics.

Case-Mix Index (CMI): The average DRG weight for all cases paid under PPS. The CMI is a measure of the relative costliness of the patients treated in each hospital or group of hospitals. (*See also* DRG.) A measure of the relative costliness of treating in an inpatient setting. An index of 1.05 means that the facility's patients are 5% more costly than average.

Case Rate: Flat fee paid for a client's treatment based on their diagnosis or presenting problem. For this fee the provider covers all of the services the client requires for a specific period of time. Also bundled rate, or flat fee-per-case. Very often used as an intervening step prior to capitation. In this model, the provider is accepting some significant risk, but does have considerable flexibility in how it meets the client's needs. Keys to success in this mode include (1) properly pricing case rate, if provider has control over it, and (2) securing a large volume of eligible clients.

Case Severity: A measure of intensity or gravity of a given condition or diagnosis for a patient. May have direct correlation with the amount of service provided and the associated costs or payments allowed.

Catastrophic Health Insurance: Policy that provides protection primarily against the higher costs of treating severe or lengthy illnesses or disabilities. Normally these are "add-on" benefits that begin coverage once the primary insurance policy reaches its maximum.

Categorically Needy: Medicaid eligibility based on defined indicators of financial need by families with children and pregnant women, and to persons who are aged, blind, or disabled. Persons not falling into these categories cannot qualify, no matter how low their income. The Medicaid statute defines over 50 distinct population groups as potentially eligible, including those for which coverage is mandatory in all states and those that may be covered at a state's option. The scope of covered services that states must provide to the categorically needy is much broader than the minimum scope of services for other groups receiving Medicaid benefits.

CCA: *See* Cost–Consequence Analysis

CCN: *See* Community Care Network

CDT: *See* Current Dental Terminology

Centers for Medicare and Medicaid Services (CMS): The Centers for Medicare and Medicaid Services (CMS) is a federal agency within the U.S. Department of Health and Human Services. Programs for which CMS is responsible include Medicare, Medicaid, State Children's Health Insurance Program (SCHIP), HIPAA, and CLIA. Formerly was HCFA. Centers for Medicare and Medicaid Services have historically maintained the UB-92 institutional EMC format specifications, the professional EMC NSF specifications, and specifications for various certifications and authorizations used by the Medicare and Medicaid programs. CMS is responsible for oversight of HIPAA administrative simplification transaction and code sets, health identifiers, and security standards. CMS also maintains the HCPCS medical code set and the Medicare Remittance Advice Remark Codes administrative code set.

Certificate of Authority (COA): Issued by state governments, it gives a health maintenance organization or insurance company its license to operate within the state.

Certificate of Coverage (COC): Outlines the terms of coverage and benefits available in a carrier's health plan.

Certificate of Need (CON): In some states, a state agency must review and approve certain proposed capital expenditures, changes in health services provided, and purchases of expensive medical equipment. Before the request goes to the state, a local review panel (the health systems agency or HSA) must evaluate the proposal and make a recommendation. CON is intended to control expansion of facilities and services by preventing excessive or duplicative development of facilities and services. Many states have sunsetted or eliminated their CON processes and requirements.

Certified Health Plan: A managed health care plan, certified by the Health Services Commission and the Office of the Insurance Commissioner to provide coverage for the uniform benefits package to state residents. Regulations vary by state, since some states require only HMOs to certify but not PPOs, IPAs, or MSOs. Increasingly, these regulations are becoming more consistent state by state.

CF: *See* Conversion Factor

Chain of Trust Agreement: Referred to in HIPAA rules, this is a contract needed to extend the responsibility to protect health care data across a series of subcontractual relationships.

CHAMPUS: Civilian Health and Medical Program of the Uniformed Services.

Charges: These are the published prices of services provided by a facility. CMS requires hospitals to apply the same schedule of charges to all patients, regardless of the expected sources or amount of payment. Controversy exists today because of the often wide disparity between published prices and contract prices. The majority of payers, including Medicare and Medicaid, are becoming managed by health plans that negotiate rates lower than published prices. Often these negotiated rates average 40% to 60% of the published rates and may be all-inclusive bundled rates.

CHC: *See* Community Health Center

CHIN: *See* Community Health Information Network

Chronic Care: Long-term care of individuals with long-standing, persistent diseases or conditions. It includes care specific to the problem as well as other measures to encourage self-care, to promote health, and to prevent loss of function.

Claim: A request by an individual (or his or her provider) to that individual's insurance company to pay for services obtained from a health care professional.

Claims-Made Policy: A form of insurance that pays claims presented to the insurer during the term of the policy or within a specific term after its expiration. It limits liability insurers' exposure to unknown future liabilities.

Claims Review: The method by which an enrollee's health care service claims are reviewed prior to reimbursement. The purpose is to validate the medical necessity of the provided services and to be sure the cost of the service is not excessive.

Claim Status Codes: A national administrative code set that identifies the status of health care claims. This code set is used in the X12N 277

Claim Status Inquiry and Response transaction and is maintained by the Health Care Code Maintenance Committee.

CLIA: *See* Clinical Laboratory Improvement Amendments

Clinical Data Repository: That component of a computer-based patient record (CPR) which accepts, files, and stores clinical data over time from a variety of supplemental treatment and intervention systems for such purposes as practice guidelines, outcomes management, and clinical research. *May also be called* a data warehouse.

Clinical Decision Support: The capability of a data system to provide key data to physicians and other clinicians in response to "flags" or triggers which are functions of embedded, provider-created rules. A system that would alert case managers that a client's eligibility for a certain service is about to be exhausted would be one example of this type of capacity. Also a key functional requirement to support clinical or critical pathways.

Clinical Laboratory Improvement Amendments (CLIA): CMS regulates all laboratory testing (except research) performed on humans in the United States through the Clinical Laboratory Improvement Amendments (CLIA). In total, CLIA covers approximately 175,000 laboratory entities. The Division of Laboratory Services, within the Survey and Certification Group, under the Center for Medicaid and State Operations, has the responsibility for implementing the CLIA program. The objective of the CLIA program is to ensure quality laboratory testing. Although all clinical laboratories must be properly certified to receive Medicare or Medicaid payments, CLIA has no direct Medicare or Medicaid program responsibilities.

Clinical or Critical Pathways: A "map" of preferred treatment/intervention activities. Outlines the types of information needed to make decisions, the timelines for applying that information, and what action needs to be taken by whom. Provides a way to monitor care "in real time." These pathways are developed by clinicians for specific diseases or events. Proactive providers are working now to develop these pathways for the majority of their interventions and developing the software capacity to distribute and store this information.

Clinic Without Walls (CWW): Similar to an independent practice association and identical to a practice without walls (PWW). Practitioners form CWWs and PWWs when they want the economies of scale and bargaining power offered by centralizing some administrative functions, but still choosing to practice separately. Many of these were formed to allow practitioners the ability to effectively contract with managed care.

Closed Access: Gatekeeper model health plan that requires covered persons to receive care from providers within the plan's coverage. Except for emergencies, the patient may only be referred to and treated by providers within the plan. A managed health care arrangement in which covered persons are required to select providers only from the plan's participating providers.

Closed Panel: Medical services are delivered in the HMO-owned health center or satellite clinic by physicians who belong to a specially formed, but legally separate, medical group that only serves the HMO. This term usually refers to a group or staff HMO models.

CMA: *See* Cost Minimization Analysis

CMI: *See* Case-Mix Index

CMP: *See* Competitive Medical Plan

CMS (formerly HCFA): *See* Centers for Medicare and Medicaid Services.

CMS-1450: The uniform institutional claim form.

CMS-1500: The uniform professional claim form.

COA: *See* Certificate of Authority

COB: *See* Coordination of Benefits

COBRA: Consolidated Omnibus Budget Reconciliation Act. A federal law under which group health plans sponsored by employers with 20 or more employees must offer continuation of coverage to employees who leave their jobs and their dependents. The employee must pay the entire premium. Coverage can be extended up to 18 months. Surviving dependents can receive longer coverage.

COC: *See* Certificate of Coverage

Coded Data: Data are separated from personal identifiers through use of a code. As long as a link exists, data are considered indirectly identifiable and not anonymous or anonymized. Coded data are not covered by the HIPAA Privacy Rule, but are protected under the Common Rule.

Code Set: Under HIPAA, this is any set of codes used to encode data elements, such as tables of terms, medical concepts, medical diagnostic codes, or medical procedure codes. This includes both the codes and their descriptions.

Coding: A mechanism for identifying and defining physicians' and hospitals' services. Coding provides universal definition and recognition of diagnoses, procedures, and level of care. Coders usually work in medical records departments, and coding is a function of billing. Medicare fraud investigators look closely at the medical record documentation, which supports codes and looks for consistency. Lack of consistency of documentation can earmark a record as "upcoded," which is considered fraud. A national certification exists for coding professionals, and many compliance programs are raising standards of quality for their coding procedures.

COI: *See* Cost of Illness Analysis

Coinsurance:

1. In property insurance, requires the policyholder to carry insurance equal to a specified percentage of the value of property to receive full payment on a loss. For health insurance, it is a percentage of each claim above the deductible paid by the policyholder. For a 20% health insurance coinsurance clause, the policyholder pays for the deductible plus 20% of his covered losses. After paying 80% of losses up to a specified ceiling, the insurer starts paying 100% of losses.

2. A cost-sharing requirement under a health insurance policy that provides that the insured will assume a portion or percentage of the costs of covered services. Health care cost which the covered person is responsible for paying, according to a fixed percentage or amount. A policy provision frequently found in major medical insurance policies under which the insured individual and the insurer share hospital and medical expenses according to a specified ratio. A type of cost sharing where the insured party and insurer share payment of the approved charge for covered services in a specified ratio after payment of the deductible. Under Medicare Part B, the beneficiary pays coinsurance of 20% of allowed charges. Many HMOs provide 100% insurance (no coinsurance) for preventive care or routing care provided "in network."

CON: *See* Certificate of Need

Common Rule: Under HIPAA, it outlines the necessity of obtaining informed consent from patients.

Community Care Network (CCN): This vehicle provides coordinated, organized, and comprehensive care to a community's population. Hospitals, primary care physicians, and specialists link preventive and treatment services through contractual and financial arrangements, producing a network that provides coordinated care with continuous monitoring of quality and accountability to the public. While the term community care network (CCN) often is used interchangeably with integrated delivery system (IDS), the CCN tends to be community based and nonprofit.

Community Health Center (CHC): An ambulatory health care program (defined under section 330 of the Public Health Service Act) usually serving a catchment area which has scarce or nonexistent health services or a population with special health needs; sometimes known as the neighborhood health center. Community health centers attempt to coordinate federal, state, and local resources into a single organization capable of delivering both health and related social services to a defined population. While such a center may not directly provide all types of health care, it usually takes responsibility to arrange all medical services needed by its patient population.

Community Health Information Network (CHIN): An integrated collection of computer and telecommunication capabilities that permit multiple providers, payers, employers, and related health care entities within a geographic area to share and communicate client, clinical, and payment information. Also known as community health management information system.

Community Rating: Setting insurance rates based on the average cost of providing health services to all people in a geographic area, without adjusting for each individual's medical history or likelihood of using medical services. A method of calculating health plan premiums using the average cost of actual or anticipated health services for all subscribers within a specific geographic area. Under the HMO Act, community rating is defined as a system of fixing rates of payment for health services which may be determined on a per person or per family basis and may vary with the number of persons in a family, but must be equivalent for all individuals and for all families of similar composition. With community rating, premiums do not vary for different groups of subscribers or with such variables as the group's claims experience, age, sex, or health status. Although there are certain exceptions, in general, federally qualified HMOs must community rate. The intent of community rating is to spread the cost of illness evenly over all subscribers rather than charging the sick more than the healthy for coverage.

Community Rating by Class (CRC) (Class Rating): For federally qualified HMOs, the community rating by class (CRC)—adjustment of community-rated premiums on the basis of such factors as age, sex, family size, marital status, and industry classification. These health plan premiums reflect the experience of all enrollees of a given class within a specific geographic area, rather than the experience of any one employer group.

Community Rating Laws: Enacted in several states on health insurance policies. Insurers are required to accept all applicants for coverage and charge all applicants the same premium for the same coverage regardless of age or health. Premiums are based on the rate determined by the geographic region's health and demographic profile.

Comorbid Condition: A medical condition that, along with the principal diagnosis, exists at admission and is expected to increase hospital length of stay by at least one day for most patients.

Competitive Bidding: Can be viewed by some as a pricing method that elicits information on costs through a bidding process to establish payment rates that reflect the costs of an efficient health plan or health care provider. Competitive bidding is also the process of offering reduced rates to health plans to obtain exclusive contracts from payers.

Complaint Ratio: A measure used by some state insurance departments to track consumer complaints against insurance companies. Generally, it is written as the number of complaints upheld against an insurance company, as a percentage of premiums written. In some states, complaints from medical providers over the promptness of payments may also be included.

Compliance: Accurately following the government's rules on Medicare billing system requirements and other federal or state regulations. A compliance program is a self-monitoring system of checks and balances to ensure that an organization consistently complies with applicable laws relating to its business activities.

Complication: A medical condition that arises during a course of treatment and is expected to increase the length of stay by at least one day for most patients.

Competitive Medical Plan (CMP): A status, established by TEFRA and granted by the federal government, to an organization that meets specific requirements, enabling that organization to obtain a Medicare risk or cost-based contract.

Composite Rate: Group rate billed to all subscribers of a given group.

Comprehensive Major Medical Insurance: A policy designed to provide the protection offered by both a basic and major medical health insurance policy. It is generally characterized by a low deductible, a coinsurance feature, and high maximum benefits.

Computer-Based Patient Record (CPR): A term for the process of replacing the traditional paper-based chart through automated electronic means; generally includes the collection of patient-specific information from various supplemental treatment systems, such as a day program and a personal care provider; its display in graphical format; and its storage for individual and aggregate purposes. Also called "digital medical record" or "electronic medical record."

Concurrent Review: Review of a procedure or hospital admission done by a health care professional (usually a nurse) other than the one providing the care, during the same time frame that the care is provided. Usually conducted during a hospital confinement to determine the appropriateness of hospital confinement and the medical necessity for continued stay. *See also* Utilization Review.

Confidentiality: The protection of individually identifiable information as required by state or federal law or by policy of the health care provider.

Consolidated Omnibus Budget Reconciliation Act (COBRA): Federal law that continues health care benefits for employees whose employment has been terminated. Employers are required to notify employees of these benefit continuation options, and failure to do so can result in penalties and fines for the employer. An act that allows workers and their families to continue their employer-sponsored health insurance for a certain amount of time after terminating employment. COBRA imposes different restrictions on individuals who leave their jobs voluntarily versus involuntarily (Department of Labor, 2002).

Consumer Health Alliance: Regional cooperatives between government and the public that will oversee the new payment system. Once all health insurance purchasing cooperatives (HIPPCs), the alliance would make sure health plans within a region conformed to federal coverage and quality standards, and oversee costs within any mandated budget.

Contingent Liability: Liability of individuals, corporations, or partnerships for accidents caused by people other than employees for whose acts or omissions the corporations or partnerships are responsible.

Continued Stay Review: A review conducted by an internal or external auditor to determine if the current place of service is still the most appropriate to provide the level of care required by the client.

Continuous Quality Improvement (CQI): An approach to health care quality management borrowed from the manufacturing sector. It builds on traditional quality assurance methods by putting in place a management structure that continuously gathers and assesses data that are then used to improve performance and design more efficient systems of care. Also known as quality improvement (QA) and total quality management (TQM).

Contract: A legal agreement between a payer and a subscribing group or individual which specifies rates, performance covenants, the relationship among the parties, schedule of benefits, and other pertinent conditions. The contract usually is limited to a 12-month period and is subject to renewal thereafter. Contracts are not required by statute or regulation, and less formal agreements may be made.

Contract Provider: Any hospital, physician, skilled nursing facility, extended care facility, individual, organization, or licensed agency that has a contractual arrangement with an insurer for the provision of services under an insurance contract.

Contract Year: A period of 12 consecutive months, commencing with each anniversary date. May or may not coincide with a calendar year.

Contributory Program: Program where the employee and the employer or the union shares the cost of group coverage.

Conversion: In group health insurance, the opportunity given the insured and any covered dependents to change his or her group insurance to some form of individual insurance, without medical evaluation, upon termination of his group insurance.

Conversion Factor (CF): The dollar amount used to multiply the relative value schedule (RVS) of a procedure to arrive at the maximum allowable for that procedure.

Conversion Factor Update: Annual percentage change to a conversion factor either set annually by the government or by the formula reflecting actual expenditure growth from two years falling below or above the original target rate. See Conversion Factor.

Conversion Privilege: The right of an individual insured under a group policy to certain kinds of individual coverage, without a medical examination, upon termination of his association with the group.

Coordination of Benefits (COB): Provision regulating payments to eliminate duplicate coverage when a claimant is covered by multiple group plans. The procedures set forth in a subscription agreement to determine which coverage is primary for payment of benefits to members with duplicate coverage. A coordination of benefits, or "nonduplication," clause in either policy prevents double payment by making one insurer the primary payer, and assuring that not more than 100% of the cost is covered. Standard rules determine which of two or more plans, each having COB provisions, pays its benefits in full and which becomes the supplementary payer on a claim. Also called cross-over.

Co-Payment, Copayment, Co-Pay: A cost-sharing arrangement in which the HMO enrollee pays a specified flat amount for a specific service (such as $10 for an office visit or $5 for each prescription drug). The amount paid must be nominal to avoid becoming a barrier to care. It does not vary with the cost of the service and is usually a flat sum amount such as $10 for every prescription or doctor visit, unlike coinsurance that is based on a percentage of the cost.

Cost–Benefit Analysis (Evaluation): An analytic method in which a program's cost is compared to the program's benefits for a period of time, expressed in dollars, as an aid in determining the best investment of resources. For example, the cost of establishing an immunization service might be compared with the total cost of medical care and lost productivity that will be eliminated as a result of more persons being immunized. Cost–benefit analysis can also be applied to specific medical tests and treatments.

Cost–Consequence Analysis (CCA): A form of analysis that compares alternative interventions or programs in which the components of incremental costs and consequences are listed without aggregation.

Cost Containment: Control of inefficiencies in the consumption, allocation, or production of health care services that contribute to higher than necessary costs. Inefficiencies are thought to exist in consumption when health services are inappropriately utilized; inefficiencies in allocation exist when health services could be delivered in less costly settings without loss of quality, and inefficiencies in production exist when the costs of producing health services could be reduced by using a different combination of resources. Cost containment is a word used freely in health care to describe most cost reduction activities by providers.

Cost Contract: An arrangement between a managed health care plan and CMS under Section 1876 or 1833 of the Social Security Act, under which the health plan provides health services and is reimbursed its costs. A TEFRA contract payment methodology option by which CMS pays for the delivery of health services to members based on the HMO's or hospital's reasonable cost. The plan or hospital receives an interim amount derived from an estimated annual budget, which may be periodically adjusted during the course of the contract to reflect actual cost experience. The expenses are audited at the end of the contract to determine the final rate the plan or provider should have been paid.

Cost-Effectiveness (Evaluation): The efficacy of a program in achieving given intervention outcomes in relation to the program costs. Follow-up studies, outcome studies, and TQM programs attempt to assess treatment efficacy, while cost-effectiveness would provide a ratio of this measurement with costs. This analysis may determine the costs and effectiveness of certain interventions compared to similar alternative interventions, determining the relative costs and degree to which they will obtain desired health outcomes.

Cost Minimization Analysis (CMA): An assessment of the least costly interventions among available alternatives that produce equivalent outcomes.

Cost of Illness (COI) Analysis: An assessment of the economic impact of an illness or condition, including treatment costs.

Cost Outlier: A case that is more costly to treat compared with other patients in a particular diagnosis-related group. Outliers also refer to any unusual occurrence of cost, cases that skew average costs, or unusual procedures.

Cost Sharing: Payment method where a person is required to pay some health costs in order to receive medical care. The general set of financing arrangements whereby the consumer must pay out-of-pocket to receive care, either at the time of initiating care, or during the provision of health care services, or both. This includes deductibles, coinsurance, and co-payments, but not the share of the premium paid by the person enrolled.

Cost Shifting: Charging one group of patients more in order to make up for underpayment by others. Most commonly, charging some privately insured patients more in order to make up for underpayment by Medicaid or Medicare.

Cost Utility Analysis: A form of effectiveness analysis where outcomes are rated in terms of utility, or quality of life.

Coverage: The guarantee against specific losses provided under the terms of an insurance policy.

Covered Benefit: A medically necessary service that is specifically provided for under the provisions of an evidence of coverage. A covered benefit must always be medically necessary, but not every medically necessary service is a covered benefit. For example, some elements of custodial or maintenance care which are excluded from coverage may be medically necessary, but are not covered.

Covered Entity: Under HIPAA, this is a health plan, a health care clearinghouse, or a health care provider who transmits any health information in electronic form in connection with a HIPAA transaction. For purposes of the HIPAA Privacy Rule, health care providers include hospitals, physicians, and other caregivers, as well as researchers who provide health care and receive, access, or generate individually identifiable health care information.

Covered Services: Services provided within a given health care plan. Health care services provided or authorized by the payer's medical staff or payment for health care services.

CPR: *See* Computer-Based Patient Record OR Customary, Prevailing, and Reasonable

CPT: *See* Current Procedural Terminology

CQI: *See* Continuous Quality Improvement

Credentialing: Review procedure where a potential or existing provider must meet certain standards in order to begin or continue participation in a given health care plan, on a panel, in a group, or in a hospital medical staff organization. The process of reviewing a practitioner's credentials (training, experience, or demonstrated ability) for the purpose of determining if criteria for clinical privileging are met. The recognition of professional or technical competence. The credentialing process may include registration, certification, licensure, professional association membership, or the award of a degree in the field. Certification and licensure affect the supply of health personnel by controlling entry into practice and influence the stability of the labor force by affecting geographic distribution, mobility, and retention of workers. Credentialing also determines the quality of personnel by providing standards for evaluating competence and by defining the scope of functions and how personnel may be used. In managed care arenas, one hears of a new basis for credentialing, referred to as financial credentialing. This refers to an organization's evaluation of a provider based on that provider's ability to provide value, or high-quality care at a reasonable cost.

Current Dental Terminology (CDT): A medical code set of dental procedures, maintained and copyrighted by the American Dental Association (ADA) and adopted by the Secretary of HHS as the standard for reporting dental services on standard transactions.

Current Procedural Terminology (CPT): A standardized mechanism of reporting services using numeric codes as established and updated annually by the AMA. A manual that assigns five-digit codes to medical services and procedures to standardize claims processing and data analysis. The coding system for physicians' services developed by the CPT Editorial Panel of the American Medical Association; basis of the Medicare coding system for physicians' services. A medical code set of physician and other services, maintained and copyrighted by the American Medical Association (AMA) and adopted by the Secretary of HHS as the standard for reporting physician and other services on standard transactions.

Customary Charge: One of the factors determining a physician's payment for a service under Medicare. Calculated as the physician's median charge for that service over a prior 12-month period.

Customary, Prevailing, and Reasonable (CPR): Current method of paying physicians under Medicare. Payment for a service is limited to the lowest of (1) the physician's billed charge for the service, (2) the physician's customary charge for the service, or (3) the prevailing charge for that service in the community. Similar to the usual, customary, and reasonable system used by private insurers.

CWW: *See* Clinic Without Walls

D

Data Aggregation: Combining of sets of protected health information by a business associate to permit data analysis.

Database Management System (DBMS): The separation of data from the computer application that allows entry or editing of data.

Data Condition: A description of the circumstances in which certain data is required.

Data Content: Under HIPAA, this is all the data elements and code sets inherent to a transaction, and not related to the format of the transaction.

Data Mapping: The process of matching one set of data elements or individual code values to their closest equivalents in another set of them. This is sometimes called a cross-walk.

Data Use Agreement (DUA): HIPAA Regulation states that a health care entity may use or disclose a "limited data set" if that entity obtains a data use agreement from the potential recipient and can only be used for research, public health, or health care operations. Relates to privacy rules of HIPAA. A satisfactory assurance between the covered entity and a researcher using a limited data set that the data will only be used for specific uses and disclosures. The data use agreement is required to include the following information: to establish that the data will be used for research, public health, or health care operations (further uses or disclosure are not permitted); to establish who is permitted to use or receive the limited data set; and to provide that the limited data set recipient will (1) not use or further disclose the information other than as permitted by the data use agreement or as required by law, (2) use appropriate safeguards to prevent use or disclosure of the information other than as provided in the agreement, (3) report to the covered entity any identified use or disclosure not provided for in the agreement, (4) ensure that any agents, including a subcontractor, to whom the limited data sets are provided agree to the same restrictions and conditions that apply to the recipient, and (5) not identify the information or contact the individuals.

Day Outlier: A patient with an atypically long length of stay compared with other patients in a particular diagnosis-related group.

Days (or Visits) per Thousand: A standard unit of measurement of utilization. Refers to an annualized use of the hospital or other institutional care. It is the number of hospital days that are used in a year for each thousand covered lives. The formula used to calculate days per thousand is as follows: (# of days/member months) × (1000 members) × (# of months). An indicator calculated by taking the total number of days (for inpatient, residential, or partial hospitalization) or visits (for outpatient) received by a specific group for a specific period of time (usually one year). A measure used to evaluate utilization management performance.

DBMS: *See* Database Management System

DCI: *See* Duplicate Coverage Inquiry

Decedents: Deceased individuals. Afforded privacy rights under the HIPAA Privacy Rule, even though not considered "human subjects" protected under the Common Rule. As is the current practice, all research protocols involving the review of medical records of deceased subjects or of living and deceased subjects require review and approval by the HRC/IRB and can be conducted without informed consent and authorization only if the protocol satisfies the criteria for a waiver. If the research includes access to the records of decedents, the investigator will be asked to document that the decedents will only be used for research and that the information is necessary for the research. The covered entity may require the investigator to provide proof of death.

Decision Support Systems: Computer technologies used in health care that allow providers to collect and analyze data in more sophisticated and complex ways. Activities supported include case mix, budgeting, cost accounting, clinical protocols and pathways, outcomes, and actuarial analysis.

Declaration: Part of a property or liability insurance policy that states the name and address of policyholder, property insured, its location and description, the policy period, premiums, and supplemental information. Referred to as the "dec page."

Deductible: The amount of loss paid by the policyholder. Either a specified dollar amount, a percentage of the claim amount, or a specified amount of time that must elapse before benefits are paid. The bigger the deductible, the lower the premium charged for the same coverage.

Deductible Carryover Credit: Charge incurred during the last 3 months of a year that may be applied to the deductible and which may be carried over into the next year.

Defensive Medicine: Doctors in recent years have admitted to and have been accused of prescribing additional tests or procedures to justify their care, strengthen support for their decisions, or simply to corroborate their diagnosis. This defensiveness is a result of lawsuits, malpractice claims, and the onslaught of external UR entities questioning care decisions. Defensive medicine is said to be one of the primary causes of the increasing cost of health care. Many physicians and the AMA fight for tort reform to reduce the need for defensive medicine. However, patient groups and patient advocates not in favor of tort reform explain that the right to sue for malpractice is a valid method of holding physicians accountable for mistakes made.

Defined Benefit Plan: A retirement plan under which pension benefits are fixed in advance by a formula based generally on years of service to the company multiplied by a specific percentage of wages, usually average earnings over that period or highest average earnings over the final years with the company.

Defined Care: An umbrella term used for defined contribution, consumer-driven and self-directed health plan arrangements and other consumer-centered initiatives.

Defined Contribution Coverage: A payment process for procurement of health benefit plans whereby employers contribute a specific dollar amount toward the costs of insurance coverage for their employees. Sometimes this includes an undefined expectation of guarantee of the specific benefits to be covered.

Defined Contribution Plan: An employee benefit plan under which the employer sets up benefit accounts and contributions are made to it by the employer and by the employee. The employer usually matches the employee's contribution up to a stated limit.

Deidentified: Under the HIPAA Privacy Rule, data are deidentified if either (1) an experienced expert determines that the risk that certain information could be used to identify an individual is "very small" and documents and justifies the determination, or (2) the data do not include any of the following 18 identifiers (of the individual or his/her relatives, household members, or employers) which could be used alone or in combination with other information to identify the subject: names, geographic subdivisions smaller than a state (including zip code), all elements of dates except year (unless the subject is greater than 89 years old), telephone numbers, FAX numbers, e-mail addresses, Social Security numbers, medical record numbers, health plan beneficiary numbers, account numbers, certificate/license numbers, vehicle identifiers including license plates, device identifiers and serial numbers, URLs, internet protocol addresses, biometric identifiers, full-face photos and comparable images, and any unique identifying number, characteristic or code; note that even if these identifiers are removed, the Privacy Rule states that information will be considered identifiable if the covered entity knows that the identity of the person may still be determined.

Department of Health and Human Services (HHS): The federal agency that oversees Medicare, Medicaid, and other federal health care programs.

Department of Justice (DOJ): The federal agency that enforces the law and handles criminal investigations. As the nation's largest law firm, the

DOJ protects citizens through effective law enforcement, crime prevention, and crime detection. It is the agency that prosecutes those in the health care system guilty of proven "fraudulent" activity.

Dependent: Person covered by someone else's health plan. In a payer's policy of insurance, a person other than the subscriber eligible to receive care because of a subscriber's contract.

Designated Mental Health Provider: Person or place authorized by a health plan to provide or suggest appropriate mental health and substance abuse care.

Designated Record Set: A health care provider's medical and billing records about individuals and any records used by the provider to make decisions about individuals. Individuals, including research subjects, have the right under the HIPAA Privacy Rule to access and amend protected health information in a designated record set.

Diagnosis-Related Groups (DRGs): An inpatient or hospital classification system used to pay a hospital or other provider for their services and to categorize illness by diagnosis and treatment. A classification scheme used by Medicare that clusters patients into 468 categories on the basis of patients' illnesses, diseases, and medical problems. Groupings of diagnostic categories are drawn from the International Classification of Diseases and modified by the presence of a surgical procedure, patient age, presence or absence of significant comorbidities or complications, and other relevant criteria. System involving classification of medical cases and payment to hospitals on the basis of diagnosis. Used under Medicare's prospective payment system to reimburse inpatient hospitals, regardless of the cost to the hospital to provide services.

Direct Contracting: Providing health services to members of a health plan by a group of providers contracting directly with an employer, thereby cutting out the middleman or third-party insurance carrier. This can be provider heaven, since the middleman—MCO—is cut out, and the provider gets some portion of the money usually made by it. The key is to price services correctly, since provider is usually at full risk in this situation. It takes a strong IDS, MSO, or AHP to do this successfully.

Directly Identifiable Health Information: Any information that includes personal identifiers. To determine what data may be considered identifiable, please see items that must be removed under the definition of Deidentified.

Direct Payment Subscriber: A person enrolled in a prepayment plan who makes individual premium payments directly to the plan rather than through a group. Rates of payment are generally higher, and benefits may not be as extensive as for the subscriber enrolled and paying as a member of the group.

Direct Sales/Direct Response: Method of selling insurance directly to the insured through an insurance company's own employees, through the mail, or via the Internet. This is in lieu of using captive or exclusive agents.

Direct Writers: Insurance companies that sell directly to the public using exclusive agents or their own employees, through the mail, or via Internet. Large insurers, whether predominately direct writers or agency companies, are increasingly using many different channels to sell insurance. In reinsurance, denotes reinsurers that deal directly with the insurance companies they reinsure without using a broker.

Disallowance: When a payer declines to pay for all or part of a claim submitted for payment.

Discharge Planning: Required by Medicare and JCAHO for all hospital patients. A procedure where aftercare services are determined for after discharge from the inpatient facility.

Disclosure: Refers to the release of identifiable health information regarding a patient or patient(s). Disclosure involves the release of information to anyone or any entity outside of the covered entity.

Discounted Fee-for-Service: A financial reimbursement system whereby a provider agrees to supply services on an FFS basis, but with the fees discounted by a certain percentage from the physician's usual and customary charges. An agreed upon rate for service between the provider and payer that is usually less than the provider's full fee. This may be a fixed amount per service, or a percentage discount. Providers generally accept such contracts because they represent a means to increase their volume or reduce their chances of losing volume.

Disease Management: A type of product or service now being offered by many large pharmaceutical companies to get them into broader health care services. Bundles use of prescription drugs with physician and allied professionals, linked to large databases created by the pharmaceutical companies, to treat people with specific diseases. The claim is that this type of service provides higher quality of care at more reasonable price than alternative, presumably more fragmented, care. The development of such products by hugely capitalized companies should be the entire indicator necessary to convince a provider of how the health care market is changing. Competition is coming from every direction—other providers of all types, payers, employers who are developing their own in-house service systems, the drug companies.

Disproportionate Share (DSH) Adjustment: A payment adjustment under Medicare's PPS for Medicaid utilization at hospitals that serve a relatively large volume of low-income patients, pregnant patients, or other patients under the Medicaid program. Disproportionate share has been a continuing topic in Congress. Some wish to eradicate it to reduce costs. Rural facilities, teaching hospitals, and hospitals in poverty areas claim that the reduction or elimination of disproportionate share payments would cause hospitals to close, move, or reduce care to the poor. DSH is a method whereby the government recognizes that hospitals treating high percentages of Medicaid payments would not be able to cover their costs and remain in service without additional government subsidy.

DME: *See* Durable Medical Equipment

DOJ: *See* Department of Justice

Domestic Insurance Company: Term used by a state to refer to any company incorporated there.

DRGs: *See* Diagnosis-Related Groups

Drug Formulary: Varying lists of prescription drugs approved by a given health plan for distribution to a covered person through specific pharmacies. Health plans often restrict or limit the type and number of medicines allowed for reimbursement by limiting the drug formulary list. The list of prescription drugs for which a particular employer or state Medicaid program will pay. Formularies are either "closed," including only certain drugs, or "open," including all drugs. Both types of formularies typically impose a cost scale requiring consumers to pay more for certain brands or types of drugs.

Drug Risk Sharing Arrangements: Provider organizations may be at partial, full, or no risk for drug costs. Providers at partial risk share in the proportion of savings or cost overruns. Groups at full risk realize all the savings or absorb all of the losses. Groups at no risk absorb none of the profits or losses. These arrangements are normally made between HMOs and providers (doctors/hospitals) in the HMO's attempt to discourage the overuse of drugs that will cause a loss of profit for the HMO. In a shared-risk arrangement, the HMO and provider share the losses and profits, thus aligning their incentives with one another.

Drug Utilization Review (DUR): Review of an insured population's drug utilization with the goal of determining how to reduce the cost of utilization. Reviews often result in recommendations to practitioners, including generic substitutions, use of formularies, use of co-payments for prescriptions, and education. In some cases, practitioners are now penalized or rewarded depending on their drug prescription–related costs and utilization. Some speculate that these incentives can adversely effect doctor decisions.

DSH: *See* Disproportionate Share Adjustment

DUA: *See* Data Use Agreement

Dual Choice (Multiple Choice, Dual Option, DC): Section 1310 of the HMO Act provides for dual choice. A choice given to employees to select between two or more health plans offered by an employer. The opportunity for an individual within an employed group to choose from two or more types of health care coverage such as an HMO and a traditional insurance plan. Many states also have legislated mandates regarding choices offered within employer packages.

Dual Eligible: A Medicare beneficiary who also receives the full range of Medicaid benefits offered in his or her state. Medicare usually pays the charges for inpatient while Medicaid will pay the co-pay for inpatient charges in hospitals. Medicare will be considered the primary insurer for inpatient care for the Care/Caid patient.

Duplicate Coverage Inquiry (DCI): Method used by an insurance company or group medical plan to inquire about the existing coverage of another insurance company or group medical plan.

Duplication of Benefits: When a person is covered under two or more health plans with the same or similar coverage.

DUR: *See* Drug Utilization Review

Durable Medical Equipment (DME): Items of medical equipment owned or rented which are placed in the home of an insured to facilitate treatment and/or rehabilitation. DME generally consist of items that can withstand repeated use. DME is primarily and customarily used to serve a medical purpose and is usually not useful to a person in the absence of illness or injury.

E

EAP: *See* Employee Assistance Program

Early and Periodic Screening, Diagnosis, and Treatment (EPSDT): The EPSDT program covers screening and diagnostic services to determine physical or mental defects in recipients under age 21, as well as health care and other measures to correct or ameliorate any defects and chronic conditions discovered.

ECF: *See* Extended Care Facility

Economic Credentialing: The use of economic criteria unrelated to quality of care or professional competency in determining an individual's qualifications for initial or continuing hospital medical staff membership or privileges. Economic credentialing has become a controversial topic involving much concern about ethics; yet economic credentialing remains the most powerful form of controlling the behavior of doctors. Other forms of control include utilization review, certification, exclusive provider panels, and more.

Economic Loss: Total financial loss resulting from the death or disability of a wage earner or from the destruction of property. Includes the loss of earnings, medical expenses, funeral expenses, the cost of restoring or replacing property, and legal expenses. It does not include noneconomic losses, such as pain caused by an injury.

EDI (Electronic Data Interchange) Translator: Used in electronic claims and medical record transmissions, this is a software tool for accepting an EDI transmission and converting the data into another format, or for converting a non-EDI data file into an EDI format for transmission. *See also* Electronic Data Interchange.

Effective Date: The date on which a policy's coverage of a risk goes into effect.

Electronic Claim: A digital representation of a medical bill generated by a provider or by the provider's billing agent for submission using telecommunications to a health insurance payer. Most claims are electronically submitted.

Electronic Data Interchange (EDI): The automated exchange of data and documents in a standardized format. In health care, some common uses of this technology include claims submission and payment, eligibility, and referral authorization. Refers to the exchange of routine business transactions from one computer to another in a standard format, using standard communications protocols.

Electronic Media Claims: A flat file format used to transmit or transport claims, such as the 192-byte UB-92 Institutional EMC format and the 320-byte Professional EMC NSF.

Electronic Medical Record (EMR): A computer-based record containing health care information. This technology, when fully developed, meets provider needs for real-time data access and evaluation in medical care. Together with clinical workstations and clinical data repository technologies, the EMR provides the mechanism for longitudinal data storage and access. A motivation for health care entities to implement this technology derives from the need for medical outcome studies, more efficient care, speedier communication among providers, and management of health plans. This record may contain some, but not necessarily all, of the information that is in an individual's paper-based medical record. One goal of HIPAA is to protect identifiable health information as the system moves from a paper-based to an electronic medical record system.

Electronic Remittance Advice: Any of several electronic formats for explaining the payments of health care claims.

Eligible Dependent: Person entitled to receive health benefits from someone else's plan.

Eligible Employee: Employee who qualifies to receive benefits.

Eligible Expenses: Charges covered under a health plan.

Eligible Person: Person who meets the qualifications of a health plan contract.

Elimination Period: Most often used to designate the waiting period in a health insurance policy. A kind of deductible or waiting period usually found in disability policies. It is counted in days from the beginning of the illness or injury.

Emergency: Sudden unexpected onset of illness or injury which requires the immediate care and attention of a qualified physician and which, if not treated immediately, would jeopardize or impair the health of the member, as determined by the payer's medical staff. Significant in that emergency may be the only acceptable reason for admission without precertification.

Emergency Center, Emergi-Center: Nonhospital-affiliated health facility that provides short-term care for minor medical emergencies or procedures needing immediate treatment; *also called* urgi-center, urgent center, or freestanding emergency medical service center.

Emergency Medical Treatment and Labor Act (EMTALA): An act pertaining to emergency medical situations. EMTALA requires hospitals to provide emergency treatment to individuals, regardless of insurance status and ability to pay.

Employee Assistance Program (EAP): A service, plan, or set of benefits that are designed for personal or family problems, including mental health, substance abuse, gambling addiction, marital problems, parenting problems, emotional problems, or financial pressures. This is usually a service provided by an employer to the employees, designed to assist employees in getting help for these problems so that they may remain on the job. EAP began with a primary drug and alcohol focus, with an emphasis on rehabilitating valued employees rather than terminating them for their substance problems. It is sometimes implemented with a disciplinary program that requires that the impaired employee participate in EAP in order to retain employment. With the advent of managed care, EAP has sometimes evolved to include case management, utilization review, and gatekeeping functions for the psychiatric and substance abuse health benefits.

Employee Retirement Income Security Act (ERISA) of 1974: Also called the Pension Reform Act, this act regulates the majority of private pension and welfare group benefit plans in the United Sates. It sets forth requirements governing, among many areas, participation, crediting of service, vesting, communication and disclosure, funding, and fiduciary conduct. It is a key legislative battleground now, because ERISA exempts most large self-funded plans from state regulation and, hence, from any reform activities undertaken at state level—which is now the arena for much health care reform.

Employer Mandate: The federal HMO Act describes conditions when federally qualified HMOs can mandate or require an employer to offer at least one federally qualified HMO plan of each type (IPA/network or group/staff). This requirement was sunsetted in 1995.

Employer's Liability: Part B of the workers' compensation policy that provides coverage for lawsuits filed by injured employees who, under certain circumstances, can sue under common law.

EMR: *See* Electronic Medical Record

EMTALA: *See* Emergency Medical Treatment and Labor Act

Encounter: A contact between an individual and the health care system for a health care service or set of services related to one or more medical conditions.

Encounter Data: Data relating to treatment or service rendered by a provider to a patient, regardless of whether the provider was reimbursed on a capitated or fee-for-service basis. Used in determining the level of service.

Enrolled Group: Persons with the same employer or with membership in an organization in common, who are enrolled collectively in a health plan. Often, there are stipulations regarding the minimum size of the group and the minimum percentage of the group that must enroll before the coverage is available. *Also called* Contract Group.

Enrollee (*Also* Beneficiary, Individual, Member): Any person eligible as either a subscriber or a dependent for service in accordance with a contract.

Enrollment: Initial process whereby new individuals apply and are accepted as members of a prepayment plan. The total number of covered persons in a health plan. Also refers to the process by which a health plan enrolls groups and individuals for membership, or the number of enrollees who sign up in any one group.

EOB: *See* Explanation of Benefits

EOC: *See* Evidence or Explanation of Coverage or Explanation of Benefits

E of I: *See* Evidence of Insurability

EPA: *See* Exclusive Provider Arrangement

EPO: *See* Exclusive Provider Organization

Episode of Care: A term used to describe and measure the various health care services and encounters rendered in connection with identified injury or period of illness.

EPSDT: *See* Early and Periodic Screening, Diagnosis, and Treatment

EQRO: *See* External Quality Review Organization

ERISA (Employee Retirement Income Security Act): Federal legislation that protects employees by establishing minimum standards for private pension and welfare plans.

Essential Community Providers: Providers such as community health centers that have traditionally served low-income populations.

Evidence-Based Medicine: Evidence-based health care is the conscientious use of current best evidence in making decisions about the care of individual patients or the delivery of health services. The term is used in quality improvement and peer review programs in hospitals and health plans.

Evidence of Insurability (E of I): Proof of a person's physical condition that affects acceptability for insurance or a health care contract.

Evidence or Explanation of Coverage (EOC) or Explanation of Benefits (EOB): A booklet provided by the carrier to the insured summarizing benefits under an insurance plan.

Excess of Loss Reinsurance: A contract between an insurer and a reinsurer, whereby the insurer agrees to pay a specified portion of a claim, and the reinsurer agrees to pay all or a part of the claim above that amount.

Excess Risk: Either specific or aggregate stop loss coverage.

Excluded Hospitals and Distinct-Part Units: Hospitals and hospital units that are specifically excluded from Medicare's prospective pay system. These commonly include children's, cancer, hospital-based outpatient care, long-term care, rehabilitation inpatient and psychiatric hospitals or units. Rehabilitation or psychiatric units of acute care hospitals are exempt if they meet certain criteria specified by HHS and are referred to as "DRG exempted." Excluded facilities are paid through submission of cost reports and TEFRA limits.

Exclusion: A provision in an insurance policy that eliminates coverage for certain risks, people, property classes, or locations. Conditions or situations not considered covered under contract or plan. Clauses in an insurance contract that deny coverage for select individuals, groups, locations, properties, or risks. Providers will negotiate for exclusions for outliers and carve-out of certain high-cost procedures, while payers will negotiate for exclusions to avoid payment of higher-cost care.

Exclusive Provider Arrangement (EPA): An indemnity or service plan that provides benefits only if care is rendered by the institutional and professional providers with which it contracts (with some exceptions for emergency and out-of-area services).

Exclusive Provider Organization (EPO): A plan that limits coverage of non-emergency care to contracted health care providers. An EPO operates similar to an HMO plan, but is usually offered as an insured or self-funded product. It sometimes looks like a managed care organization that is organized similarly to a PPO in that physicians do not receive capitated payments, but the plan only allows patients to choose medical care from network providers. If a patient elects to seek care outside of the network, then he or she will usually not be reimbursed for the cost of the treatment. An EPO uses a small network of providers and has primary care physicians serving as care coordinators (or gatekeepers). Typically, an EPO has financial incentives for physicians to practice cost-effective medicine by using either a prepaid per capita rate or a discounted fee schedule, plus a bonus if cost targets are met. Most EPOs are forms of POS, plans because they pay for some out-of-network care.

Exclusive Remedy: Part of the social contract that forms the basis for workers' compensation statutes under which employers are responsible for work-related injury and disease, regardless of whether it was the employee's fault, and in return the injured employee gives up the right to sue when the employer's negligence causes the harm.

Exclusivity Clause: A part of a contract which prohibits physicians, providers, or other care entities from contracting with more than one managed care organization. Exclusive contracts are common in staff-model HMOs and IPAs but becoming less common in other health plan contracting.

Expansion: Some HMOs compute plan expansion as part of the capitation rate in order to provide the necessary capital for growth.

Expense Ratio: Percentage of each premium dollar that goes to insurers' expenses including overhead, marketing, and commissions.

Experience: A term used to describe the relationship of premium to claims for a plan, coverage, or benefits for a stated time period. It is usually expressed as a ratio or percent.

Experience-Rated Premium: A premium which is based upon the anticipated claims experience of, or utilization of service by, a contract group according to its age, sex, constitution, and any other attributes expected to affect its health service utilization, and which is subject to periodic adjustment in line with actual claims or utilization experience.

Experience Rating: The process of setting rates partially or in whole on evaluating previous claims experience for a specific group or pool of groups.

The rating system by which the plan determines the capitation rate or premium rate is determined by the experience of the individual group enrolled, based on actual or anticipated health care use by the specific group of insureds. Each group will have a different rate based on utilization. This system tends to penalize small groups with high utilization. A method of adjusting health plan premiums based on the historical utilization data and distinguishing characteristics of a specific subscriber group, such as determining the premium based on a group's claims experience, age, sex or health status. Experience rating is not allowed for federally qualified HMOs.

Explanation of Benefits (EOB): A statement sent to covered individuals explaining services provided, amount to be billed, and payments made. A summary of benefits provided subscribers by the carrier.

Exposure: Possibility of loss.

Extended Care Facility (ECF): A nursing or convalescent home offering skilled nursing care and rehabilitation services on a 24-hour basis.

Extension of Benefits: Insurance policy provision that allows medical coverage to continue past termination of employments.

External Quality Review Organization (EQRO): States are required to contract with an entity that is external to and independent of the state and its HMO and HIO contractors to perform an annual review of the quality of services furnished by each HMO or HIO contractor.

F

Favorable Selection: Selection of subscribers or covered lives based on data that shows a tendency for utilization of health services in that population group to be lower than expected or estimated.

Federal Bureau of Investigation (FBI): As an agency under the DOJ, the FBI investigates violations of federal criminal law and provides law enforcement assistance to federal, state, local, and international agencies. The FBI has investigated hospitals for fraud and abuse.

Federally Qualified Health Center (FQHC): A federal payment option that enables qualified providers in medically underserved areas to receive cost-based Medicare and Medicaid reimbursement and allows for the direct reimbursement of nurse practitioners, physician assistants, and certified nurse midwives. Many outpatient clinics and specialty outreach services are qualified under this provision that was enacted in 1989.

Federally Qualified HMO: A prepaid health plan that has met strict federal standards and has been granted qualification status. A federally qualified

HMO is eligible for loans and loan guarantees not available to non-qualified plans. Employers of 25 or more workers were, until recently, required to offer a federally qualified HMO if the plan requested to be included in the company's health benefits program.

Federal Medicaid Managed Care Waiver Program: The process used by states to receive permission to implement managed care programs for their Medicaid or other categorically eligible beneficiaries.

Federal Qualification: A status designated by CMS after conducting an extensive evaluation of an HMO's organization and operations. An organization must be federally qualified or be designated as a competitive medical plan (CMP) to be eligible to participate in Medicare and cost and risk contracts. Federal designation that allows an organization to participate in certain Medicare cost and risk contracts.

Fee Disclosure: Physicians and caregivers discussing their charges with patients prior to treatment.

Fee-for-Service (FFS): Traditional method of payment for health care services, where specific payment is made for specific services rendered. Usually people speak of this in contrast to capitation, DRG, or per diem discounted rates, none of which are similar to the traditional fee-for-service method of reimbursement. Under a fee-for-service payment system, expenditures increase if the fees themselves increase, if more units of service are provided, or if more expensive services are substituted for less expensive ones. This system contrasts with salary, per capita, or other prepayment systems, where the payment to the physician is not changed with the number of services actually used. Payment may be made by an insurance company, the patient, or a government program such as Medicare or Medicaid. With respect to the physicians or other suppliers of service, this refers to payment in specific amounts for specific services rendered—as opposed to retainer, salary, or other contract arrangements. In relation to the patient, it refers to payment in specific amounts for specific services received, in contrast to the advance payment of an insurance premium or membership fee for coverage, through which the services or payment to the supplier are provided.

Fee Schedule: A listing of accepted fees or established allowances for specified medical procedures. As used in medical care plans, it usually represents the maximum amounts the program will pay for the specified procedures.

FFS: *See* Fee-for-Service

Fiduciary: Relating to, or founded upon, a trust or confidence. A legal term. A fiduciary relationship exists where an individual or organization has an explicit or implicit obligation to act in behalf of another person's or organization's interests in matters which affect the other person or organization. This fiduciary is also obligated to act in the other person's best interest with total disregard for any interests of the fiduciary. Traditionally, it was generally believed that a physician had a fiduciary relationship with patients. This is being questioned in the era of managed care as the public becomes aware of the other influences that are effecting physician decisions. Doctors are provided incentives by managed care companies to provide less care, by pharmaceutical companies to order certain drugs, and by hospitals to refer to their hospitals. With the pervasive monetary incentives influencing doctor decisions, consumer advocates are concerned because the patient no longer has an unencumbered fiduciary.

Fiduciary Bond: A type of surety bond, sometimes called a probate bond, which is required of certain fiduciaries, such as executors and trustees, that guarantees the performance of their responsibilities.

Fiduciary Liability: Legal responsibility of a fiduciary to safeguard assets of beneficiaries. A fiduciary, for example a pension fund manager, is required to manage investments held in trust in the best interest of beneficiaries. Fiduciary liability insurance covers breaches of fiduciary duty such as misstatements or misleading statements, errors, and omissions.

File-and-Use States: States where insurers must file rate changes with their regulators, but do not have to wait for approval to put them into effect.

Financial Responsibility Law: A state law requiring that all automobile drivers show proof that they can pay damages up to a minimum amount if involved in an auto accident. Varies from state to state, but can be met by carrying a minimum amount of auto liability insurance.

First-Dollar Coverage: Insurance coverage with no front-end deductible, where coverage begins with the first dollar of expense incurred by the insured for any covered benefit.

First-Party Coverage: Coverage for the policyholder's own property or person. In no-fault auto insurance, it pays for the cost of injuries. In no-fault states with the broadest coverage, the personal injury protection (PIP) part of the policy pays for medical care, lost income, funeral expenses, and where the injured person is not able to provide services such as child care, for substitute services.

Fiscal Intermediary: The agent (e.g., Blue Cross) that has contracted with providers of service to process claims for reimbursement under health care coverage. In addition to handling financial matters, it may perform other functions such as providing consultative services or serving as a center for communication with providers and making audits of providers' needs. This entity may also be referred to as TPA or third-party administrator. A private organization, usually an insurance company, that serves as an agent for the Health Care Financing Administration (CMS), which is part of HHS, that determines the amount of payment due to hospitals and other providers and pays them for the Medicare services they have provided. Intermediaries make initial coverage determinations and handle the early stages of beneficiary appeals.

Fiscal Soundness: The requirement that managed care organizations have sufficient operating funds, on hand or available in reserve, to cover all expenses associated with services for which they have assumed financial risk.

Fixed Costs: Costs that do not change with fluctuations in census or in utilization of services.

Flat Fee-per-Case: Flat fee paid for a client's treatment based on their diagnosis and/or presenting problem. For this fee the provider covers all of the services the client requires for a specific period of time. This method often characterizes "second generation" managed care systems. After the MCOs squeeze out costs by discounting fees, they often come to this method. If a provider is still standing after discount blitz, this approach can be good for provider and clients, since it permits a lot of flexibility for provider in meeting client needs. DRGs are an example of flat fees paid by diagnosis.

Flexible Benefit Plan: Program offered by some employers in which employees may choose among a number of health care benefit options.

Flexible Spending Account (FSA): A plan that provides employees a choice between taxable cash and nontaxable benefits for unreimbursed health care expenses or dependent care expenses. This plan qualifies under Section 125 of the IRS Code.

Formatting and Protocol Standards: Data exchange standards which are needed between CPR systems, as well as CPT and other provider systems, to ensure uniformity in methods for data collection, data storage, and data presentation. Proactive providers are current in their knowledge of these standards and work to ensure their information systems conform to the standards.

Formulary: An approved list of prescription drugs; a list of selected pharmaceuticals and their appropriate dosages felt to be the most useful and cost-effective for patient care. Organizations often develop a formulary under the aegis of a pharmacy and therapeutics committee. In HMOs, physicians are often required to prescribe from the formulary.

FQHC: *See* Federally Qualified Health Center

Fraud:

1. Intentional misrepresentations that can result in criminal prosecution, civil liability, and administrative sanctions.
2. Intentional lying or concealment by policyholders to obtain payment of an insurance claim that would otherwise not be paid, or lying or misrepresentation by the insurance company managers, employees, agents, and brokers for financial gain.

Freedom of Choice: A principle of Medicaid that allows a recipient the freedom to choose among participating Medicaid providers. This term is also used by indemnity plans to indicate that subscribers may use the providers of their choice.

Free-Look Period: A period of up to one month during which the purchaser of an annuity can cancel the contract with no penalty. Rules vary by state.

Frequency: Number of times a loss occurs. One of the criteria used in calculating premium rates.

Fronting: A procedure in which a primary insurer acts as the insurer of record by issuing a policy, but then passes the entire risk to a reinsurer in exchange for a commission. Often, the fronting insurer is licensed to do business in a state or country where the risk is located, but the reinsurer is not. The reinsurer in this scenario is often a captive or an independent insurance company that cannot sell insurance directly in a particular country.

FSA: *See* Flexible Spending Account

Functional Health Status: Refers to a patient's ability to perform typical daily physical and social/role functions, plus other measures of self-perceived health status such as well-being, vitality, and mental health.

Funding Level: Amount of revenue required to finance a medical care program.

Funding Method: System for employers to pay for a health benefit plan. Most common methods are prospective and/or retrospective premium payment, shared risk arrangement, self-funded, or refunding products.

G

GAAP/Generally Accepted Accounting Principles: Used in financial statements that publicly held companies prepare for the Securities and Exchange Commission.

Gag Clause: A provision of a contract between a managed care organization and a health care provider that restricts the amount of information a provider may share with a beneficiary or that limits the circumstances under which a provider may recommend a specific treatment option.

Gatekeeper: A primary care physician, utilization review, case management, local agency, or managed care entity responsible for determining when and what services a patient can access and receive reimbursement for. An arrangement in which a primary care provider serves as the patient's agent, arranges for and coordinates appropriate medical care and other necessary and appropriate referrals. A PCP is involved in overseeing and coordinating all aspects of a patient's medical care. In order for a patient to receive a specialty care referral or hospital admission, the PCP must preauthorize the visit, unless there is an emergency. The term gatekeeper is also used in health care business to describe anyone (EAP, employer-based case manager, UR entity, etc.) that makes the decision of where a patient will receive services.

Gatekeeping: The process by which a primary care physician directly provides primary care and coordinates all diagnostic testing and specialty referrals required for a patient's medical care. Referrals and procedures usually are preauthorized by gatekeepers except in cases of emergency care.

Generally Accepted Accounting Principles (GAAP): Generally accepted accounting principles (GAAP) accounting is used in financial statements that publicly held companies prepare for the Securities and Exchange Commission.

Genetics: The study of how particular traits are passed from parents to children. Identifiable genetic information receives the same level of protection as other health care information under the HIPAA Privacy Rule. Of note for genetic researchers, the rule defines "identifiable" information to include information from the individual as well as relatives. Thus researchers considering whether to deidentify data should review the definition of deidentified information closely.

Global Budgeting: Limits placed on categories of health spending. A method of hospital cost containment in which participating hospitals must share a prospectively set budget. Method for allocating funds among hospitals may vary, but the key is that the participating hospitals agree to an aggregate cap on revenues that they will receive each year. Global budgeting may also be mandated under a universal health insurance system.

Global Fee: A total charge for a specific set of services, such as obstetrical services that encompass prenatal, delivery, and postnatal care. Managed care organizations will often seek contracts with hospitals that contain set global fees for certain sets of services. Outliers and carve-outs will be those services not included in the global negotiated rates.

GPWW: *See* Group Practice Without Walls

Grace Period: Period past the due date of a premium during which coverage may not be cancelled.

Gramm-Leach-Bliley Act: Financial services legislation, passed by Congress in 1999, that removed Depression-era prohibitions against the combination of commercial banking and investment banking activities. It allows insurance companies, banks, and securities firms to engage in each others' activities and own one another.

Grievance Procedures: The process by which an insured can air complaints and seek remedies.

Gross Charges per 1000: An indicator calculated by taking the gross charges incurred by a specific group for a specific period of time, dividing it by the average number of covered members or lives in that group during the same period, and multiplying the result by 1000. This is calculated in the aggregate and by modality of treatment (e.g., inpatient, residential, partial hospitalization, and outpatient). A measure used to evaluate utilization management performance.

Gross Costs per 1000: An indicator calculated by taking the gross costs incurred for services received by a specific group for a specific period of time, dividing it by the average number of covered members or lives in that group during the same period, and multiplying the result by 1000. This is calculated in the aggregate and by modality of treatment (e.g., inpatient, residential, partial hospitalization, and outpatient). A measure used to evaluate utilization management performance. This is the key concept for the provider. What matters is our cost and, in managed care, we must control this indicator and make sure it is below our collections per 1000.

Group Insurance: A single policy covering a group of individuals, usually employees of the same company or members of the same association and their dependents. Coverage occurs under a master policy issued to the employer or association. Any insurance policy or health services contract by which groups of employees (and often their dependents) are covered under a single policy or contract, issued by their employer or other group entity.

Group Model HMO, Group Network HMO: An HMO that contracts with one or more independent group practices to provide services to its members in one or more locations. Health care plan involving contracts with physicians organized as a partnership, professional corporation, or other legal association. It can also refer to an HMO model in which the HMO contracts with one or more medical groups to provide services to members. In either case, the payer or health plan pays the medical group, which, in turn, is responsible for compensating physicians. The medical group may also be responsible for paying or contracting with hospitals and other providers.

Group Practice: A group of persons licensed to practice medicine in the state, who, as their principal professional activity, and as a group responsibility, engage or undertake to engage in the coordinated practice of their profession primarily in one or more group practice facilities, and who in their connection share common overhead expenses if and to the extent such expenses are paid by members of the group, medical and other records, and substantial portions of the equipment and the professional, technical, and administrative staffs. Group practices use the acronyms PA, IPA, MSO, and others. Group practices are far more common now than a decade ago, because physicians seek to lower costs, increase contracting power, and share payer contracts.

Group Practice Without Walls (GPWW): Similar to an independent practice association, this type of physician group represents a legal and formal entity where certain services are provided to each physician by the entity, and the physician continues to practice in his/her own facility. It can include marketing, billing and collection, staffing, management, and the like. *Also called* Clinic Without Walls.

Guaranteed Eligibility: A defined period of time (3 to 6 months) that all patients enrolled in prepaid health programs are considered eligible for Medicaid, regardless of their actual eligibility for Medicaid. A state may apply to HCFA for a waiver to incorporate this into their contracts.

Guaranteed Issue: Requirement that health plans offer coverage to all businesses during some period each year.

Guaranty Fund: The mechanism by which solvent insurers ensure that some of the policyholder and third-party claims against insurance companies that fail are paid. Such funds are required in all 50 states, the District of Columbia, and Puerto Rico, but the type and amount of claim covered by the fund varies from state to state. Some states pay policyholders' unearned premiums—the portion of the premium for which no coverage was provided because the company was insolvent. Some have deductibles. Most states have no limits on workers' compensation payments. Guaranty funds are supported by assessments on insurers doing business in the state.

H

HCFA 1500: The Health Care Financing Administration's standard form for submitting provider service claims to third-party companies or insurance carriers. HCFA is now called CMS, *see* CMS.

Health: The state of complete physical, mental, and social well-being and not merely the absence of disease or infirmity. It is recognized, however, that health has many dimensions (anatomical, physiological, and mental) and is largely culturally defined. The relative importance of various disabilities will differ depending upon the cultural milieu and the role of the affected individual in that culture. Most attempts at measurement have been assessed in terms or morbidity and mortality.

Health and Human Services (HHS): The Department of Health and Human Services that is responsible for health-related programs and issues. Formerly HEW, the Department of Health, Education, and Welfare. The Office of Health Maintenance Organizations (OHMO) is part of HHS, and detailed information on most companies is available here through the Freedom of Information Act.

Health Benefits Package: The services and products a health plan offers.

Health Care, Healthcare: Care, services, and supplies related to the health of an individual. Health care includes preventive, diagnostic, therapeutic, rehabilitative, maintenance, or palliative care, and counseling, among other services. Health care also includes the sale and dispensing of prescription drugs or devices.

Health Care Clearinghouse: A public or private entity that does either of the following (entities, including but not limited to, billing services, repricing companies, community health management information systems or community health information systems, and "value-added" networks and switches, are health care clearinghouses if they perform these functions): (1) processes or facilitates the processing of information received from another entity in a nonstandard format or containing nonstandard data content into standard data elements or a standard transaction; (2) receives a standard transaction from another entity and processes or facilitates the processing of information into nonstandard format or nonstandard data content for a receiving entity. This term is used in the HIPAA rules.

Health Care Financing Administration (HCFA): The federal government agency within the Department of Health and Human Services which directs and oversees the Medicare and Medicaid programs (Titles XVIII and XIX of the Social Security Act) and conducts research to support those programs. It is now called CMS, and generally it oversees the states' administrations of Medicaid, while directly administering Medicare.

Health Care Operations: Institutional activities that are necessary to maintain and monitor the operations of the institution. Examples include but are not limited to conducting quality assessment and improvement activities; developing clinical guidelines; case management; reviewing the competence or qualifications of health care professionals; education and training of students, trainees, and practitioners; fraud and abuse programs; business planning and management; and customer service. Under the HIPAA Privacy Rule, these are allowable uses and disclosures of identifiable information "without specific authorization." Research is not considered part of health care operations.

Health Care Provider: Providers of medical or health care or researchers who provide health care are health care providers. Normally health care providers are clinics, hospitals, doctors, dentists, psychologists, and similar professionals.

Healthcare Provider Taxonomy Codes: An administrative code set that classifies health care providers by type and area of specialization. The code set will be used in certain adopted transactions. (Note: A given provider may have more than one Healthcare Provider Taxonomy Code.)

Health Employer Data and Information Set (HEDIS): A set of HMO performance measures that are maintained by the National Committee for Quality Assurance. HEDIS data is collected annually and provides an informational resource for the public on issues of health plan quality. (*See also* Health Plan Employer Data and Information Set.)

Health Information: Information in any form (oral, written, or otherwise) that relates to the past, present, or future physical or mental health of an individual. That information could be created or received by a health care provider, a health plan, a public health authority, an employer, a life insurer, a school, a university, or a health care clearinghouse. All health information is protected by state and federal confidentiality laws and by HIPAA privacy rules.

Health Insurance: Financial protection against the health care costs of the insured person. May be obtained in a group or individual policy.

Health Insurance Portability and Accountability Act of 1996 (HIPAA): A federal law that allows persons to qualify immediately for comparable health insurance coverage when they change their employment relationships. This legislation sets a precedent for federal involvement in insurance regulation. It sets minimum standards for regulation of the small group insurance market and for a set group in the individual insurance market in the area of portability and availability of health insurance. As a result of this law, hospitals, doctors, and insurance companies are now required to share patient medical records and personal information on a wider basis. This wide-based sharing of medical records has led to privacy rules, greater computerization of records, and consumer concerns about confidentiality. In addition, HIPAA required the creation of a federal law to protect personally identifiable health information; if that did not occur by a specific date (which it did not), HIPAA directed the

Department of Health and Human Services (DHHS) to issue federal regulations with the same purpose. DHHS has issued HIPAA privacy regulations (the HIPAA Privacy Rule) as well as other regulations under HIPAA. HIPAA gives HHS the authority to mandate the use of standards for the electronic exchange of health care data; to specify what medical and administrative code sets should be used within those standards; to require the use of national identification systems for health care patients, providers, payers (or plans), and employers (or sponsors); and to specify the types of measures required to protect the security and privacy of personally identifiable health care information. Also known as the Kennedy–Kassebaum Bill, the Kassebaum–Kennedy Bill, K2, or Public Law 104-191.

Health Insurance Purchasing Cooperatives (HIPC): Public or private organizations that secure health insurance coverage for the workers of all member employers. The goal of these organizations is to consolidate purchasing responsibilities to obtain greater bargaining clout with health insurers, plans, and providers, to reduce the administrative costs of buying, selling, and managing insurance policies. Private cooperatives are usually voluntary associations of employers in a similar geographic region who band together to purchase insurance for their employees. Public cooperatives are established by state governments to purchase insurance for public employees, Medicaid beneficiaries, and other designated populations.

Health Level Seven (HL7): A data interchange protocol for health care computer applications that simplifies the ability of different vendor-supplied IS systems to interconnect. Although not a software program in itself, HL7 requires that each health care software vendor program HL7 interfaces for its products.

Health Maintenance Organization (HMO): HMOs offer prepaid, comprehensive health coverage for both hospital and physician services. The HMO is paid monthly premiums or capitated rates by the payers, which include employers, insurance companies, government agencies, and other groups representing covered lives. The HMO must meet the specifications of the federal HMO act as well as meeting many rules and regulations required at the state level. There are four basic models: group model, individual practice association, network model, and staff model. An HMO contracts with health care providers (e.g., physicians, hospitals, and other health professionals). The members of an HMO are required to use participating or approved providers for all health services, and generally all services will need to meet further approval by the HMO through its utilization program. Members are enrolled for a specified period of time. An HMO may turn around and subcapitate to other groups. For example, it may carve-out certain benefit categories, such as mental health, and subcapitate these to a mental health HMO. Or the HMO may subcapitate to a provider, provider group, or provider network. HMOs are the most restrictive form of managed care benefit plans, because they restrict the procedures, providers, and benefits.

Health Manpower Shortage Area (HMSA): An area or group that the U.S. Department of Health and Human Services designates as having an inadequate supply of health care providers. HMSAs can include (1) an urban or rural geographic area, (2) a population group for which access barriers can be demonstrated to prevent members of the group from using local providers, or (3) medium- and maximum-security correctional institutions and public or nonprofit private residential facilities.

Health Oversight Agency: Under HIPAA rules, this refers to a person or entity at any level of the federal, state, local, or tribal government that oversees the health care system or requires health information to determine eligibility or compliance or to enforce civil rights laws.

Health Plan: An entity that assumes the risk of paying for medical treatments (i.e., uninsured patient, self-insured employer, payer, or HMO).

Health Plan Employer Data and Information Set (HEDIS): A set of performance measures designed to standardize the way health plans report data to employers. HEDIS currently measures five major areas of health plan performance: quality, access and patient satisfaction, membership and utilization, finance, and descriptive information on health plan management. HEDIS was initially developed in 1991 by the National Committee for Quality Assurance.

Health Professional Shortage Area (HPSA): A geographic area, population group, or medical facility that HHS determines to be served by too few health professionals of particular specialties. Physicians who provide services in HPSAs qualify for the Medicare bonus payments. This may also include repayment of medical school loans or other incentives. These reports are published annually by HHS and can be of assistance to providers or groups wishing to recruit physicians to particular areas.

Health Resources and Services Administration (HRSA): HRSA is a component of the U.S. Department of Health and Human Services. Included in HRSA responsibilities is administration of the Ryan White Care funds with a budget of about $1 billion/year to support a continuum of care services for persons with HIV infection.

Health Service Agreement (HSA): Detailed explanation of procedures and benefits provided to an employer by a health plan.

Health Status: The state of health of a specified individual, group, or population. It may be measured by obtaining proxies such as people's subjective assessments of their health; by one or more indicators of mortality and morbidity in the population, such as longevity or maternal and infant mortality; or by using the incidence or prevalence of major diseases (communicable, chronic, or nutritional). Conceptually, health status is the proper outcome measure for the effectiveness of a specific population's medical care system, although attempts to relate effects of available medical care to variations in health status have proved difficult.

HEDIS: *See* Health Plan Employer Data and Information Set or Health Employer Data and Information Set

HHS: *See* Department of Health and Human Services or Health and Human Services

HIPAA: *See* Health Insurance Portability and Accountability Act of 1996

HIPC: *See* Health Insurance Purchasing Cooperatives

HL7: *See* Health Level Seven

HMO: *See* Health Maintenance Organization

HMSA: *See* Health Manpower Shortage Area

Hold Harmless Clause: A clause frequently found in managed care contracts whereby the HMO and the physician hold each other not liable for malpractice or corporate malfeasance if either of the parties is found to be liable. Many insurance carriers exclude this type of liability from coverage. It may also refer to language that prohibits the provider from billing patients if their managed care company becomes insolvent. State and federal regulations may require this language.

Home Health Care: Full range of medical and other health related services such as physical therapy, nursing, counseling, and social services that are delivered in the home of a patient by a provider.

Horizontal Integration, Horizontal Consolidation: Merging of two or more firms at the same level of production in some formal, legal relationship. In hospital networks, this may refer to the grouping of several hospitals, the grouping of outpatient clinics with the hospital, or a geographic network of various health care services. Integrated systems seek to integrate both vertically with some organizations and horizontally with others. When local health plans (or local hospitals) merge. This practice was popular in the late 1990s and was used to expand regional business presence. *See* Vertical Integration.

Hospice: Facility or program providing care for the terminally ill.

Hospital: Any institution duly licensed, certified, and operated as a hospital. In no event shall the term "hospital" include a convalescent facility, nursing home, or any institution or part thereof which is used principally as a convalescence facility, rest facility, nursing facility, or facility for the aged.

Hospital Affiliation: A contractual agreement between a health plan and one or more hospitals whereby the hospital provides the inpatient services offered by the health plan.

Hospital Alliances: Groups of hospitals joined together to share services and develop group-purchasing programs to reduce costs. May also refer to a spectrum of contracts, agreements, or handshake arrangements for hospitals to work together in developing programs, serving covered lives or contracting with payers or health plans. *See also* Network, Integrated Delivery System, or PHO.

Hospital Audit Companies: Retrospective audit providers that typically achieve a 15% to 20% savings of billed claims.

Hospital Days (per 1000): A measurement of the number of days of hospital care HMO members use in a year. It is calculated as follows: total number of days spent in a hospital by members divided by total members. This information is available through HHS, OHMO, and a variety of sources.

HPSA: *See* Health Professional Shortage Area

HRSA: *See* Health Resources and Service Administration

HSA: *See* Health Service Agreement

Human Subject: Under HIPAA rules, this term refers to a living subject participating in research about whom directly or indirectly identifiable health information or data are obtained or created.

I

IBNR: *See* Incurred But Not Reported Losses

ICD-9-CM: *See* International Classification of Diseases, Ninth Revision, Clinical Modification

IDS: *See* Integrated Delivery System

Incentives: Profit sharing arrangements offered by HMOs and managed care plans that permit hospitals, providers, subcontractors, and physicians to share in amounts earned from plan savings through reduced hospital and specialty referral usage. Normally, clinicians involved in profit sharing will increase personal income or profit by reducing the quantity of care, supplies, or services provided to patients. Consumers sometimes view these incentives as suspect, claiming profit sharing between health plans and providers results in reduction of quality of service. Federal fraud and abuse rules may affect the types of incentive plans that health centers and physicians may enter into. Managed care plans view incentives as necessary methods to align the physicians' (and sometimes hospitals') incentives with the incentives of the managed care plans.

Incidence: In epidemiology, the number of cases of disease, infection, or some other event having their onset during a prescribed period of time in relation to the unit of population in which they occur. Incidence measures morbidity or other events as they happen over a period of time. Examples include the number of accidents occurring in a manufacturing plant during a year in relation to the number of employees in the plant, or the number of cases of mumps occurring in a school during a month in relation to the number of pupils enrolled in the school. It usually refers only to the number of new cases, particularly of chronic diseases. Hospitals also track certain risk management or quality problems with a system called incidence reporting.

Incurred But Not Reported Losses (IBNR): Losses that are not filed with the insurer or reinsurer until years after the policy is sold. Some liability claims may be filed long after the event that caused the injury to occur. Asbestos-related diseases, for example, do not show up until decades after the exposure. IBNR also refers to estimates made about claims already reported, but where the full extent of the injury is not yet known, such as a workers' compensation claim where the degree to which work-related injuries prevents a worker from earning what he or she earned before the injury unfolds over time. Insurance companies regularly adjust reserves for such losses as new information becomes available.

Incurred Claims: All claims with dates of service within a specified period.

Incurred Claims Loss Ratio: Incurred claims divided by premiums.

Incurred Losses: Losses occurring within a fixed period, whether or not adjusted or paid during the same period.

Indemnify: To make good a loss through compensation or reimbursement. "To make whole."

Indemnity: Health insurance benefits provided in the form of cash payments rather than services. Insurance program in which the covered person is reimbursed for covered expenses. An indemnity insurance contract usually defines the maximum amounts that will be paid for covered services. Indemnity insurance plans may have a PPO option, UR and case management features, or include a network or other preferred provider restrictions, but will not have an HMO plan. Indemnity is the traditional form of insurance. Normally when one thinks of indemnity health coverage, one is thinking of the type of plan that does not require "precertification" and does not restrict the physicians, drugs, or hospitals that will be paid for. Indemnity coverage usually has higher premiums. Indemnity insurance plans are the classic plans—where few restrictions are in place. With these plans, members are normally able to use the providers of their choice and are able to make independent decisions about the type of care they wish to receive. Usually these plans include co-payments, deductibles, and maximums, but rarely require case management certification or approvals. Managed care, particularly HMO and capitation, has evolved away from the indemnity method. Yet, many people are still covered under indemnity plans.

Indemnity Carrier: Usually an insurance company or insurance group that provides marketing, management, claims payment, and review, and agrees to assume risk for its subscribers at some predetermined rate.

Indemnity Plan (Indemnity Health Insurance): A plan that reimburses physicians for services performed, or beneficiaries for medical expenses incurred. Such plans are contrasted with group health plans, which provide service benefits through group medical practice.

Independent Practice Association (IPA) or Organization (IPO): A delivery model in which the HMO contracts with a physician organization, which in turn contracts with individual physicians. The IPA physicians practice in their own offices and continue to also see their FFS patients. The HMO reimburses the IPA on a capitated basis; however, the IPA may reimburse the physicians on an FFS or capitated basis.

Indirectly Identifiable Health Information: Data that do not include personal identifiers, but link the identifying information to the data through use of a code. These data are still considered identifiable by the HIPAA Common Rule.

Individually Identifiable Health Information: A term used in health care to describe a subset of health information that identifies the individual or can reasonably be used to identify the individual. State and federal confidentiality laws as well as HIPAA have standards and rules regarding the protection of individually identifiable health information of patients.

Individual Plans: A type of insurance plan for individuals and their dependents who are not eligible for coverage through employer group coverage.

Individual (Independent) Practice Association (IPA): An organized form of prepaid medical practice in which participating physicians remain in their independent office settings, seeing both enrollees of the IPA and private-pay patients. Participating physicians may be reimbursed by the IPA on a fee-for-service basis or a capitation basis. Sometimes thought of as an HMO model in which the HMO contracts with a physician organization that in turn contracts with individual physicians. The IPA physicians provide care to HMO members from their private offices and continue to see their fee-for-service patients.

Informed Consent: Refers to requirements (by HIPPA, Medicare, state, and federal laws) that health care providers and researchers explain the purposes, risks, benefits, confidentiality protections, and other relevant aspects of the provision of medical care, a specific procedure, or participation in medical research. Informed consent is also required for the authorization of release or disclosure of individually identifiable health care information, under HIPAA.

Inpatient Care: Care given a registered bed patient in a hospital, nursing home, or other medical or postacute institution.

In-Plan Services: Services that are covered under the state Medicaid plan and included in the patient's managed care contract, or are furnished by a participating provider.

Insolvency: Insurer's inability to pay debts. Insurance insolvency standards and the regulatory actions taken vary from state to state. When regulators deem an insurance company is in danger of becoming insolvent, they can take one of three actions: place a company in conservatorship or rehabilitation, if the company can be saved, or liquidation if salvage is deemed impossible. The difference between the first two options is one of degree—regulators guide companies in conservatorship but direct those in rehabilitation. Typically the first sign of problems is inability to pass the financial tests regulators administer as a routine procedure.

Institutional Review Board (IRB): A group of medical professionals formed together for the purpose of providing peer review to protect the rights of human subjects in medical research and clinical trials. HIPAA privacy regulations require an IRB also to protect the privacy rights of research subjects in specific ways.

Insurable Risk: Risks for which it is relatively easy to get insurance and that meet certain criteria. These include being definable, accidental in nature, and part of a group of similar risks large enough to make losses predictable. The insurance company also must be able to come up with a reasonable price for the insurance.

Insurance: A system to make large financial losses more affordable by pooling the risks of many individuals and business entities and transferring them to an insurance company or other large group in return for a premium.

Insurance Pool: A group of insurance companies that pool assets, enabling them to provide an amount of insurance substantially more than can be provided by individual companies to ensure large risks such as nuclear power stations. Pools may be formed voluntarily or mandated by the state to cover risks that cannot obtain coverage in the voluntary market such as coastal properties subject to hurricanes.

Insurance Regulatory Information System (IRIS): Uses financial ratios to measure insurers' financial strength. Developed by the National Association of Insurance Commissioners. Each individual state insurance department chooses how to use IRIS.

Insurance Score: Insurance scores are confidential rankings based on credit information. This includes whether the consumer has made timely payments on loans, the number of open credit card accounts, and whether a bankruptcy filing has been made. An insurance score is a measure of how well consumers manage their financial affairs, not of their financial assets. It does not include information about income or race.

Studies have shown that people who manage their money well tend also to manage their most important asset, their home, well. And people who manage their money responsibly also tend to handle driving a car responsibly. Some insurance companies use insurance scores as an insurance underwriting and rating tool.

Integrated Benefits: Coverage where the distinction between job-related and nonoccupational illnesses or injuries is eliminated and workers' compensation and general health coverage are combined. Legal obstacles exist, however, because the two coverages are administered separately. Previously called 24-hour coverage.

Integrated Delivery System (IDS), Integrated Services Network (ISN): Many different, but similar, definitions exist for IDS. IDS, as an entity, does not have to abide by strict regulations, as does an HMO. When an IDS offers a health plan, however, it must then abide by the requirements of the state and federal government for health plans, insurance companies, or HMOs. Without owning a health plan product, an IDS will usually abide by the regulations that govern its separate businesses, that is, regulations governing hospitals, clinics, and physicians. An IDS can be a financial or contractual arrangement between health providers (usually hospitals and doctors) to offer a comprehensive range of health care services through a separate legal entity operating, at least for these purposes, as a single health care delivery system. IDS can be a network of organizations, usually including hospitals and physician groups, that provides or arranges to provide a coordinated continuum of services to a defined population and is held both clinically and fiscally accountable for the outcomes of the populations served. IDS can also be a health care provider organization which vertically integrates physician, hospital, and usually, also health plan businesses in some manner, in order to establish a full continuum of care, seamless of delivery of services, and the ability to manage care under new reimbursement arrangements. *Also called* delivery system, vertically integrated system, horizontally integrated system, health delivery network, accountable health plan, and other names.

Intensive Care Management: Intensive community services for individuals with severe and persistent mental illness that are designed to improve planning for their service needs. Services include outreach, evaluation, and support.

Interface: A means of communication between two computer systems, two software applications, or two modules. Real-time interface is a key element in health care information systems due to the need to access patient care information and financial information instantaneously and comprehensively. Such real-time communication is the key to managing health care in a cost-effective manner, because it provides the necessary decision-making information for clinicians, providers, and payers.

Internal Medicine: Generally, that branch of medicine that is concerned with diseases that do not require surgery, specifically, the study and treatment of internal organs and body systems. It encompasses many sub-specialties; internists, the doctors who practice internal medicine, often serve as family physicians to supervise general medical care.

International Classification of Diseases, Ninth Revision, Clinical Modification (ICD-9-CM, ICD-10-CM): This is the universal coding method used to document the incidence of disease, injury, mortality, and illness. A diagnosis and procedure classification system designed to facilitate collection of uniform and comparable health information. The ICD-9-CM was issued in 1979. This system is used to group patients into DRGs, prepare hospital and physician billings, and prepare cost reports. Classification of disease by diagnosis codified into six-digit numbers.

Intervention Strategy: A generic term used in public health to describe a program or policy designed to have an impact on an illness or disease. Hence a mandatory seat belt law is an intervention designed to reduce automobile-related fatalities.

IPA: *See* Independent Practice Association/Individual Practice Association or Independent Practice Organization

IRB: *See* Institutional Review Board

IRIS: *See* Insurance Regulatory Information System

ISN: (Integrated Services Network) *See* Integrated Delivery System

J

JCAHO: *See* Joint Commission on the Accreditation of Healthcare Organizations

J-Codes: A subset of the HCPCS Level II code set with a high-order value of "J" that has been used to identify certain drugs and other items.

Job-Lock: Laws have now been enacted by congress that include continuance of benefits (COBRA) and other requirements which eliminate preexisting clauses for those individuals who change coverage plans but have maintained continuance of coverage overall. The inability of individuals to change jobs because they would lose crucial health benefits.

Joint Commission on the Accreditation of Healthcare Organizations (JCAHO): Formerly called JCAH, or Joint Commission on Accreditation of Hospitals, this is the peer review organization which provides the primary review of hospitals and health care providers. Many insurance companies require providers to have this accreditation in order to seek third-party payment, although many small hospitals cannot afford the cost of accreditation. JCAHO usually surveys organizations once every 3 years, sending in a medical and administrative team to review policies, patient records, professional credentialing procedures, governance, and quality improvement programs. JCAHO revises its "standards" annually.

L

Large Claim Pooling: System that isolates claims above a certain level and charges them to a pool funded by charges of all groups who share the pool. The system is designed to help stabilize significant premium fluctuations.

Large Urban Area: An urban statistical region with population of one million or more.

LATA: *See* Local Access Transport Area

Law of Large Numbers: The theory of probability on which the business of insurance is based. Simply put, this mathematical premise says that the larger the group of units insured, the more accurate the predictions of loss will be.

LEC: *See* Local Exchange Carrier

Legacy Systems: Computer applications, both hardware and software, which have been inherited through previous acquisition and installation. Most often, these systems run business applications that are not integrated with each other. Newer systems which stress open design and distributed processing capacity are gradually replacing such systems.

Legend Drug: Drug that the law says can only be obtained by prescription.

Length of Stay (LOS): The duration of an episode of care for a covered person. The number of days an individual stays in a hospital or inpatient facility. May also be reviewed as "average length of stay (ALOS)."

LEP: *See* Limited English Proficiency

Liability Insurance: Insurance for what the policyholder is legally obligated to pay because of bodily injury or property damage caused to another person.

Licensing: A process most states employ, which involves the review and approval of applications from HMOs prior to beginning operation in certain areas of the state. Areas examined by the licensing authority include fiscal soundness, network capacity, MIS, and quality assurance. The applicant must demonstrate it can meet all existing statutory and regulatory requirements prior to beginning operations.

Lifetime Limit: A cap on the benefits paid under a policy. Many policies have a lifetime limit of $1 million, which means that the insurer agrees to cover up to $1 million in covered services over the life of the policy.

Limited Data Set: Under HIPAA, this term refers to a set of data that may be used for research, public health, or health care operations without an authorization or waiver of authorization. The limited data set is defined as PHI that excludes the following direct identifiers of the individual or of relatives, employers, or household members of the individual: names; postal address information (other than town or city, state, and zip code); telephone and fax numbers; electronic mail addresses; social security numbers; medical record numbers; health plan beneficiary numbers; account numbers; certificate/license numbers; vehicle identifiers and serial numbers, including license plates; device identifiers and serial numbers; Web universal resource locators (URLs); Internet protocol (IP) address; biometric identifiers, including finger and voice prints; full-face photos, and comparable images. A covered entity must enter into a data use agreement with the recipient of a limited data set. It should be noted that, although a limited data set is subject to only select provisions of the HIPAA Privacy Rule, it may be covered by the Common Rule.

Limited English Proficiency (LEP): A term used to describe when a person speaks a language other than English and has limited proficiency with the language, as to comprehension, reading, and spoken word.

Limiting Charge: The maximum amount that a nonparticipating physician is permitted to charge a Medicare beneficiary for a particularly defined procedure or bundled service. These limits are published by the individual state intermediaries for Medicare and CMS and are usually combined in reports with the allowed charges and regional payment schedules. In 1993, the limiting charge was set at 115% of the Medicare-allowed charge. However, this does not reflect what the physician will be paid.

Limits: Maximum amount of insurance that can be paid for a covered loss.

Line: Type or kind of insurance, such as personal lines.

Liquidation: Enables the state insurance department as liquidator or its appointed deputy to wind up the insurance company's affairs by selling its assets and settling claims upon those assets. After receiving the liquidation order, the liquidator notifies insurance departments in other states and state guaranty funds of the liquidation proceedings. Such insurance company liquidations are not subject to the Federal Bankruptcy Code but to each state's liquidation statutes.

Liquor Liability: Coverage for bodily injury or property damage caused by an intoxicated person who was served liquor by the policyholder.

Local Access Transport Area (LATA): A defined region in which a telephone and long distance carrier operates. Important concept for those CHINs that depend upon phone lines. When creating communications networks, you try to avoid crossing boundaries of these, if possible, since costs escalate dramatically when there is a need to communicate over more than one LATA.

Local Codes: A generic term for code values that are defined for a state or other local division or for a specific payer. Commonly used to describe HCPCS Level III Codes.

Local Exchange Carrier (LEC): The telephone company that provides and supports the local connection to the public switched telephone network. In many areas of the United States, the LEC is one of the seven Regional Bell Operating Companies (RBOCs) or "Baby Bells." These LECs become partners for organizations seeking to develop a CHIN or, more conservatively, simply seeking to integrate their information system across many sites within a region.

Lock-In: A contractual provision by which members are required to use certain health care providers in order to receive coverage (except in cases of urgent or emergent need).

Long-Term Care (LTC): A set of health care, personal care, and social services required by persons who have lost, or never acquired, some degree of functional capacity (e.g., the chronically ill, aged, disabled, or retarded) in an institution or at home, on a long-term basis. The term is often used more narrowly to refer only to long-term institutional care such as that provided in nursing homes, homes for the retarded, and mental hospitals. Ambulatory services such home health care, which can also be provided on a long-term basis, are seen as alternatives to long-term institutional care.

Long-Term Care Insurance: Coverage that, under specified conditions, provides skilled nursing, intermediate care, or custodial care for a patient (generally over age 65) in a nursing facility or his or her residence.

LOS: *See* Length of Stay

Loss: A reduction in the quality or value of a property, or a legal liability.

Loss Adjustment Expenses: The sum insurers pay for investigating and settling insurance claims, including the cost of defending a lawsuit in court.

Loss Costs: The portion of an insurance rate used to cover claims and the costs of adjusting claims. Insurance companies typically determine their rates by estimating their future loss costs and adding a provision for expenses, profit, and contingencies.

Loss of Use: A provision in homeowners and renters insurance policies that reimburses policyholders for any extra living expenses due to having to live elsewhere while their home is being restored following a disaster.

Loss Ratio: Percentage of each premium dollar an insurer spends on claims (*see also* Medical Loss Ratio).

Loss Reserves: The company's best estimate of what it will pay for claims, which is periodically readjusted. They represent a liability on the insurer's balance sheet.

LTC: *See* Long-Term Care

M

MAAC: *See* Maximum Allowable Actual Charge

Major Medical Expense Insurance: Policies designed to help offset the heavy medical expenses resulting from catastrophic or prolonged illness or injury. They generally provide benefits payments for 75% to 80% of most types of medical expenses above a deductible paid by the insured.

Malpractice Insurance: Insurance against the risk of suffering financial damage due to professional misconduct or lack of ordinary skill. Malpractice requires that the patient prove some injury and that the injury was the result of negligence on the part of the professional. A practitioner is liable for damages or injuries caused by malpractice.

Managed Behavioral Health Program: A program of managed care specific to psychiatric or behavioral health care. This usually is a result of a "carve-out" by an insurance company or managed care organization (MCO). Reimbursement may be in the form of subcapitation, fee for service, or capitation.

Managed Care:

1. Arrangement between an employer or insurer and selected providers to provide comprehensive health care at a discount to members of the insured group and coordinate the financing and delivery of health care. Managed care uses medical protocols and procedures agreed on by the medical profession to be cost-effective, also known as medical practice guidelines.

2. Systems and techniques used to control the use of health care services. Includes a review of medical necessity, incentives to use certain providers, and case management. The body of clinical, financial, and organizational activities designed to ensure the provision of appropriate health care services in a cost-efficient manner. Managed care techniques are most often practiced by organizations and professionals that assume risk for a defined population (e.g., health maintenance organizations), but this is not always the case. Managed care is a broad term and encompasses many different types of organizations, payment mechanisms, review mechanisms, and collaborations. Managed care is sometimes used as a general term for the activity of organizing doctors, hospitals, and other providers into groups in order to enhance the quality and cost-effectiveness of health care. Managed care organizations (MCO) include HMO, PPO, POS, EPO, PHO, IDS, AHP, IPA, etc. Usually when one speaks of a managed care organization, one is speaking of the entity that manages risk, contracts with providers, is paid by employers or patient groups, or handles claims processing. Managed care has effectively formed a "go-between," brokerage, or third-party arrangement by existing as the gatekeeper between payers and providers and patients. The term managed care is often misunderstood, as it refers to numerous aspects of health care management, payment, and organization. It is best to ask the speaker to clarify what he or she means when using the term "managed care." In the purest sense, all people working in health care and medical insurance can be thought of as "managing care." Any system of health payment or delivery arrangements where the plan attempts to control or coordinate use of health services by its enrolled members in order to contain health expenditures, improve quality, or both. Arrangements often involve a defined delivery system of providers with some form of contractual

arrangement with the plan. *See* Health Maintenance Organization, Independent Practice Association, Preferred Provider Organization.

Managed Care Organization (MCO): A health plan that seeks to manage care. Generally, this involves contracting with health care providers to deliver health care services on a capitated (per member per month) basis. For specific types of managed care organizations, *see also* Health Maintenance Organization and Independent Practice Association.

Managed Care Plan: A health plan that uses managed care arrangements and has a defined system of selected providers that contract with the plan. Enrollees have a financial incentive to use participating providers that agree to furnish a broad range of services to them. Providers may be paid on a prenegotiated basis.

Managed Competition: A health insurance system that bands together employers, labor groups, and others to create insurance purchasing groups. Employers and other collective purchasers would make a specified contribution toward insurance purchase for the individuals in their group; the employer's set contribution acts as an incentive for insurers and providers to compete. This term first surfaced as a result of Bill Clinton's health reform package in the early 1990s.

Managed Health Care Plan: An arrangement that integrates financing and management with the delivery of health care services to an enrolled population. It employs or contracts with an organized system of providers that delivers services and frequently shares financial risk.

Management Information System (MIS): The common term for the computer hardware and software that provides the support of managing the plan.

Management Services Organization (MSO): Usually an entity owned by a hospital, physician group, PHO, or IDS that provides management services and administrative systems to one or more medical practices. The management services organization provides administrative and practice management services to physicians. A hospital, hospitals, or investors may typically own an MSO. Large group practices may also establish MSOs to sell management services to other physician groups.

Mandated Benefits: Benefits that health plans are required by law to provide.

Mandated Providers: Providers whose services must be included in coverage offered by a health plan. State or federal law can require these mandates.

Manual: A book published by an insurance or bonding company or a rating association or bureau that gives rates, classifications, and underwriting rules.

Manual Rates: Rates based on a health plan's average claims data and adjusted for certain factors, such as group demographics or industry.

Market Area: The targeted geographic area or areas of greatest market potential. The market area does not have to be the same as the postacute facility's catchment area.

Market Basket Index: A common term in the field of economics. In health care business, this refers to a ratio or index of the annual change in the prices of goods and services providers used to produce health services. Different market baskets exist for PPS-based hospital inputs and capital inputs, DRG-exempt facility operating inputs (such as SNF, home health agency, and renal dialysis facility). Also called input price index.

Market Share: A certain percentage of the market area or targeted market population. Usually used to describe a forecasted goal or a past penetration of the market.

Master Patient/Member Index: An index or file with a unique identifier for each patient or member that serves as a key to a patient's or member's health record.

Maximum Allowable Actual Charge (MAAC): A limitation on billed charges for Medicare services provided by nonparticipating physicians. For physicians with charges exceeding 115% of the prevailing charge for nonparticipating physicians, MAACs limit increases in actual charges to 1% a year. For physicians whose charges are less than 115% of the prevailing, MAACs limit actual charge increases so they may not exceed 115%.

Maximum Defined Data Set: Under HIPAA, this is all of the required data elements for a particular standard based on a specific implementation specification. An entity creating a transaction is free to include whatever data any receiver might want or need. The recipient is free to ignore any portion of the data that is not needed to conduct their part of the associated business transaction, unless the inessential data is needed for coordination of benefits.

Maximum Out-of-Pocket Expenses: Limit on total number of co-payments or limit on total cost of deductibles and coinsurance under a benefit plan.

McCarran–Ferguson Act: A 1945 Act of Congress exempting insurance businesses from federal commerce laws and delegating regulatory authority to the states. The act grants insurers a limited exemption from federal antitrust legislation.

MCE: *See* Medical Care Evaluation Scale

MCO: *See* Managed Care Organization

MCR: *See* Medicare Cost Report

Mediation: Nonbinding procedure in which a third party attempts to resolve a conflict between two other parties.

Medicaid (Title XIX): Government entitlement program for the poor, blind, aged, disabled, or members of families with dependent children (AFDC). Each state has its own standards for qualification. A federally aided, state-operated and administered program that provides medical benefits for certain indigent or low-income persons in need of health and medical care. The program, authorized by Title XIX of the Social Security Act, is basically for the poor. It does not cover all of the poor, however, but only persons who meet specified eligibility criteria. Subject to broad federal guidelines, states determine the benefits covered, program eligibility, rates of payment for providers, and methods of administering the program. All states but Arizona have Medicaid programs.

Medical Allied Manpower: This category includes some sixty occupations or specialties that can be divided into two large categories based on time required for occupational training. The first category includes those occupations that require at least a baccalaureate degree, for example, clinical laboratory scientists and technologists, dietitians and nutritionists, health educators, medical record librarians, and occupational speech and rehabilitation therapists. The second group includes those occupations that require less than a baccalaureate degree, such as aides for each of the above categories, as well as physician assistants and radiological technicians.

Medical Care Evaluation Studies (MCE): The name given to a generic form of health care review in which problems in the quality of the delivery and organization of health care services are addressed and monitored. A program based on MCEs is recommended as a way of meeting the federal government's requirements for an internal quality assurance program for federally qualified HMOs.

Medical Code Sets: Codes that characterize a medical condition or treatment. These code sets are usually maintained by professional societies and public health organizations. Compare to administrative code sets.

Medical Group Practice: The American Group Practice Association, the American Medical Association, and the Medical Group Management Association define medical group practice as provision of health care services by a group of at least three licensed physicians engaged in a formally organized and legally recognized entity sharing equipment, facilities, common records, and personnel involved in both patient care and business management.

Medical Informatics: Medical informatics is the systematic study, or science, of the identification, collection, storage, communication, retrieval, and analysis of data about medical care services to improve decisions made by physicians and managers of health care organizations. Medical informatics will be as important to physicians and medical managers as the rules of financial accounting are to auditors.

Medical Loss Ratio (MLR): Cost ratio of total benefits used compared to revenues received. Usually referred to by a ratio, such as 0.96—which means that 96% of premiums were spent on purchasing medical services. The goal is to keep this ratio below 1.00—preferably in the 0.80 ranges, since the MCO's or insurance company's profit comes from premiums. Currently, successful HMOs do have MLRs in the 0.70 to 0.80 range. The ratio between the cost to deliver medical care and the amount of money that was taken in by a plan. Insurance companies often have a medical loss ratio of 96% or more. Tightly managed HMOs may have medical loss ratios of 75% to 85%, although the overhead (or administrative cost ratio) is concomitantly higher.

Medically Necessary, Medical Necessity, Medical Necessary Services: Services or supplies which meet the following tests: they are appropriate and necessary for the symptoms, diagnosis, or treatment of the medical condition; they are provided for the diagnosis or direct care and treatment of the medical condition; they meet the standards of good medical practice within the medical community in the service area; they are not primarily for the convenience of the plan member or a plan provider; and they are the most appropriate level or supply of service which can safely be provided.

Medically Needy: Persons who are categorically eligible for Medicaid and whose income, less accumulated medical bills, is below state income limits for the Medicaid program. Often seen as a problem among the "working poor" or among the senior population.

Medical Management Information System (MMIS): A data system that allows payers and purchasers to track health care expenditure and utilization patterns. May also be referred to as Health Information System (HIS), Health Information Management (HIM), or Information System (IS).

Medical Payments Insurance: A coverage in which the insurer agrees to reimburse the insured and others up to a certain limit for medical or funeral expenses as a result of bodily injury or death by accident. Payments are without regard to fault.

Medical Review, Medical Review Criteria: Screening of health care utilization and the criteria used for this screening. Medical reviews are usually conducted by insurance companies, third-party payers, review organizations and case managers. This is the underlying basis for reviewing the quality and appropriateness of care provided to selected cases.

Insurance companies rely heavily on medical review and their own criteria as cost control. Through medical review, payers are able to limit or reduce the utilization of health care services. Medical review may sometimes put patients at odds with their insurance companies or hospitals and doctors in conflict with payers.

Medical Savings Account (MSA): An account in which individuals can accumulate contributions to pay for medical care or insurance. Some states give tax-preferred status to MSA contributions, but such contributions are still subject to federal income taxation. MSAs differ from medical reimbursement accounts, sometimes called flexible benefits or Section 115 accounts, in that they need not be associated with an employer. MSAs are not currently recognized in federal statute. President George W. Bush promoted MSAs heavily in his 2004 presidential campaign as a method to provide coverage for the uninsured. However, MSAs are unlikely to meet that need due to the disparity between income levels and health care costs.

Medical Services Organization (MSO): An organized group of physicians, usually from one hospital, into an entity able to contract with others for the provision of services.

Medical Underwriting: The use of historical or current medical health status information to evaluate an applicant to a health benefit plan for coverage.

Medical Utilization Review: The practice used by insurance companies to review claims for medical treatment.

Medicare: Federal program for people 65 or older that pays part of the costs associated with hospitalization, surgery, doctors' bills, home health care, and skilled-nursing care.

Medicare (Title XVIII): A federal program for the elderly and disabled, regardless of financial status. It is not necessary, as with Medicaid, for Medicare recipients to be poor. A U.S. health insurance program for people aged 65 and over, for persons eligible for social security disability payments for two years or longer, and for certain workers and their dependents who need kidney transplantation or dialysis. Monies from payroll taxes and premiums from beneficiaries are deposited in special trust funds for use in meeting the expenses incurred by the insured. It consists of two separate but coordinated programs: hospital insurance (Part A) and supplementary medical insurance (Part B). Medicare covers more than 34 million Americans (16% of population) at an annual estimated cost of more than $133 billion.

Medicare Approved Charge: The amount Medicare approves for payment to a physician. Typically, Medicare pays 80% of the approved charge, and the beneficiary pays the remaining 20%. Physicians may bill beneficiaries for an additional amount (the balance) not to exceed 15% of the Medicare approved charge.

Medicare Contractor: A Medicare Part A Fiscal Intermediary (institutional), a Medicare Part B Carrier (professional), or a Medicare Durable Medical Equipment Regional Carrier (DMERC).

Medicare Cost Report (MCR): An annual report required of all institutions participating in the Medicare program. The MCR records each institution's total costs and charges associated with providing services to all patients, the portion of those costs and charges allocated to Medicare patients, and the Medicare payments received.

Medicare Economic Index (MEI): An index that tracks changes over time in physician practice costs. From 1975 through 1991, increases in prevailing charge screens were limited to increases in the MEI.

Medicare Provider Analysis and Review (MEDPAR) File: A CMS data file that contains charge data and clinical characteristics, such as diagnoses and procedures, for every hospital inpatient bill submitted to Medicare for payment.

Medicare Remittance Advice Remark Codes: A national administrative code set for providing either claim-level or service-level Medicare-related messages that cannot be expressed with a Claim Adjustment Reason Code. This code set is used in the X12 835 Claim Payment and Remittance Advice transaction.

Medicare Risk Contract: An agreement by an HMO or competitive medical plan to accept a fixed dollar reimbursement per Medicare enrollee, derived from costs in the fee-for-service sector, for delivery of a full range of prepaid health services.

Medicare Supplemental Policy: A policy that pays for the cost of services not covered by Medicare, such as coinsurance and deductibles.

Medigap: Private health insurance plans that supplement Medicare benefits by covering some costs not paid for by Medicare. Medigap plans are supplements to Medicare insurance. Medigap plans vary from state to state; standardized Medigap plans *also may be known as* Medicare Select plans.

Medigap/MedSup: Policies that supplement federal insurance benefits particularly for those covered under Medicare.

MEDPAR: *See* Medicare Provider Analysis and Review File

MEI: *See* Medicare Economic Index

Member: Used synonymously with the terms enrollee and insured. A member is any individual or dependent who is enrolled in and covered by a managed health care plan.

Mental Health Parity: Mental health parity refers to providing the same insurance coverage for mental health treatment as that offered for medical and surgical treatments. The Mental Health Parity Act was passed in 1996 and established parity in lifetime benefit limits and annual limits.

Mental Health Provider: Psychiatrist, social worker, hospital, or other facility licensed to provide mental health services.

MET: *See* Multiple Employer Trust

MEWA: *See* Multiple Employer Welfare Arrangement

Midlevel Practitioner: Nurse practitioners, certified nurse-midwives, and physicians' assistants who have been trained to provide medical services that otherwise might be performed by a physician. Midlevel practitioners practice under the supervision of a doctor of medicine or osteopathy who takes responsibility for the care they provide. Physician extender is another term for these personnel. It is important to note that, in many states now, nurse practitioners are not required to practice under the supervision of an MD or DO.

Minimum Necessary: A HIPAA Privacy Rule standard requiring that, when protected health information is used or disclosed, only the information that is needed for the immediate use or disclosure should be made available by the health care provider or other covered entity. This standard does not apply to uses and disclosures for treatment purposes (so as not to interfere with treatment) or to uses and disclosures that an individual has authorized, among other limited exceptions. Justification regarding what constitutes the minimum necessary will be required in some situations (e.g., disclosures with a waiver of authorization and nonroutine disclosures).

MIS: *See* Management Information System

Miscellaneous Expenses: Hospital charges, other than room and board, such as those for X-rays, drugs, laboratory fees, and other ancillary services.

MLR: *See* Medical Loss Ratio

MMIS: *See* Medical Management Information System

Modified Community Rating: Rating of medical service usage in a given area, adjusted for data such as age, sex, etc.

Modified Fee-for-Service: System that pays providers fees for services provided, with certain maximum fees for each service.

Morbidity: The extent of illness, injury, or disability in a defined population. It is usually expressed in general or specific rates of incidence or prevalence.

Mortality: Death. Used to describe the relation of deaths to the population in which they occur. The mortality rate (death rate) expresses the number of deaths in a unit of population within a prescribed time and may be expressed as crude death rates (total deaths in relation to total population during a year) or as death rates specific for diseases and, sometimes, for age, sex, or other attributes (e.g., number of deaths from cancer in white males in relation to the white male population during a given year).

MSA: *See* Medical Savings Account

MSO: One of the following: medical staff organization, an organized group of physicians, usually from one hospital, into an entity able to contract with others for the provision of services; or management (or medical) services organization, an entity formed by, for example, a hospital, a group of physicians, or an independent entity, to provide business-related services such as marketing and data collection to a grouping of providers like an IPA, PHO, or CWW. This second definition is becoming the almost exclusive usage.

Multiple Employer Trust (MET): A legal trust established by a plan sponsor that brings together a number of small, unrelated employers for the purpose of providing group medical coverage on an insured or self-funded basis. Not quite a health plan purchasing cooperative, but along the same lines. More market oriented and usually smaller in scale. Redefined as a MEWA by the Multiple Employer Welfare Arrangement Act of 1982.

Multiple Employer Welfare Arrangement (MEWA): As defined in 1983 Erlenborn ERISA Amendment, an employee welfare benefit plan or any other arrangement providing any of the benefits of an employee welfare benefit plan to the employees of two or more employers. MEWAs that do not meet the ERISA definition of employee benefit plan and are not certified by the U.S. Department of Labor may be regulated by states. MEWAs that are fully insured and certified must only meet broad state insurance laws regulating reserves.

Multiple Option Plan: Health care plan that lets employees or members choose their own plan from a group of options, such as HMO, PPO, or major medical plan.

Multispecialty Group: A group of doctors who represent various medical specialties and who work together in a group practice.

Municipal Liability Insurance: Liability insurance for municipalities.

Mutual Holding Company: An organizational structure that provides mutual companies with the organizational and capital-raising advantages of stock insurers, while retaining the policyholder ownership of the mutual.

Mutual Insurance Company: A company owned by its policyholders that returns part of its profits to the policyholders as dividends. The insurer uses the rest as a surplus cushion in case of large and unexpected losses.

N

Named Peril: Peril specifically mentioned as covered in an insurance policy.

National Claims History (NCH) System: A CMS data reporting system that combines both Part A and Part B claims in a common file. The NCH system became fully operational in 1991.

National Committee for Quality Assurance (NCQA): A nonprofit organization created to improve patient care quality and health plan performance in partnership with managed care plans, purchasers, consumers, and the public sector. NCQA was formed in 1979 by the managed care industry and became independent in 1990. NCQA review is voluntary for health plans, but most plans seek its accreditation. The object of NCQA review and accreditation is to provide information to purchasers and patients and to encourage plans to compete based on quality and value rather than solely on price and provider network.

National Council for Prescription Drug Programs: An ANSI-accredited group that maintains a number of standard formats for use by the retail pharmacy industry, some of which have been adopted as HIPAA standards.

National Drug Code (NDC): A medical code set maintained by the Food and Drug Administration that contains codes for drugs that are FDA-approved. The secretary of HHS adopted this code set as the standard for reporting drugs and biologics on standard transactions. Classification system for drug identification, similar to UPC code.

National Health Insurance: Proposal by politicians to make government the single payer for all health care, similar to Great Britain or Canada. Providers like some aspects of this idea because it provides for "universal coverage" for all citizens. However, businesses and providers (as businesses themselves) dislike the idea of the government administering a program that they will either have to fund or be funded by. Proposals for national health insurance are surely to be debated by politicians for many years to come.

National Practitioner Data Bank: A computerized data bank maintained by the federal government that contains information on physicians against whom malpractice claims have been paid or certain disciplinary actions have been taken. Hospitals and other agencies pay a fee to access these records. Many regulatory agencies now require hospitals to utilize the NPDB prior to credentialing physicians at their facilities.

National Provider Identifier: A system for uniquely identifying all providers of health care services, supplies, and equipment. A term proposed by the secretary of HHS as the standard identifier for health care providers.

NCH: *See* National Claims History System

NCQA: *See* National Committee for Quality Assurance

NDC: *See* National Drug Code

Neonatal Intensive Care Unit (NEO ICU): A hospital unit with special equipment for the care of premature and seriously ill newborn infants.

Network: An affiliation of providers through formal and informal contracts and agreements. Networks may contract externally to obtain administrative and financial services. A list of physicians, hospitals, and other providers who provide health care services to the beneficiaries of a specific managed care organization.

Network-Model HMO: This type of HMO contracts with more than one physician group and may contract with single or multispecialty groups as well as hospitals and other health care providers. A health plan that contracts with multiple physician groups to deliver health care to members. Generally limited to large single- or multispecialty groups. Distinguished from group-model plans that contract with a single medical group, IPAs that contract through an intermediary, and direct-contract-model plans that contract with individual physicians in the community.

No-Fault: Auto insurance coverage that pays for each driver's own injuries, regardless of who caused the accident. No-fault varies from state to state. It also refers to an auto liability insurance system that restricts lawsuits to serious cases. Such policies are designed to promote faster reimbursement and to reduce litigation.

No-Fault Medical: A type of accident coverage in homeowners policies.

Nonadmitted Insurer: Insurers licensed in some states, but not others. States where an insurer is not licensed call that insurer nonadmitted. They sell coverage that is unavailable from licensed insurers within the state.

Nonparticipating Physician (or Provider): A provider, doctor, or hospital that does not sign a contract to participate in a health plan, usually which requires reduced rates from the provider. In the Medicare program, this refers to providers who are therefore not obligated to accept assignment on all Medicare claims. In commercial plans, nonparticipating providers are *also called* out-of-network providers or out-of-plan providers. If a beneficiary receives service from an out-of-network provider, the health plan (other than Medicare) will pay for the service at a reduced rate or will not pay at all.

Nonplan Provider: A health care provider without a contract with an insurer. Same as nonparticipating provider.

No-Pay, No-Play: The idea that people who do not buy coverage should not receive benefits. Prohibits uninsured drivers from collecting damages from insured drivers. In most states with this law, uninsured drivers may not sue for noneconomic damages such as pain and suffering. In other states, uninsured drivers are required to pay the equivalent of a large deductible ($10,000) before they can sue for property damages and another large deductible before they can sue for bodily harm.

Nosocomial Infections: Infections that are acquired while a patient is in a hospital are referred to as nosocomial infections; a term derived from "nosos" the Greek word for "disease." Often nosocomial infections become apparent while the patient is still in the hospital, but in some cases symptoms may not show up until after the affected patient is discharged. About one patient in ten acquires an infection as a direct result of being hospitalized. Infection control can be very cost-effective. Approximately one third of nosocomial infections are preventable.

Notice of Loss: A written notice required by insurance companies immediately after an accident or other loss. Part of the standard provisions defining a policyholder's responsibilities after a loss.

NPLANID: A term used by CMS for a proposed standard identifier for health plans. CMS had previously used the terms PayerID and PlanID for the health plan identifier.

Nurse Practitioner (NP): A registered nurse qualified and specially trained to provide primary care, including primary health care in homes and in ambulatory care facilities, long-term care facilities, and other health care institutions. Normally, NPs are licensed and possess master's degrees. Nurse practitioners generally function under the supervision of a physician but not necessarily in his/her or her presence. In some states, NPs are able to provide basic medical services without requiring MD or DO supervision. They are either salaried or reimbursed on a fee-for-service basis. They are sometimes considered "midlevel practitioners."

Nursing Home Insurance: A form of long-term care policy that covers a policyholder's stay in a nursing facility.

O

Occupancy Rate: A measure of inpatient health facility use, determined by dividing available bed days by patient days. It measures the average percentage of a hospital's beds occupied and may be institution-wide or specific for one department or service.

Occupational Disease: Abnormal condition or illness caused by factors associated with the workplace. Like occupational injuries, this is covered by workers' compensation policies.

Occupational Health: OSHA, county health departments, and regulatory bodies oversee occupational health hazards in workplaces, including hospitals. Occupational health programs include the employer activities undertaken to protect and promote the health and safety of employees in the workplace, including minimizing exposure to hazardous substances, evaluating work practices and environments to reduce injury, and reducing or eliminating other health threats. Many health providers offer occupational health consultations as well as occupational health screenings, treatments, and case management. Employers and health providers often enter agreements whereby health providers will provide these services as well as manage the related workers' compensation case management and rehabilitation programs. Employers seek to remain in compliance with regulations and reduce costs associated with employee injury and benefit utilization. Often, EAPs and drug prevention or drug testing programs are also combined under this category.

Occurrence Policy: Insurance that pays claims arising out of incidents that occur during the policy term, even if they are filed many years later.

Office for Civil Rights: This office is part of HHS. Its HIPAA responsibilities include oversight of the privacy requirements.

Office of Inspector General (OIG): The office responsible for auditing, evaluating, and criminal and civil investigating for HHS, as well as imposing sanctions, when necessary, against health care providers.

Ombudsperson or Ombudsman: A person within a managed care organization or a person outside of the health care system (such as an appointee of the state) who is designated to receive and investigate complaints from beneficiaries about quality of care, inability to access care, discrimination, and other problems that beneficiaries may experience with their managed care organization. This individual often functions as the beneficiary's advocate in pursuing grievances or complaints about denials of care or inappropriate care. Organizations are mostly able to designate a member of their own staff as ombudsman.

Open Access: A term describing a member's ability to self-refer for specialty care. Open access arrangements allow a member to see a participating provider without a referral from another doctor. Health plan members' abilities, rights, or invitation to self-refer for specialty care. *Also called* open panel.

Open Competition States: States where insurance companies can set new rates without prior approval, although the state's commissioner can disallow them if they are not reasonable and adequate or are discriminatory.

Open Enrollment Period: A period during which subscribers in a health benefit program have an opportunity to select among health plans being offered to them, usually without evidence of insurability or waiting periods. A period of time which eligible subscribers may elect to enroll in, or transfer between, available programs providing health care coverage. Under an open enrollment requirement, a plan must accept all who apply during a specific period each year.

Open Panel: A term describing a member's ability to self-refer for specialty care. Open access arrangements allow a member to see a participating provider without a referral from another doctor. Health plan members' abilities, rights, or invitation to self-refer for specialty care. *Also called* Open Access.

Organized Care System: Often used to discuss a more evolved form of IDSs and CCNs, this relatively new term describes the result of mergers and alliances between and among physicians, health systems, and managed care organizations. These systems often have the same performance imperatives as IDSs and CCNs: improve health status, integrate delivery, demonstrate value, improve efficiency of care delivery and prevention, and meet patient and community needs.

Outcome: A clinical outcome is the result of medical or surgical intervention or nonintervention, or the results of a specific health care service or benefit package. The valued results of care as experienced primarily by the patient but also by physicians and all other participants in the processes contributing to the outcomes.

Outcomes Management: Providers and payers alike wish to find a method of managing care in a way that would produce the best outcomes. Managed care organizations are increasingly interested in learning to manage the outcome of care rather than just managing the cost of care. It is thought that, through a database of outcomes experience, caregivers will know better which treatment modalities result in consistently better outcomes for patients. Outcomes management may lead to the development of clinical protocols. A clinical outcome is the result of medical or surgical intervention or nonintervention. Managed services organizations are now attempting to better manage clinical outcomes for their enrollees to increase the satisfaction of patients and payers while holding down costs.

Outcomes Measurement: System used to systematically track clinical treatment and responses to that treatment. The methods for measuring outcomes are quite varied among providers. Much disagreement exists regarding the best practice or tools to utilize to measure outcomes. In fact, much disagreement exists in the medical field about the definition of outcome itself. A tool to assess the impact of health services in terms of improved quality and/or longevity of life and functioning.

Outcomes Research: Research on measures of changes in patient outcomes, that is, patient health status and satisfaction, resulting from specific medical and health interventions. Attributing changes in outcomes to medical care requires distinguishing the effects of care from the effects of the many other factors that influence patients' health and satisfaction. With the elimination of the physician's fiduciary responsibility to the patient, outcomes data is gaining increasing importance for patient advocacy and consumer protection. Outcomes research will also be used in the future by payers to identify potential partners on the basis of good outcomes.

Outlier: A patient whose length of stay or treatment cost differs substantially from the stays or costs of most other patients in a diagnosis-related group. Under DRG reimbursement, outliers are given exceptional treatment subject to peer review and organization review.

Outlier Thresholds: The day and cost cutoff points that separate inlier patients from outlier patients.

Out-of-Area Benefits: Benefits supplied to a patient by a payer or managed care organization when the patient needs services while outside the geographic area of the network. MCOs often attempt to negotiate a case-by-case discount with providers when patients utilize their services while "out of area."

Out-of-Network Benefits: With most HMOs, a patient cannot have any services reimbursed if provided by a hospital or doctor who is not in the network. With PPOs and other managed care organizations, there may exist a provision for reimbursement of "out-of-network" providers. Usually this will involve higher co-pay or a lower reimbursement.

Out-of-Network Provider: A health care provider with whom a managed care organization does not have a contract to provide health care services. Because either the beneficiary must pay all of the costs of care from an out-of-network provider or their cost-sharing requirements are greatly increased, depending on the particular plan a beneficiary is in, out-of-network providers are generally not financially accessible to Medicaid beneficiaries.

Out-of-Pocket Expenses, Out-of-Pocket Costs: Costs borne by the member that are not covered by health care plan. Portion of health services or health costs that must be paid for by the plan member, including deductibles, co-payments, and coinsurance. In the age of managed care, out-of-pocket expenses can also refer to the payment of services not covered by or approved for reimbursement by the health plan.

Out-of-Pocket Limit: A cap placed on out-of-pocket costs, after which benefits increase to provide full coverage for the rest of the year. It is a stated dollar amount set by the insurance company, in addition to regular premiums.

Outpatient Care: Care given a person who is not bedridden. Also called ambulatory care. Many surgeries and treatments are now provided on an outpatient basis, while previously they had been considered reason for inpatient hospitalization. Some say this is the fastest growing segment of health care.

P

Paid Claims Loss Ratio: Paid claims divided by premiums.

Part A Medicare: Refers to the inpatient portion of benefits under the Medicare program, covering beneficiaries for inpatient hospital, home health, hospice, and limited skilled nursing facility services. Beneficiaries are responsible for deductibles and co-payments. Part A services are financed by the Medicare HI Trust Fund, which consists of Medicare tax payments. Part B, on the other hand, refers to outpatient coverage.

Part B Medicare: Refers to the outpatient benefits of Medicare. Medicare Supplementary Medical Insurance (SMI) under Part B of Title XVII of the Social Security Act covers Medicare beneficiaries for physician services, medical supplies, and other outpatient treatment. Beneficiaries are responsible for monthly premiums, co-payments, deductibles, and balance billing. Part B services are financed by a combination of enrollee premiums and general tax revenues.

Partial Capitation: A contract between a payer and a subcapitor, provider, or other payer whereby payments made are a combination of capitated premiums and fee-for-service payments. The proportion of the ratios determines the amount of risk. Sometimes certain outliers are paid as fee for service (difficult childbirth, cardiac care, cancer), while routine care (preventative, family, simple surgeries and common diagnoses) are capitated.

Partial Hospitalization Program (PHP): Acute level of psychiatric treatment normally provided for four or more hours per day. Normally includes group therapies and activities with homogeneous patient populations. Is used as a referral step-down from inpatient care or as an alternative to inpatient care. Unlike intensive outpatient or simple outpatient services, PHP provides an attending psychiatrist, onsite nursing, and social work. Reimbursed by payers at a rate that is roughly one-half of inpatient psychiatric hospitalization day rate. Patients do not spend the night at the partial hospital.

Partial Risk Contract: A contract between a purchaser and a health plan, in which only part of the financial risk is transferred from the purchaser to the plan. Forms of this are often seen in "self-funded" plans, competitive bidding arrangements, and new health plans.

Participating Physician or Participating Provider:

1. Simply refers to a provider under a contract with a health plan. A physician or hospital that has agreed to provide services for a set payment provided by a payer, or who agrees to other arrangements, or who agrees to provide services to a set of covered lives or defined patients. Also refers to a provider or physician who signs an agreement to accept assignment on all Medicare claims for one year.

2. A primary care physician in practice in the payer's managed care service area who has entered into a contract.

3. Any provider licensed in the state of provision and contracted with an insurer. Usually this refers to providers who are a part of a network. That network would be a panel of participating providers. Payers assemble their own provider panels.

Patient Liability: The dollar amount that an insured is legally obligated to pay for services rendered by a provider. These may include co-payments, deductibles, and payments for uncovered services.

Patient Origin Study: A study, generally undertaken by an individual health program or health planning agency, to determine the geographic distribution of the residences of the patients served by one or more health programs. Such studies help define catchment and medical trade areas and are useful in locating and planning the development of new services.

Payer (Usually Third-Party Payer): The public or private organization that is responsible for payment for health care expenses. Payers may be insurance companies or self-insured employers.

PBM: *See* Pharmacy Benefit Manager

PCCM: *See* Primary Care Case Management

PCN: *See* Primary Care Network

PCP (Primary Care Physician): Often acts as the primary gatekeeper in health plans. That is, often the PCP must approval referrals to specialists. Particularly in HMOs and some PPOs, all members must choose or are assigned a PCP.

PCP Capitation: A reimbursement system for health care providers of primary care services who receive a prepayment every month. The payment amount is based on age, sex, and plan of every member assigned to that physician for that month.

PCP: *See* Primary Care Physician or Primary Care Provider

PCR: *See* Physician Contingency Review

Peer Review: The mechanism used by the medical staff to evaluate the quality of total health care provided by the managed care organization. The evaluation covers how well all health personnel perform services and how appropriate the services are to meet the patients' needs. Evaluation of health care services by medical personnel with similar training. Generally, the evaluation by practicing physicians or other professionals of the effectiveness and efficiency of services ordered or performed by other members of the profession (peers). Frequently, peer review refers to the activities of the professional review organizations, and also to review of research by other researchers. This is the most common method utilized in managed care for monitoring the utilization by physicians. In other words, other physicians will review the decisions made by a physician. Much controversy has surfaced in this area in recent years. Some physicians are reluctant to be reviewed by physicians over the phone or by having their written records read. Some consumers suspect that peer review is not true peer review, since both the providers and the reviewers often have personal financial incentives to reduce or increase medical care. See Fiduciary. Nonetheless, peer review is utilized in all managed care settings.

Peer Review Organization (PRO): An organization established by the Tax Equity and Fiscal Responsibility Act (TEFRA) of 1982 to review quality of care and appropriateness of admissions, readmissions, and discharges for Medicare and Medicaid. These organizations are held responsible for maintaining and lowering admission rates, reducing lengths of stay, while insuring against inadequate treatment. PROs can conduct review of medical records and claims to evaluate the appropriateness of care provided. PROs also exist within private carriers and providers. Peer review itself is a process whose confidentiality in private organizations is protected by law. This allows hospitals and groups to conduct internal investigation and monitoring of care decisions and outcomes without the production of related documents in court proceedings. Providers have fought for these protections.

Per Diem Rates: A form of payment for services in which the provider is paid a daily fee for specific services or outcomes, regardless of the cost of provision. Per diem rates are paid without regard to actual charges and may vary by level of care, such as medical, surgical, intensive care, skilled care, psychiatric, etc. Per diem rates are usually flat all-inclusive rates.

Performance Gap: The occurrence, trend, or incident that shows that a clinician's performance falls short of expected performance levels, particularly when the clinician ignores accumulated scientific evidence supporting other clinical interventions or when the clinician does not reach benchmarked targets.

Performance Measurement: Measures and results that describe the health care being provided and the outcomes. Performance may be stated in terms of health outcome, quality of care, timeliness, correctness, percentage of goals attained or percentage of mistakes made. Performance measures may also indicate whether a health plan or provider has appropriately provided certain services expected to lead to desirable outcomes. Closely related to continuous quality of improvement (CQI) and utilization review (UR).

Performance Standards: Standards set by the MCO or payer that the provider will need to meet in order to maintain its credentialing, renew its contract, or avoid penalty. These will vary from payer to payer and contract to contract. Standards an individual provider is expected to meet, especially with respect to quality of care. The standards may define volume of care delivered per time period. Thus, performance standards for obstetricians/gynecologists may specify some or all of the following: office hours and office visits per week or month, on-call days, deliveries per year, gynecological operations per year, etc.

Per Member Per Month (PMPM): Applies to a revenue or cost for each enrolled member each month. The number of units of something divided by member months. Often used to describe premiums or capitated payments to providers, but can also refer to the revenue or cost for each enrolled member each month. Many calculations, other than cost or premium, use PMPM as a descriptor.

Personal Injury Protection (PIP) Coverage: Portion of an auto insurance policy that covers the treatment of injuries to the driver and passengers of the policyholder's car.

Personal Representative: A person authorized under state or other law to act on behalf of the individual in making health-related decisions. Examples include a court-appointed guardian with medical authority, a health care agent under a health care proxy, and a parent acting on behalf of an unemancipated minor (with exceptions where state law gives minors the right to make health decisions). For a decedent, the personal representative may be an executor, administrator, or other authorized person.

Per Thousand Members Per Year (PTMPY): A common way of reporting utilization. The most common example of hospital utilization, expressed as days PTMPY.

Pharmacy Benefit Manager (PBM): PBMs are third-party administrators of prescription drug benefits.

PHO: *See* Physician–Hospital Organization

PHP: *See* Partial Hospitalization Program OR Prepaid Health Plan

Physician Attestation: The requirement that the attending physician certify, in writing, the accuracy and completion of the clinical information used for DRG assignment.

Physician Contingency Reserve (PCR): Portion of a claim deducted and held by a health plan before payment is made to a capitated physician. Revenue that is withheld from a provider's payment to serve as an incentive for providing less expensive service. A typical withhold is approximately 20% of the claim. This amount can be paid back to the provider following analysis of his/her practice and service utilization patterns.

Physician Current Procedural Terminology (CPT): List of services and procedures performed by providers, with each service/procedure having a unique five-digit identifying code. CPT is the health care industry's standard for reporting of physician services and procedures. Used in billing and records.

Physician–Hospital Organization (PHO): An organization representing hospitals and physicians as an agent. A legal entity formed by a hospital and a group of physicians to further mutual interests and to achieve market objectives. A PHO generally combines physicians and a hospital into a single organization for the purpose of obtaining payer contracts. A contracted arrangement among physicians and hospital(s) wherein a single entity, the PHO, agrees to provide services to insurers' subscribers. The PHO serves as a collective negotiating and contracting unit. A PHO may be structured to share the risk of contracting between hospital(s) and doctors. PHOs may also own, operate, or subcontract MSOs, health plans, or providers. A PHO can manage risk. It is typically owned and governed jointly by a hospital and shareholder physicians.

Physician Organization: This term describes physician linkages and alliances that allow physicians to manage risk and capitation. Information systems, physician relationships, and financial integration allow these organizations to be more integrated than the traditional solo practice or IPA relationship between health care providers and/or managed care organizations that are working to develop a "seamless" continuum of health care services. Sometimes physician organizations are simply group practices or professional organizations without intention of acting as a contracting entity.

Physician Payment Review Commission: Established by Congress in 1986 to advise it on reforms of Medicare policies for paying physicians. Submits a report to congress annually.

Physician Practice Management Company (PPMC): A company that provides management and administrative support, often with capital for clinical expansion. The usual management fee is 15% to 30% of net revenue minus the nonprovider related clinic expenses.

PIP: *See* Personal Injury Protection Coverage

Plan Administration: A term often used to describe the management unit with responsibility to run and control a managed care plan—includes accounting, billing, personnel, marketing, legal, purchasing, possibly underwriting, management information, facility maintenance, and servicing of accounts. This group normally contracts for medical services and hospital care. If an insurance company is the underwriter, it may serve as its own administrator or may contract to a third-party administrator. Self-insured plans do the same.

Plan Document: The document that contains all of the provisions, conditions, and terms of operation of a pension or health or welfare plan. This document may be written in technical terms as distinguished from a summary plan description (SPD) that, under ERISA, must be written in a manner calculated to be understood by the average plan participant.

Plan Sponsor: An entity that sponsors a health plan. This can be an employer, a union, or some other entity.

Play or Pay: Proposal to make employers provide health care coverage for employees or pay a special government tax.

PMPM: *See* Per Member Per Month

Point-of-Service (POS) Plan: Health insurance policy that allows the employee to choose between in-network and out-of-network care each time medical treatment is needed. Generally the level of coverage is reduced for services associated with the use of nonparticipating providers. Managed care plan that specifies that those patients who go outside of the plan for services may pay more out-of-pocket expenses. A health insurance benefits program in which subscribers can select between different delivery systems (i.e., HMO, PPO, and fee-for-service) when in need of health care services and at the time of accessing the services, rather than making the selection between delivery systems at time of open enrollment at place of employment. Typically, the costs associated with receiving care from the in-network or approved providers are less than when care is rendered by noncontracting providers. Or the costs are less if provided by approved providers in either the HMO or PPO rather than out-of-network or out-of-plan providers. This is a method of influencing patients to use certain providers without restricting their freedom of choice too severely.

Policy: A written contract for insurance between an insurance company and policyholder stating details of coverage.

Pooling: Combining risks for groups into one risk pool.

Portability: Requirement that health plans guarantee continuous coverage without waiting periods for persons moving between plans. The ability for an individual to transfer from one health insurer to another health insurer with regard to preexisting conditions or other risk factors. This is a new protection for beneficiaries involving the issuance of a certificate of coverage from a previous health plan to be given to the new health plan. Under this requirement, a beneficiary who changes jobs is guaranteed coverage with the new plan, without a waiting period or having to meet additional deductible requirements. Primarily, this refers to the requirement that insurers waive any preexisting condition exclusion for beneficiaries previously covered through other insurance.

POS: *See* Point-of-Service Plan

PPMC: *See* Physician Practice Management Company

PPO: *See* Preferred Provider Organization

PPS: *See* Prospective Payment System

PPS (Prospective Payment System) Inpatient Margin: A measure that compares DRG-based operating and capital payments with Medicare-allowable inpatient operating and capital costs. It is calculated by subtracting total Medicare-allowable inpatient operating and capital costs from total PPS operating and capital payments and dividing by total PPS operating and capital payments.

PPS (Prospective Payment System) Operating Margin: A measure that compares PPS operating payments with Medicare-allowable inpatient operating costs. This measure excludes Medicare costs and payments for capital, direct medical education, organ acquisition, and other categories not included among Medicare-allowable inpatient operating costs. It is calculated by subtracting total Medicare-allowable inpatient operating costs from total PPS operating payments and dividing by total PPS operating payments.

PPS (Prospective Payment System) Year: A designation referring to hospital cost reporting periods that begin during a given federal fiscal year, reflecting the number of years since the initial implementation of PPS. For example, PPS1 refers to hospital fiscal years beginning during federal fiscal year 1984, which was the first year of PPS. For a hospital with a fiscal year beginning July 1, PPS 1 covers the period from July 1, 1984, through June 30, 1985.

Practical Nurses: Practical nurses, also known as vocational nurses, provide nursing care and treatment of patients under the supervision of a licensed physician or registered nurse. Licensure as a licensed practical nurse (LPN) or in California and Texas as a licensed vocational nurse (LVN) is required.

Practice Parameters, Practice Guidelines: Systematically developed statements to standardize care and to assist in practitioner and patient decisions about the appropriate health care for specific circumstances. Practice guidelines are usually developed through a process that combines scientific evidence of effectiveness with expert opinion. Practice guidelines are also referred to as clinical criteria, protocols, algorithms, review criteria, and guidelines. The American Medical Association defines practice parameters as strategies for patient management, developed to assist physicians in clinical decision making. Practice parameters may also be referred to as practice options, practice guidelines, practice policies, or practice standards.

Preadmission Review, Preadmission Certification, Precertification, or Preauthorization: Review of "need" for inpatient care or other care before admission. This refers to a decision made by the payer, MCO, or insurance company prior to admission. The payer determines whether or not the payer will pay for the service. Most managed care plans require precertification. This is a method of controlling and monitoring utilization by evaluating the need for service prior to the service being rendered. The practice of reviewing claims for inpatient admission prior to the patient entering the hospital in order to assure that the admission is medically necessary. A method of monitoring and controlling utilization by evaluating the need for medical service prior to it being performed. The process of notification and approval of elective inpatient admission and identified outpatient services before the service is rendered. An administrative procedure whereby a health provider submits a treatment plan to a third party before treatment is initiated. The third party usually reviews the treatment plan, monitoring one or more of the following: patient's eligibility, covered service, amounts payable, application of appropriate deductibles, co-payment factors and maximums. Under some programs, for instance, predetermination by the third party is required when covered charges are expected to exceed a certain amount. *Similar processes*: preauthorization, precertification, preestimate of cost, pretreatment estimate, and prior authorization.

Preauthorization: A cost-containment feature of many group medical policies whereby the insured must contact the insurer prior to a hospitalization or surgery and receive authorization for the service.

Preexisting Condition: A medical condition developed prior to issuance of a health insurance policy that may result in the limitation in the contract on coverage or benefits. Some policies exclude coverage of such conditions for a period of time or indefinitely. Federally qualified HMOs cannot limit coverage for preexisting conditions. New statutes in 1997 and 1998 altered the freedom other health plans have enjoyed in setting preexisting time limits. Certification of prior coverage may mean new insurers would need to waive preexisting clauses for some subscribers.

Preferred Provider Organization (PPO): Some combination of hospitals and physicians that agrees to render particular services to a group of people, perhaps under contract with a private insurer. A health care delivery system that contracts with providers of medical care to provide services at discounted fees to members. Members may seek care from nonparticipating providers, but generally are financially penalized for doing so by the loss of the discount and subjection to co-payments and deductibles. The services may be furnished at discounted rates, and the insured population may incur out-of-pocket expenses for covered services received outside the PPO if the outside charge exceeds the PPO payment rate. A PPO can also be a legal entity, or it may be a function of an already formed health plan, HMO, or PHO. The entity may have a health benefit plan that is also referred to as a PPO. PPOs are a common method of managing care while still paying for services through an indemnity plan. Most PPO plans are point-of-service plans, in that they will pay a higher percentage for care provided by providers in the network. Many insurers will offer PPOs as well as HMOs. Generally PPOs will offer more choice for the patient and will provide higher reimbursement to the providers.

Premium: Amount paid to a carrier for providing coverage under a contract. Money paid out in advance for insurance coverage.

Prepaid Capitation: A prospectively paid, fixed, annual, quarterly, or monthly premium per person or per family that covers specified benefits. A cost-containment alternative to fee-for-service usually employed by HMOs.

Prepaid Group Practice: Prepaid group practice plans involve multispecialty associations of physicians and other health professionals, who contract to provide a wide range of preventive, diagnostic, and treatment services on a continuing basis for enrolled participants.

Prepaid Health Plan (PHP): Entity that either contracts on a prepaid, capitated risk basis to provide services that are not risk-comprehensive services, or contracts on a nonrisk basis. Additionally, some entities that meet the above definition of HMOs are treated as PHPs through special statutory exemptions.

Prepayment: A method of paying for the cost of health care services in advance of their use. A method providing in advance for the cost of predetermined benefits for a population group, through regular periodic payments in the form of premiums, dues, or contributions, including those contributions that are made to a health and welfare fund by employers on behalf of their employees.

Prevailing Charge, Prevailing Fee: One of the factors determining a physician's payment for a service under Medicare, or other plan, set at a percentile of customary charges of all physicians in the locality.

Prevalence: The number of cases of disease, infected persons, or persons with some other attribute, present at a particular time and in relation to the size of the population from which drawn. It can be a measurement of morbidity at a moment in time (e.g., the number of cases of hemophilia in the country as of the first of the year).

Preventive Care: Health care that emphasizes prevention, early detection, and early treatment, thereby reducing the costs of health care in the long run. Health care that seeks to prevent or foster early detection of disease and morbidity and focuses on keeping patients well in addition to healing them when they are sick.

Pricer, or Repricer: A person, an organization, or a software package that reviews procedures, diagnoses, fee schedules, and other data and determines the eligible amount for a given health care service or supply. Additional criteria can then be applied to determine the actual allowance, or payment, amount.

Primary Care: Basic or general health care usually rendered by general practitioners, family practitioners, internists, obstetricians, and pediatricians—who are often referred to as primary care practitioners or PCPs. Professional and related services administered by an internist, family practitioner, obstetrician-gynecologist or pediatrician in an ambulatory setting, with referral to secondary care specialists, as necessary.

Primary Care Case Management (PCCM): This is a Freedom of Choice Waiver program, under the authority of Section 1915(b) of the Social Security Act. States contract directly with primary care providers who agree to be responsible for the provision and/or coordination of medical services to Medicaid recipients under their care. Currently, most PCCM programs pay the primary care physician a monthly case management fee in addition to receiving fee-for-services payment.

Primary Care Network (PCN): A group of primary care physicians who share the risk of providing care to members of a given health plan.

Primary Care Physician (PCP): A "generalist" such as a family practitioner, pediatrician, internist, or obstetrician. In a managed care organization, a primary care physician is accountable for the total health services of enrollees including referrals, procedures, and hospitalization.

Primary Care Provider (PCP): The provider that serves as the initial interface between the member and the medical care system. The PCP is usually a physician, selected by the member upon enrollment, who is trained in one of the primary care specialties, who treats and is responsible for coordinating the treatment of members assigned to his/her plan.

Primary Company: In a reinsurance transaction, the insurance company that is reinsured.

Primary Coverage: Plan that pays its expenses without consideration of other plans, under coordination of benefits rules.

Primary Physician Capitation: The amount paid to each physician monthly for services based on the age, sex and number of the members selecting that physician.

Principal Diagnosis: The medical condition that is ultimately determined to have caused a patient's admission to the hospital. The principal diagnosis is used to assign every patient to a diagnosis-related group. This diagnosis may differ from the admitting and major diagnoses.

Prior Approval States: States where insurance companies must file proposed rate changes with state regulators and gain approval before they can go into effect.

Prior Authorization: A formal process requiring a provider to obtain approval to provide particular services or procedures before they are done. This is usually required for nonemergency services that are expensive or likely to be abused or overused. A managed care organization will identify those services and procedures that require prior authorization, without which the provider may not be compensated.

Privacy: For purposes of the HIPAA Privacy Rule, privacy means an individual's interest in limiting who has access to personal health care information.

Privacy Board: A board of members authorized by the HIPAA Privacy Rule to approve a waiver of authorization for use and/or disclosure of identifiable health information. For research purposes, the institutional review board may also function as the privacy board.

Privacy Notice: Institution-wide notice describing the practices of the covered entity regarding protected health information. Health care providers and other covered entities must give the notice to patients and research subjects and should obtain signed acknowledgements of receipt. Internal and external uses of protected health information are explained. It is the responsibility of the researcher to provide a copy of the privacy notice to any subject who has not already received one. If the researcher does provide the notice, the researcher should also obtain the subject's written acknowledgement of receipt. These have become more common and visible in hospitals and physician offices due to HIPAA requirements.

PRO: *See* Peer Review Organization

Product Liability: A section of tort law that determines who may sue and who may be sued for damages when a defective product injures someone. No uniform federal laws guide manufacturer's liability, but under strict liability, the injured party can hold the manufacturer responsible for damages without the need to prove negligence or fault.

Product Liability Insurance: Protects manufacturers' and distributors' exposure to lawsuits by people who have sustained bodily injury or property damage through the use of the product.

Professional Review Organization: An organization that reviews the services provided to patients in terms of medical necessity professional standards and appropriateness of setting.

Professional Standards Review Organization (PSRO): A physician-sponsored organization charged with reviewing the services provided patients who are covered by Medicare, Medicaid, and maternal and child health programs. The purpose of the review is to determine if the services rendered are medically necessary; provided in accordance with professional criteria, norms, and standards; and provided in the appropriate setting.

Profile: Aggregated data in formats that display patterns of health care services over a defined period of time.

Profile Analysis or Profiling: Review and analysis of profiles to identify and assess patterns of health care services. Expressing a pattern of practice as a rate—some measure of utilization (of costs or services) or outcome (as functional status, morbidity, or mortality) aggregated over time for a defined population of patients. This is used to compare with other practice patterns. May be used for physician practices, health plans, or geographic areas.

Proof of Loss: Documents showing the insurance company that a loss occurred.

Property/Casualty Insurance: Covers damage to or loss of policyholders' property and legal liability for damages caused to other people or their property. Property/casualty insurance, which includes auto, homeowners, and commercial insurance, is one segment of the insurance industry. The other sector is life/health. Outside the United States, property/casualty insurance is referred to as nonlife or general insurance.

Prospective Payment System (PPS): A payment method that establishes rates, prices, or budgets before services are rendered and costs are incurred. Providers retain or absorb at least a portion of the difference between established revenues and actual costs. (1) The Medicare system used to pay hospitals for inpatient hospital services; based on the DRG classification system. (2) Medicare's acute care hospital payment method for inpatient care. Prospective per-case payment rates are set at a level intended to cover operating costs in an efficient hospital for treating a typical inpatient in a given diagnosis-related group. Payments for each hospital are adjusted for differences in area wages, teaching activity, care to the poor, and other factors. Hospitals may also receive additional payments to cover extra costs associated with atypical patients (outliers) in each DRG. Capital costs, originally excluded from PPS, are being phased into the system. In 2001, capital payments were changed to a fully prospective, per-case basis.

Protected Health Information: Under HIPAA, this refers to individually identifiable health information transmitted or maintained in any form.

Provider: Usually refers to a hospital or doctor who "provides" care. A health plan, managed care company, or insurance carrier is not a health care provider. Those entities are called payers. The lines are blurred sometimes, however, when providers create or manage health plans. At that point, a provider is also a payer. A payer can be provider if the payer owns or manages providers, as with some staff-model HMOs.

Provider Excess: Specific or aggregate stop loss coverage extended to a provider instead of a payer or employer.

Provider Services Organization (PSO): Defined by CMS as a public or private entity that is established or organized by a health care provider or group of affiliated providers, that provides a substantial proportion of the services under its Medicare contract directly through the provider or group of affiliated providers, and in which the provider or affiliated providers directly or indirectly share substantial financial risk and have at least a majority financial interest. Similar to the concept of MSO, *see* Medical Services Organization, or Management Services Organization.

PSO: *See* Provider Services Organization

PSRO: *See* Professional Standards Review Organization

Psychotherapy Notes: These include notes recorded by the health care provider who is a mental health professional during a counseling session, either in a private session or in a group. These notes are separate from documentation placed in the medical chart and do not include prescriptions. Specific patient authorization is required for use and disclosure of psychotherapy notes.

PTMPY: *See* Per Thousand Members Per Year

Public Health Authority: A federal, state, local, or tribal person or organization that is required to conduct public health activities.

Purchaser: This entity not only pays the premium, but also controls the premium dollar before paying it to the provider. Included in the category of purchasers or payers are patients, businesses, and managed care organizations. While patients and businesses function as ultimate purchasers, managed care organizations and insurance companies serve a processing or payer function.

Purchasing Group: An entity that offers insurance to groups of similar businesses with similar exposures to risk.

Q

Quality: Quality is, according to the Institute of Medicine (IOM), the degree to which health services for individuals and populations increase the likelihood of desired health outcomes and are consistent with current professional knowledge. Quality can be defined as a measure of the degree to which delivered health services meet established professional standards and judgments of value to consumers. Quality may also be seen as the degree to which actions taken or not taken maximize the probability of beneficial health outcomes and minimize risk and other untoward outcomes, given the existing state of medical science and art. Quality is frequently described as having three dimensions: quality of input resources, quality of the process of services delivery (the use of appropriate procedures for a given condition), and quality of outcome of service use (actual improvement in condition or reduction of harmful effects). Quality programs are commonly called QA, TQM, QI, CQI—all referring to the process of monitoring quality in systematic ways.

Quality Assurance (QA): Activities and programs intended to assure the quality of care in a defined medical setting. Such programs include peer or utilization review components to identify and remedy deficiencies in quality. The program must have a mechanism for assessing its effectiveness and may measure care against preestablished standards. Also called quality improvement. A formal methodology and set of activities designed to access the quality of services provided. Quality assurance includes formal review of care, problem identification, corrective actions to remedy any deficiencies, and evaluation of actions taken.

Quality Assurance Reform Initiative (QARI): A process developed by the Health Care Financing Administration (now called CMS) to develop a health care quality improvement system for Medicaid managed care plans. The Quality Assurance Reform Initiative was unveiled in 1993 to assist states in the development of continuous quality improvement systems, external quality assurance programs, internal quality assurance programs, and focused clinical studies.

Quality Improvement (QI): Also called performance improvement (PI), QI is a management technique to assess and improve internal operations. QI focuses on organizational systems rather than individual performance and seeks to continuously improve quality rather than reacting when certain baseline statistical thresholds are crossed. The process involves setting goals, implementing systematic changes, measuring outcomes, and making subsequent appropriate improvements. QI implies that concurrent systems are used to continuously improve quality, rather than reacting when certain baseline statistical thresholds are crossed. Quality improvement programs usually use tools such as cross-functional teams, task forces, statistical studies, flow charts, process charts, Pareto charts, etc. This is the more commonly used term in health care, replacing QA.

Quality Management (QM): Used interchangeably with quality assurance (QA), quality management usually involves an internal review process that audits the quality of care delivered and implements corrective actions to remedy any deficiencies identified in the quality of direct patient care, administrative services, or support services. The process can employ peer review, outcomes assessment, and utilization management techniques to assess and improve the quality of care. The level of care may be measured against preestablished standards.

R

Rate Band: The allowable variation in insurance premiums as defined in state regulations. Acceptable variation may be expressed as a ratio from highest to lowest (e.g., 3:1) or as a percent from the community rate (e.g., ±20%). Usually based on risk factors such as age, gender, occupation, or residence.

Rate Regulation: The process by which states monitor insurance companies' rate changes, done either through prior approval or open-competition models.

Rate Review: Review by a government or private agency of a hospital's budget and financial data, performed for the purpose of determining the reasonableness of the hospital rates and evaluating proposed rate increases.

Rating Agencies: Six major credit agencies determine insurers' financial strength and viability to meet claims obligations. They are A.M. Best

Co.; Duff & Phelps Inc.; Fitch, Inc.; Moody's Investors Services; Standard & Poor's Corp.; and Weiss Ratings, Inc. Factors considered include company earnings, capital adequacy, operating leverage, liquidity, investment performance, reinsurance programs, and management ability, integrity, and experience. A high financial rating is not the same as a high consumer satisfaction rating.

Rating Bureau: The insurance business is based on the spread of risk. The more widely risk is spread, the more accurately loss can be estimated. An insurance company can more accurately estimate the probability of loss on 100,000 homes than on ten. Years ago, insurers were required to use standardized forms and rates developed by rating agencies. Today, large insurers use their own statistical loss data to develop rates. But small insurers, or insurers focusing on special lines of business, with insufficiently broad loss data to make them actuarially reliable, depend on pooled industry data collected by such organizations as the Insurance Services Office (ISO), which provides information to help develop rates such as estimates of future losses and loss adjustment expenses like legal defense costs.

RBRBS: *See* Resource-Based Relative Value Scale

Real Value: Measurement of an economic amount corrected for change in price over time (inflation), thus expressing a value in terms of constant prices. A common term in economics.

Receivables: Amounts owed to a business for goods or services provided.

Referral: The process of sending a patient from one practitioner to another for health care services. Health plans may require that designated primary care providers authorize a referral for coverage of specialty services.

Referral Center (*Also Called* Triage, Call Center, 24-Hour Certification, or 1-800): This is a mechanism established by health plans to direct patients to approved hospitals and doctors. Often the Referral Center serves a UR function and certified or precertifies the care. These centers are also used by hospitals to refer patients to certain doctors, reduce use of the emergency room, or provide follow-up patient contact. Managed care organizations utilize these centers as their central hub of communications with patients and providers at the time of service.

Referral Pool: An amount set aside to pay for noncapitated services provided by a PCP, services provided by a referral specialist and/or emergency services.

Referral Services: Medical services arranged for by the physician and provided outside the physician's office other than hospital services.

Refinement: The correction of relative values in Medicare's relative value scale that was initially set incorrectly.

Registered Nurses (RNs): Registered nurses are responsible for carrying out the physician's instructions. They supervise practical nurses and other auxiliary personnel who perform routine care and treatment of patients. Registered nurses provide nursing care to patients or perform specialized duties in a variety of settings from hospital and clinics to schools and public health departments. A license to practice nursing is required in all states. For licensure as an RN, an applicant must have graduated from a school of nursing approved by the state board for nursing and have passed a state board examination.

Reinsurance:

1. Insurance bought by insurers. A reinsurer assumes part of the risk and part of the premium originally taken by the insurer, known as the primary company. Reinsurance effectively increases an insurer's capital and therefore its capacity to sell more coverage. The business is global, and some of the largest reinsurers are based abroad. Reinsurers have their own reinsurers, called retrocessionaires. Reinsurers do not pay policyholder claims. Instead, they reimburse insurers for claims paid.

2. An insurance arrangement whereby the MCO or provider is reimbursed by a third party for costs exceeding a preset limit, usually an annual maximum. A method of limiting the risk that a provider or managed care organization assumes by purchasing insurance that becomes effective after set amount of health care services have been provided. This insurance is intended to protect a provider from the extraordinary health care costs that just a few beneficiaries with extremely extensive health care needs may incur. Insurance purchased by an insurance company or health plan from another insurance company to protect itself against losses. A contract by which an insurer procures a third party to insure it against loss or liability by reason of such original insurance. The practice of an HMO or insurance company of purchasing insurance from another company to protect itself against part or all the losses incurred in the process of honoring the claims of policyholders. *Also called* "risk control" insurance. *See also* Risk and Stop Loss.

Relative Value Scale (RVS): An index assigning various weights to various medical services. Each weight represents a relative amount to be paid for each service. The RVS used in the development of the Medicare Fee Schedule for physicians consists of three cost components: physician work, practice expense, and malpractice expense.

Relative Value Unit (RVU): The unit of measure for a relative value scale. RVUs must be multiplied by a dollar conversion factor to become payment amounts. This is a common term in economics. RVUs are often used in physician practice management to compare performance of doctors within a group.

Renewal: Continuance of coverage for a new policy term.

Renters Insurance: A form of insurance that covers a policyholder's belongings against perils such as fire, theft, windstorm, hail, explosion, vandalism, riots, and others. It also provides personal liability coverage for damage the policyholder or dependents cause to third parties. It also provides additional living expenses, known as loss-of-use coverage, if a policyholder must move while his or her dwelling is repaired. It also can include coverage for property improvements. Possessions can be covered for their replacement cost or the actual cash value that includes depreciation.

Report Card: An accounting of the quality of services, compared among providers over time. The report card measures and compares providers on predetermined, measurable quality and other outcome indicators. Hospitals and insurance companies may publish their report card results if favorable. Generally, consumers use report cards to choose a health plan or provider, while policy makers may use report card results to determine overall program effectiveness, efficiency, and financial stability.

Research: When used by HIPAA, this term refers to a systematic investigation, including research development, testing, and evaluation, designed to develop or contribute to general knowledge.

Reserves:

1. A company's best estimate of what it will pay for claims.
2. Monies earmarked by health plans to cover anticipated claims and operating expenses. A fiscal method of withholding a certain percentage of premium to provide a fund for committed but undelivered health care and such uncertainties as longer hospital utilization levels than expected, over-utilization of referrals, accidental catastrophes, and the like. A percentage of the premiums support this fund. Businesses other than health plans also manage reserves. For example, hospitals document reserves as that portion of the accounts receivable that they hope to collect but have some doubt about their ability to collect. Rather than book these amounts as income, hospitals will "reserve" these amounts until paid.

Resource-Based Relative Value Scale (RBRVS): A schedule of values assigned to health care services that give weight to procedures based upon resources needed by the provider to effectively deliver the service or perform that procedure. Unlike other relative value scales, RBRVS ignores historical charges and includes factors such as time, effort, technical skill, practice cost, and training cost. Established as part of the Omnibus Reconciliation Act of 1989, Medicare payment rules for physician services were altered by establishing an RBRVS fee schedule. This payment methodology has three components: a relative value for each procedure, a geographic adjustment factor, and a dollar conversion factor. A Medicare weighting system to assign units of value to each CPT code (procedure) performed by physicians and other providers.

Retention: The amount of risk retained by an insurance company that is not reinsured.

Retrocession: The reinsurance bought by reinsurers to protect their financial stability.

Retrospective Rating (Retro):

1. Insurance coverage that provides for premium determination at the end of the coverage period, subject to a minimum and maximum based upon actual experience.
2. A method of permitting the final premium for a risk to be adjusted, subject to an agreed-upon maximum and minimum limit based on actual loss experience. It is available to large commercial insurance buyers.

Retrospective Review Process: System for analyzing medical necessity and appropriateness of services rendered. A review that is conducted after services are provided to a patient. The review focuses on determining the appropriateness, necessity, quality, and reasonableness of health care services provided. Becoming seen as the least desirable method; supplanted by concurrent reviews.

Revenue Share: The proportion of a practice's total revenue devoted to a particular type of expense. For example, the practice expense revenue share is that proportion of revenue used to pay for practice expense.

RHC: *See* Rural Health Clinic

Risk: The chance or possibility of loss. For example, physicians may be held at risk if hospitalization rates exceed agreed upon thresholds. Potential financial liability, particularly with respect to who or what is legally responsible for that liability. With insurance, the patient and insurance company share risk, but the company's risk is limited by the policy's dollar limitations. In HMOs, the patient is at risk only for co-payments and the cost of noncovered services. The HMO, however, with its income fixed, is at risk for whatever volume of care is entailed, however costly it turns out to be. Providers may also bear risk if they are paid a fixed amount (capitation) by the HMO. The sharing of risk is often employed as a utilization control mechanism within the HMO setting. Risk is also defined in insurance terms as the possibility of loss associated with a given population.

Risk-Adjusted Capitation: An actuarial term, this refers to methodology of payment to providers which reflects fixed payment amounts per member per month and then is adjusted further to take into account the lower or higher costs of providing care to individuals or groups of individuals, based on health status or characteristics.

Risk Adjuster: A measure used to adjust payments made to carriers or payers on behalf of a group of enrollees in order to compensate for spending, which is expected to be lower or higher than average, based on the health status or demographic characteristics of the enrollees. An actuarial result of analysis.

Risk Adjustment: A system of adjusting rates paid to managed care providers to account for the differences in beneficiary demographics, such as age, gender, race, ethnicity, medical condition, geographic location, at-risk population (i.e., homeless), etc. A process by which premium dollars are shifted from a plan with relatively healthy enrollees to another with sicker members. It is intended to minimize any financial incentives health plans may have to select healthier than average enrollees. In this process, health plans that attract higher-risk providers and members would be compensated for any differences in the proportion of their members that require high levels of care compared to other plans. A statistical method of paying managed care organizations different capitated payments based on the composition and relative healthiness of their beneficiaries. This procedure would generally compensate providers of HIV services with a higher capitated payment than providers of other (often less costly) health care services. In a competitive and voluntary health insurance market, like that in the United States, health plans have a strong financial incentive to attract the healthiest enrollees, while excluding sicker, higher-risk enrollees. This incentive encourages health plans to compete on the basis of risk selection rather than on the basis of cost efficiency and quality of health care. In the private insurance market, risk adjustment is a corrective tool designed to reorient the incentives for health plans and enrollees, reducing the negative consequences of enrolling high-risk users by compensating plans according to the health risk of plans' enrollees.

Risk Assessment: Anticipating the cost of providing health care to groups of enrollees. Actuarial assessments examine utilization history, demographics, health characteristics, environmental attributes, and other sociological, economic, and market characteristics. Risk assessment can also include, less commonly, the identification of etiology of health problems.

Risk-Bearing Entity: An organization that assumes financial responsibility for the provision of a defined set of benefits by accepting prepayment for some or all of the cost of care. A risk-bearing entity may be an insurer, a health plan, or self-funded employer, or a PHO or other form of PSN. Health plans (except under employer self-insured programs) usually are risk bearing. Providers and provider organizations, if capitated, can also be risk bearing. There are two types of risk: insurance risk and business risk, each calculated and considered separately.

Risk Contract: A risk contract is broadly any contract that results in any party assuming insurance or business risk. Normally this means, in health care, that if the employer, health plan, or provider assumes risk, it is agreeing to cover the expense of increased utilization beyond the projected costs or payment provided. Normally risk is assumed by the health plan or insurance carrier but can be carried by the provider in capitated arrangements or by the employer in self-insured arrangements. A contract payment methodology between HCFA and an HMO or CMP that requires the delivery of (at least) all covered services to members as medically necessary in return for a fixed monthly payment rate from the government and (often) a premium paid by the enrollee. The HMO is then liable for those contractually offered services without regard to cost. (*Note*: Medicaid beneficiaries enrolled in risk contracts are not required to pay premiums.)

Risk Corridor: A financial arrangement between a payer of health care services, such as a state Medicaid agency, and a provider, such as a managed care organization, that spreads the risk for providing health care services. Risk corridors protect the provider from excessive care costs for individual beneficiaries by instituting stop loss protections, and they protect the payer by limiting the profits that the provider may earn.

Risk Factor: Any characteristic, behavior, or condition which, based on history, utilization, or theory, is thought to directly influence susceptibility to a specific health problem, increase costs, or result in increased utilization.

Risk Load: In underwriting, a factor that is multiplied into the rate to offset some adverse parameter of the group.

Risk Management: Management of the varied risks to which a business firm or association might be subject. It includes analyzing all exposures to gauge the likelihood of loss and choosing options to better manage or minimize loss. These options typically include reducing and eliminating the risk with safety measures, buying insurance, and self-insurance.

Risk Measure: The expected per capita costs of health care services to a defined group in a specific future period.

Risk Pool: A pool of money that is at risk for being used for defined expenses. Commonly, if the pool money that is put at risk is not expended by the end of the year, some or all of it is returned to those managing the risk. Two different definitions are in use: (1) a pool of funds set aside as reserves to be used for defined expenses (under capitation, if all of the risk pool is not used by the end of the contract year, it is usually disseminated to participating providers) and (2) legislatively created programs that group individuals who cannot secure coverage in the private market (funding comes from government or assessment on insurers).

Risk Selection: Occurrence when a disproportionate share of high or low users of care join a health plan.

Risk Sharing: The distribution of financial risk among parties furnishing a service. For example, if a hospital and a group of physicians from a corporation provide health care at a fixed price, a risk-sharing arrangement would entail both the hospital and the group being held liable if expenses exceed revenues. A method by which medical insurance premiums are shared by plan sponsors and participants, in contrast to traditional indemnity plans in which insurance premiums belonged solely to insurance company that assumed all risk of using these premiums. Key to this approach is that the premiums are the only payment providers receive; this provides powerful incentive to be parsimonious with care.

Rural Health Clinic (RHC): A public or private hospital, clinic, or physician practice designated by the federal government as in compliance with the Rural Health Clinics Act (Public Law 95-210). The practice must be located in a Medically Underserved area or a Health Professions Shortage Area and use a physician assistant and/or nurse practitioners to deliver services. A rural health clinic must be licensed by the state and provide preventive services. These providers are usually qualified for special compensations, reimbursements, and exemptions.

Rural Health Clinics Act: Establishes a reimbursement mechanism to support the provision of primary care services in rural areas. Public Law 95-210 was enacted in 1977 and authorizes the expanded use of physician assistants, nurse practitioners, and certified nurse practitioners; extends Medicare and Medicaid reimbursement to designated clinics; and raises Medicaid reimbursement levels to those set by Medicare.

RVS: *See* Relative Value Scale

RVU: *See* Relative Value Unit

S

Sanction: Reprimand that gives binding force to a law or rule, or secures obedience to it, as the penalty for breaking it, or a reward for carrying it out. The government and its agencies can sanction hospitals, providers, and health plans. Health plans sometimes seek to sanction hospitals and physicians. Medical staffs sometimes seek sanctions against their members.

SAP: *See* Statutory Accounting Principles

SCH: *See* Sole Community Hospital

Schedule: A list of individual items or groups of items that are covered under one policy or a listing of specific benefits, charges, credits, assets, or other defined items.

SCHIP: *See* State Children's Health Insurance Program or Plan.

SCR: *See* Standard Class Rate

Secondary Care: Services provided by medical specialists who generally do not have first contact with patients (e.g., cardiologist, urologists, dermatologists). In the United States, however, there has been a trend toward self-referral by patients for these services, rather than referral by primary care providers. This is quite different from the practice in England, for example, where all patients must first seek care from primary care providers and are then referred to secondary and/or tertiary providers, as needed.

Secondary Coverage: Health plan that pays costs not covered by primary coverage under coordination of benefits rules. Any insurance that supplements Medicare coverage. The three main sources for secondary insurance are employers, privately purchased Medigap plans, and Medicaid.

Section 1115 Medicaid Waiver: The Social Security Act grants the secretary of HHS broad authority to waive certain laws relating to Medicaid for the purpose of conducting pilot, experimental, or demonstration projects which are "likely to promote the objectives" of the program. Section 1115 demonstration waivers allow states to change provisions of their Medicaid programs, including eligibility requirements, the scope of services available, the freedom to choose a provider, a provider's choice to participate in a plan, the method of reimbursing providers, and the statewide application of the program. Health plans and capitated providers can seek waivers through their state intermediaries.

Section 1915(B) Medicaid Waiver: Section 1915(b) waivers allow states to require Medicaid recipients to enroll in HMOs or other managed care plans in an effort to control costs. The waivers allow states to implement a primary care case-management system; require Medicaid recipients to choose from a number of competing health plans, provide additional benefits in exchange for savings resulting from recipients' use of cost-effective providers, and limit the providers from which beneficiaries can receive nonemergency treatment. The waivers are granted for 2 years, with 2-year renewals. Often referred to as a "freedom-of-choice waiver."

Self-Funding: Employer or organization assumes complete responsibility for health care losses of its covered employees. This usually includes setting up a fund against which claim payments are drawn, and claims processing is often handled through an administrative services contract with an independent organization. In this case, the employer does not pay premiums to an insurance carrier, but rather pays administrative costs to the insurance company or health plan and, in essence, treats them as a third-party administrator (TPA) only. However, the employee may not be able to detect any difference because the plan description, and membership cards may carry the name of the insurance company not the employer. *Same as* self-insurance.

Self-Insurance: The concept of assuming a financial risk oneself, instead of paying an insurance company to take it on. Every policyholder is a self-insurer in terms of paying a deductible and co-payments. Large firms often self-insure frequent, small losses such as damage to their fleet of vehicles or minor workplace injuries. However, to protect injured employees state laws set out requirements for the assumption of work-ers' compensation programs. Self-insurance also refers to employers who assume all or part of the responsibility for paying the health insurance claims of their employees. Firms that self-insure for health claims are exempt from state insurance laws mandating the illnesses that group health insurers must cover.

When an employer is self-insured, this means that the payer or man-aged care company manages the employer's funds rather than requiring the employer to pay premiums. Many employers choose to self-insure because they are then exempted from certain insurance laws and also think that they will spend less money in the short run. Employers assume the risks involved and also have full rights to all insurance claim information. Typically, the self-insured employer is a large employer. The employees or patients will not be able to discern if their employer is self-insured easily, since all paperwork or benefits cards usually contain the name of the insurance company.

Sentinel Event: Adverse health events that may have been avoided through appropriate care or alternate interventions. Providers are required to alert JCAHO and often state licensing authorities of all sentinel events, including a review of risk factors, preventative measures, and case analysis.

Severity: Size of a loss. One of the criteria used in calculating premiums rates.

Shadow Pricing: Within a given employer group, pricing of premiums by HMO based upon the cost of indemnity insurance coverage, rather than strict adherence to community rating or experience rating criteria.

Shared Risk Pool for Referral Services: In capitation, the pool established for the purpose of sharing the risk of costs for referral services among all participating providers. Commonly, this involves a group or specialty category of physicians and is based on utilization. Sometimes, risk pools are established in partnered or limited partner or foundation capitation systems, whereby both providers and health plans share risk in a limited way.

Shared Savings: A provision of most prepaid health care plans where at least part of the providers' income is directly linked to the financial performance of the plan. If costs are lower than projections, a percentage of these savings are referred to the providers.

Single-Stream Funding: The consolidation of multiple sources of funding into a single stream. This is a key approach used in progressive mental health systems to ensure that "funds follow consumers."

Site-of-Service Differential: The difference in the monies paid when the same service is performed in a different practice setting or by a different provider. One example would be an examination in an emergency room versus in a family doctor's office.

Skilled Nursing Facility (SNF): A licensed institution, as defined by Medicare, which is primarily engaged in the provision of skilled nursing care. SNFs are usually DRG- or PPS-exempt and are located within hospitals, but sometimes are located in rehab facilities or nursing homes.

Small Group Market: The insurance market for products sold to groups that are smaller than a specified size, typically employer groups. The size of groups included usually depends on state insurance laws and thus varies from state to state, with 50 employees the most common size.

SMI: *See* Supplemental Medical Insurance

SNF: *See* Skilled Nursing Facility

Sole Community Hospital (SCH): A hospital which (1) is more than 50 miles from any similar hospital, (2) is 25 to 50 miles from a similar hospital and isolated from it at least one month a year as by snow, or is the exclusive provider of services to at least 75% of its service area populations, (3) is 15 to 25 miles from any similar hospital and is isolated from it at least one month a year, or (4) has been designated as an SCH under previous rules. The Medicare DRG program makes special optional payment provisions for SCHs, most of which are rural, including providing that their rates are set permanently so that 75% of their payment is hospital-specific and only 25% is based on regional DRG rates.

Solo Practice, Solo Practitioner: A physician who practices alone or with others but does not pool income or expenses. This form of practice is becoming increasingly less common as physicians band together for contracting, overhead costs, and risk sharing.

Solvency: Insurance companies' ability to pay the claims of policyholders. Regulations to promote solvency include minimum capital and surplus requirements, statutory accounting conventions, limits to insurance company investment and corporate activities, financial ratio tests, and financial data disclosure.

SPD: *See* Summary Plan Description

Specific Stop Loss: The form of excess risk coverage that provides protection for the employer against high claims on any one individual. This is protection against abnormal severity of a single claim rather than abnormal frequency of claims in total.

Spend Down: A term used in Medicaid for persons whose income and assets are above the threshold for the state's designated medically needy criteria, but are below this threshold when medical expenses are factored in. The amount of expenditures for health care services, relative to income, that qualifies an individual for Medicaid in states that cover categorically eligible, medically indigent individuals. Eligibility is determined on a case-by-case basis.

Spider Graphs/Charts: A technique or tool developed by Ernst & Young to combine analyses of a market's level of managed care evolution with an internal readiness review.

SSI: *See* Social Security Income

Stacking: Practice that increases the money available to pay auto liability claims. In states where this practice is permitted by law, courts may allow policyholders who have several cars insured under a single policy, or multiple vehicles insured under different policies, to add up the limit of liability available for each vehicle.

Staff-Model HMO: A model in which the HMO hires its own physicians. All premiums and other revenues accrue to the HMO, which, in turn, compensates physicians. Very much like the group model, except the doctors are employees of the HMO. Generally, all ambulatory health services are provided under one roof in the staff model.

Standard Class Rate (SCR): Base revenue requirement per member multiplied by demographic information to determine monthly premium rates.

Standing Referral: A referral to a specialist provider that covers routine visits to that provider. It is a common practice to permit the gatekeeper to make referrals for only a limited number of visits (often three or fewer). In cases where the medical condition requires regular visits to a specialist, this type of referral eliminates the need to return to the gatekeeper each time the initial referral expires.

State Children's Health Insurance Plan (SCHIP): Under Title XXI of the Balanced Budget Act of 1997, the availability of health insurance for children with no insurance or for children from low-income families was expanded by the creation of SCHIP. SCHIPs operate as part of a state's Medicaid program.

State Children's Health Insurance Program (SCHIP): Although Medicaid has made great strides in enrolling low-income children, significant numbers of children remain uninsured. From 1988 to 1998, the proportion of children insured through Medicaid increased from 15.6% to 19.8%. At the same time, however, the percentage of children without health insurance increased from 13.1% to 15.4%. The increase in uninsured children is mostly the result of fewer children being covered by employer-sponsored health insurance. The Balanced Budget Act of 1997 created a new children's health insurance program called the State Children's Health Insurance Program. This program gave each state permission to offer health insurance for children, up to age 19, who are not already insured. SCHIP is a state-administered program, and each state sets its own guidelines regarding eligibility and services.

Statutory Accounting Principles (SAP): More conservative standards than under GAAP accounting rules, they are imposed by state laws that emphasize the present solvency of insurance companies. SAP helps ensure that the company will have sufficient funds readily available to meet all anticipated insurance obligations by recognizing liabilities earlier or at a higher value than GAAP and assets later or at a lower value. For example, SAP requires that selling expenses be recorded immediately rather than amortized over the life of the policy.

Stop Loss Insurance: Insurance purchased by an insurance company or health plan from another insurance company to protect itself against losses. Reinsurance purchased to protect against the single overly large claim or the excessively high aggregated claim during a set period. Stop loss may also be used by providers when purchasing malpractice, workers' compensation, and liability coverages.

Structured Settlement: Legal agreement to pay a designated person, usually someone who has been injured, a specified sum of money in periodic payments, usually for his or her lifetime, instead of in a single lump-sum payment.

Subcapitation:

1. An arrangement whereby a capitated health plan pays its contracted providers on a capitated basis.
2. An arrangement that exists when an organization being paid under a capitated system contracts with other providers on a capitated basis, sharing a portion of the original capitated premium. Can be done under carve-out, with the providers being paid on a PMPM basis.

Subrogation: The legal process by which an insurance company, after paying a loss, seeks to recover the amount of the loss from another party who is legally liable for it.

Subscriber: Employment group or individual that contracts with an insurer for medical services. Usually synonymous with enrollee, covered individual, or member.

Subscriber Contract: A written agreement that describes the individual's health care policy. *Also called* subscribe certificate or member certificate.

Summary Plan Description (SPD): In self-funded plans, a written explanation of the eligibility for and benefits available to employees required by ERISA.

Superfund: A federal law enacted in 1980 to initiate cleanup of the nation's abandoned hazardous waste dump sites and to respond to accidents that release hazardous substances into the environment. The law is officially called the Comprehensive Environmental Response, Compensation, and Liability Act.

Supplemental Insurance: Any private health insurance plan held by a Medicare beneficiary or commercial beneficiary, including Medigap policies and postretirement health benefits. Supplemental insurance usually pays the deductible or co-pay and sometimes will pay the entire bill when the primary carrier's benefits are exhausted.

Supplemental Medical Insurance (SMI): Part B of the Medicare program. Part B normally covers the outpatient services, as opposed to Part A, which covers inpatient services. This voluntary program requires payment of a monthly premium, which covers 25% of program costs. Beneficiaries are responsible for a deductible and coinsurance payments for most covered services.

Supplemental Security Income (SSI): A federal cash assistance program for low-income aged, blind, and disabled individuals, established by Title XVI of the Social Security Act. States may use SSI income limits to establish Medicaid eligibility.

Supplemental Services: Optional services a health plan covers or provides.

Surplus Lines Tax: A tax imposed by state law when coverage is placed with an insurer not licensed or admitted to transact business in the state where the risk is located. Unlike premium tax for admitted insurers, the surplus lines tax is not included in the premium and must be collected from the policyholder and remitted to the state.

T

Tax Equity and Fiscal Responsibility Act of 1982 (TEFRA): The federal law that created the current risk and cost contract provisions under which health plans contract with HCFA. Legislation that created the target rate of increase cost-based limits on reimbursements for inpatient operating costs. These limits are considered per Medicare discharges total amounts. A facility's target amount is derived from costs in its base year (first full fiscal year of operation with application to CMS as same) updated to the current fiscal year by the annual allowable rate of increase. Medicare payments for operating costs generally may not exceed the facility's target amount and still be paid by CMS. These provisions apply to hospitals and units excluded from PPS and DRG. When cost reports fall short of the TEFRA limit, certain paybacks are provided. If costs exceed TEFRA, facilities can submit an exception report and may or may not be provided additional payment. Many facilities that established TEFRA limits in the early 1980s are finding they consistently exceed their TEFRA limits. Units normally under the TEFRA rules are psychiatric units, rehab units, freestanding specialty hospitals, oncology outpatient clinics, and others.

Telehealth, Telemedicine, E-Health: The use of telecommunications (i.e., wire, Internet, radio, optical, or electromagnetic channels transmitting text, X-ray, images, records, voice, data, or video) to facilitate medical diagnosis, patient care, patient education, or medical learning. Many rural areas are finding uses for telehealth and telemedicine in providing oncology, home health, emergency, radiology and psychiatry services, among others. Telehealth services have been used between providers, to provide supervision of one another, and to provide evaluation of patients. Medicaid and Medicare provide some limited reimbursement for certain services provided to patients via telecommunication. Telehealth is likely to serve greater purposes and populations in the future.

Termination Date: Date that a group contract expires or an individual is no longer eligible for benefits.

Terrorism Coverage: Included as a part of the package in standard commercial insurance policies before September 11, 2001, virtually free of charge. Since September 11, terrorism coverage prices have increased substantially to reflect the current risk.

Tertiary Care: Services provided by highly specialized providers such as neurosurgeons, thoracic surgeons, and intensive care units. These services often require highly sophisticated technology and facilities.

Therapeutic Alternatives/Therapeutic Equivalents: Drug products that provide the same pharmacological or chemical effect in equivalent doses.

Third-Party Administrator (TPA): An independent organization that provides administrative services including claims processing and underwriting for other entities, such as insurance companies or employers. Often insurance companies will contract as TPAs with other insurance companies or health plans. TPAs are not always insurance companies. TPAs are organizations with expertise and capability to administer all or a portion of the claims process. Self-insured employers will often contract with TPAs to handle their insurance functions. Insurance companies will sometimes outsource the claims, UR, or membership functions to a TPA. Sometimes TPAs will only manage provider networks, only claims, or only UR. Hospitals or provider organizations desiring to set up their own health plans will often outsource certain responsibilities to TPAs. TPAs are prominent players in the managed care industry.

Third-Party Coverage: Liability coverage purchased by the policyholder as a protection against possible lawsuits filed by a third party. The insured and the insurer are the first and second parties to the insurance contract.

Third-Party Payer: Any organization, public or private, that pays or insures health or medical expenses on behalf of beneficiaries or recipients. An individual pays a premium for such coverage in all private and in some public programs; the payer organization then pays bills on the individual's behalf. Such payments are called third-party payments and are distinguished by the separation among the individual receiving the service (the first party), the individual or institution providing it (the second party), and the organization paying for it (third party).

Third-Party Payment: Payment by a financial agent such as an HMO, insurance company, or government rather than direct payment by the patient for medical care services. The payment for health care when the beneficiary is not making payment, in whole or in part, in his own behalf.

Title XVIII (Medicare): The title of the Social Security Act that contains the principal legislative authority for the Medicare program and, therefore, a common name for the program.

Title XIX (Medicaid): The title of the Social Security Act that contains the principal legislative authority for the Medicaid program and, therefore, a common name for the program.

Tort: A legal term denoting a wrongful act resulting in injury or damage on which a civil court action, or legal proceeding, may be based.

Tort Law: The body of law governing negligence, intentional interference, and other wrongful acts for which civil action can be brought, except for breach of contract, which is covered by contract law.

Tort Reform: Legislative limits or changes or judicial reform of the rules governing medical malpractice lawsuits and other lawsuits. Tort simply refers to lawsuit. Reform implies that limits can be placed on individual rights to sue or on the amounts or situations for which they can seek relief. Tort is considered to be by some as the primary cause of the rising costs of health care. Reform, then, would lower health care costs. On the other hand, patient advocates are against tort reform, claiming that the health care industry and managed care industries require monitoring and that lawsuits keep health care providers and payers in check. Congress debates tort reform each session, but to date, few restrictions have been placed on tort cases.

Total Budget: Otherwise known as a "global" budget, a cap on overall health spending.

Total Margin: A measure that compares total hospital revenue and expenses for inpatient, outpatient, and nonpatient care activities. The total margin is calculated by subtracting total expenses from total revenue and dividing by total revenue.

Total Quality Management (TQM): Related to quality management, TQM identifies required system elements to measure, design, and select processes that consistently deliver superior outcomes. These fundamentals make up the basis for TQM.

TPA: *See* Third-Party Administrator

TQM: *See* Total Quality Management

Tracking of Disclosures: The HIPAA Privacy Rule gives individuals the right to request an accounting of disclosures of protected health information over the previous six years. If an individual authorizes uses or disclosures for research, the disclosures do not need to be tracked, but disclosures must be tracked if the researcher receives an IRB-approved waiver of authorization. The accounting of disclosures generally must include the date of the disclosure, the name of the entity or person (and address if known) who received the protected health information, a brief description of the information disclosed, and a brief statement of the purpose of the disclosure. The rule allows for an alternative tracking option for research involving 50 or more people.

Transaction: Usually refers to the exchange of information for administrative or financial purposes such as health insurance claims or payment. Under HIPAA, this is the exchange of information between two parties to carry out financial or administrative activities related to health care.

Transfer: Movement of a patient between hospitals or between units in a given hospital. In Medicare, a full DRG rate is paid only for transferred patients that are defined as discharged. In managed care, transfers are often suggested by UR entities to move patients to lower-cost care facilities.

Transparency: A term used to explain the way information on financial matters, such as financial reports and actions of companies or markets, are communicated so that they are easily understood and frank.

Travel Insurance: Insurance to cover problems associated with traveling, generally including trip cancellation due to illness, emergency care, repatriation of remains, lost luggage, and other incidents.

Treatment: The provision of health care by one or more health care providers. Treatment includes any consultation, referral, or other exchanges of information to manage a patient's care. The HIPAA Privacy Notice explains that the HIPAA Privacy Rule allows the provider and its affiliates to use and disclose protected health information for treatment purposes without specific authorization.

Treatment Episode: The period of treatment between admission and discharge from a modality (e.g., inpatient, residential, partial hospitalization, and outpatient) or the period of time between the first procedure and last procedure on an outpatient basis for a given diagnosis. Many health care statistics and profiles use this unit as a base for comparisons.

Trending: Methods of estimating future costs of health services by reviewing past trends in cost and utilization of these services.

Triage: Triage is the act of categorizing patients according to acuity and by determining which need services first. Most commonly occurs in emergency rooms, but can occur in any health care setting. Classification of ill or injured persons by severity of condition. Designed to maximize and create the most efficient use of scarce resources of medical personnel and facilities. Managed care organizations, health plans, and provider systems are setting up programs or clinics called "triage centers." These centers serve as an extension of the utilization review process, as diversions from emergency room care or as case management resources. These triage centers also serve to steer patients away from more costly care (for example, a child with a cold is steered away from an emergency room). Triage can also be handled on the telephone and may be called a preauthorization center, crisis center, call center, or information line.

Triage Providers: Medical personnel who classify ill or injured persons by severity of condition. When providers or insurance companies manage triage on the telephone, this service may be referred to as preauthorization center, crisis center, call center or information line. Providers may also manage triage in emergency rooms, walk-in centers, disaster scenes, or outreach centers.

Triple-Option Plan: A plan (usually offered by a single carrier or a joint venture between two or more carriers) that gives subscribers or employees a choice among HMO, PPO, and traditional indemnity plans.

U

UB-92—Uniform Billing Code of 1992: Bill form used to submit hospital insurance claims for payment by third parties. Similar to HCFA 1500, but reserved for the inpatient component of health services. An electronic format of the CMS-1450 paper claim form that has been in general use since 1993. (Now revised to UB-04.)

UCR: *See* Usual, Customary, and Reasonable Charges

UM: *See* Utilization Management

Unbundling: The practice of providers billing for a package of health care procedures on an individual basis when a single procedure could be used to describe the combined service.

Uncompensated Care: Service provided by physicians and hospitals for which no payment is received from the patient or from third-party payers. Some costs for these services may be covered through cost-shifting. Not all uncompensated care results from charity care. It also includes bad debts from persons who are not classified as charity cases but who are unable or unwilling to pay their bill.

Underinsurance: The result of the policyholder's failure to buy sufficient insurance. An underinsured policyholder may only receive part of the cost of replacing or repairing damaged items covered in the policy.

Underinsured: People with public or private insurance policies that do not cover all necessary health care services, resulting in out-of-pocket expenses that exceed their ability to pay.

Underwriting: Process of selecting, classifying, analyzing, and assuming risk according to insurability. The insurance function bearing the risk of adverse price fluctuations during a particular period. Analysis of a group that is done to determine rates or to determine whether the group should be offered coverage at all.

Uninsured: People who lack public or private health insurance.

Uninsured Motorist Coverage: Portion of an auto insurance policy that protects a policyholder from uninsured and hit-and-run drivers.

Universal Access: The right and ability to receive a comprehensive, uniform, and affordable set of confidential, appropriate, and effective health services. Universal service is a reality in countries with national medicine programs or socialized health care, such as the United Kingdom, Canada, France, and most countries in the world. Few countries have the private insurance programs as the primary form of health care, as in the United States.

Universal Coverage: A type of government sponsored health plan that would provide health care coverage to all citizens. This is an aspect of President Clinton's original health plan in the mid 1990s and is an attribute of national health insurance plans similar to those offered in other countries such as the United Kingdom or Canada. While government-sponsored health care is not likely to be universal, politicians in Washington continuously discuss the concept of providing health care to all Americans. Expect to see more and more discussion of modified universal coverage ideas in the years to come.

Update Factor: The year-to-year increase in base payment amounts for PPS and excluded hospitals and dialysis facilities. The update factors generally are legislated by congress after considering annual recommendations provided by ProPAC and HHS.

UR: *See* Utilization Review, Case Management

Urgent Services: Benefits covered in an evidence of coverage that are required in order to prevent serious deterioration of an insured's health that results from an unforeseen illness or injury.

Use: Under HIPAA, this term refers to the employment, application, utilization, examination, analysis, or sharing of individually identifiable health information within a covered entity.

U.S. per Capita Cost (USPCC): The national average cost per Medicare beneficiary, calculated annually by CMS's Office of the Actuary.

Usual, Customary, and Reasonable (UCR) Charges: The amount a health plan will recognize for payment for a particular medical procedure. It is typically based on what is considered "reasonable" for that procedure in your service area. Commonly charged fees for health services in a certain area. The use of fee screens to determine the lowest value of provider reimbursement based on (1) the provider's usual charge for a given procedure, (2) the amount customarily charged for the service by other providers in the area (often defined as a specific percentile of all charges in the community), and (3) the reasonable cost of services for a given patient after medical review of the case. Most health plans provide reimbursement for usual and customary charges, although no universal formula has been established for these rates.

Utilization: Use of services and supplies. Utilization is commonly examined in terms of patterns or rates of use of a single service or type of service such as hospital care, physician visits, and prescription drugs. Measurement of utilization of all medical services in combination is usually done in terms of dollar expenditures. Use is expressed in rates per unit of population at risk for a given period, such as the number of admissions to the hospital per 1,000 persons over age 65 per year, or the number of visits to a physician per person per year for an annual physical.

Utilization Management (UM): The process of evaluating the necessity, appropriateness, and efficiency of health care services against established guidelines and criteria. Evaluation of the necessity, appropriateness, and efficiency of the use of health care services, procedures, and facilities. UM usually includes new actions or decisions based on the overall analysis of the utilization.

Utilization Review (UR), Case Management: A formal review of utilization for appropriateness of health care services delivered to a member on a prospective, concurrent, or retrospective basis. In a hospital, this includes review of the appropriateness of admissions, services ordered and provided, length of a stay, and discharge practices, both on a concurrent and retrospective basis. A peer review group or a public agency can do utilization review. UR is a method of tracking, reviewing, and rendering opinions regarding care provided to patients. Usually UR involves the use of protocols, benchmarks, or data with which to compare specific cases to an aggregate set of cases. Those cases falling outside the protocols or range of data are reviewed individually. Managed care organizations will sometimes refuse to reimburse or pay for services that do not meet their own sets of UR standards. UR involves the review of patient records and patient bills primarily but may also include telephone conversations with providers. The practices of precertification, re-certification, retrospective review, and concurrent review all describe UR methods. UR is one of the primary tools utilized by IDS, MCO, and health plans to control overutilization, reduce costs, and manage care.

Utilization Risk: The risk that actual service utilization might differ from utilization projections.

V

Variable-Contribution Health Plan: In contrast to a fixed-contribution plan, a variable contribution involves employers committing to a specified level of benefits funding for their employees, regardless of the actual benefit price. Employers are thus locked into variable contribution arrangements because they are committed to funding a certain benefit structure without knowing what the future costs may be if premiums are raised.

Vertical Disintegration: A practice of selling off health plan subsidiaries or provider activities. Vertical disintegration was a trend in the late 1990s.

Vertical Integration: Organization of production whereby one business entity controls or owns all stages of the production and distribution of goods or services. In health care, vertical integration can take many forms, but generally implies that physicians, hospitals, and health plans have combined their organizations or processes in some manner to increase efficiencies, increase competitive strength, or improve quality of care. Integrated delivery systems or health care networks are generally vertically integrated.

Vital Statistics: Statistics relating to births (natality), deaths (mortality), marriages, health, and disease (morbidity). Vital statistics for the United States are published by the National Center for Health Statistics. Vital statistics can be obtained from CDC, state health departments, county health departments, and other agencies. An individual patient's vital statistics in a health care setting may also refer simply to blood pressure, temperature, height and weight, etc.

Volume and Intensity of Services: The quantity of health care services per enrollee, taking into account both the number and the complexity of the services provided.

Volume Performance Standard (VPS) System: The VPS provides a mechanism to adjust fee updates for the Medicare Fee Schedule based on how annual increases in actual expenditures compare with previously determined performance standard rates of increase.

Volume Performance Standards (VPS): A mechanism to adjust updates to fee-for-service payment rates based on actual aggregate.

W

Waiting Periods: The length of time an individual must wait to become eligible for benefits for a specific condition after overall coverage has begun.

Waiver:

1. The surrender of a right or privilege. In life insurance, a provision that sets certain conditions, such as disablement, which allow coverage to remain in force without payment of premiums.
2. Approval that the Centers for Medicare and Medicaid Services (CMS, formerly called HCFA), the federal agency that administers the Medicaid program, may grant to state Medicaid programs to exempt them from specific aspects of Title XIX, the federal Medicaid law. Most federal waivers involve loss of freedom of choice regarding which providers beneficiaries may use, exemption from requirements that all Medicaid programs be operated throughout an entire state, or exemption from requirements that any benefit must be available to all classes of beneficiaries (which enables states to experiment with programs only available to special populations).

Waiver of Authorization: Under HIPAA, under limited circumstances, a waiver of the requirement for authorization for use or disclosure of private health information may be obtained from the IRB by the researcher. A waiver of authorization can be approved only if specific criteria have been met.

War Risk: Special coverage on cargo in overseas ships against the risk of being confiscated by a government in wartime. It is excluded from standard ocean marine insurance and can be purchased separately. It often excludes cargo awaiting shipment on a wharf or on ships 15 days after arrival in port.

Wellness: A dynamic state of physical, mental, and social well-being; a way of life which equips the individual to realize the full potential of his or her capabilities and to overcome and compensate for weaknesses; a lifestyle which recognizes the importance of nutrition, physical fitness, stress reduction, and self-responsibility. Wellness has been viewed as the result of four key factors over which an individual has varying degrees of control: human biology, environment, health care organization, and lifestyle. Preventive medicine associated with lifestyle and preventive care can reduce health care utilization and costs. "Wellness" programs became popular with the advent of managed care in the 1980s, with the philosophy and business idea that health plans needed to emphasize keeping their beneficiaries well. However, there has been a drop-off in these programs since the 1990s as health plans recognize the difficulty in assessing efficacy, and they found that subscribers tend to change plans regularly, thus reducing benefit of keeping one population "well."

Withhold: Portion of a claim deducted and held by a health plan before payment is made to a capitated physician. A form of compensation whereby a health plan withholds payment to a provider until the end of a period, at which time the plan distributes any surplus based on some measure of provider efficiency or performance. That portion of the monthly capitated payment to providers withheld by the MCO to create an incentive for efficient or reduced utilization of care or services. A provider that exceeds their withhold amount does not receive a dispersion at the end of the contract period.

Withhold Pool: The aggregate amount withheld from all providers' capitation payments as an amount to cover excess expenditures of his or a group's referral or other pool.

Workers' Compensation: A state-mandated program providing insurance coverage for work-related injuries and disabilities. Several states have either enacted or are considering changes to the workers' compensation laws to allow employers to cover occupational injuries and illnesses within their own existing group medical plans. Some employers pay premiums to the state or to insurance companies for this coverage. Others are self-funded and use third-party case management or administrative services to manage the processes.

Z

Zero-Sum Budgeting: A "deficit-neutral" budget process in which new expenditures are paid through cuts in existing programs or increases in revenue. The end result is the same bottom line and no increase in the deficit (if governmental) or debt (if referring to private or public corporation or company).

Index

A

Access, 199
Accident insurance, 199
Accountable Health Plan (AHP), 199–200
Accounting; *see also* Finances
  principles, 245
  receivables, 294
  statutory principles, 305
Accreditation, 24, 50, 109, 127, 157
Activities of daily living (ADLs), 200
Activity-based costing (ABC), 200
Actuarial analyses, 1, 204, 230, 298
Acute care, 201, 207, 239, 291
Adjudication, 24
Adjusted community rate (ACR), 6
Administrative services organization (ASO),
  31
Admitted company, 204
Adverse event, 100
Adverse selection, 147, 204
Aetna U.S. Healthcare, 27
Aetna v. Davila, 41, 42
Affiliation, 18
Affinity sales, 204
Agency companies, 205, 233
Agency for Health Care Policy and Research
  (AHCPR), 205
Agents
  exclusive, 205
  independent, 205
Agreements, *see* Contract law
Aid to Families with Dependent Children
  (AFDC), 46
Alien insurance company, 206
All patient diagnosis-related group (APDRG),
  206–207
All-payer systems, 207

All-products contracts, 21, 126
  and kickbacks, 26
  language of, 22–23
  outlawing, 27
  problems with, 23–26
  regulatory violations, 25, 26, 27
Alternate delivery systems, 207
Alternative dispute resolution (ADR), 85
Alternative markets, 207
Ambulatory care, 207
American Medical Association (AMA), 13,
  24
Ancillary services, 207
ANSI (American National Standards
  Institute), 208, 273
Antitrust laws, 15, 17, 25, 26
Any willing provider laws, 208
Appeals, 30, 32, 33
  timing, 35–36
Approvals
  of charges, 209
  of health care facilities, 209
  for treatment, 209
Arbitration, 85, 89, 150, 192
Archer MSAs, 56
Arizona Health Care Cost Containment
  System (AHCCCS), 46, 47
Assignment of benefits, 41, 69, 78
Assisted living, 209
Audits, provider treatment, 209–210
Authorizations, 1, 31, 177–178
  consumer directed health plans (CDHPs),
  61
  under HIPAA, 210
  prior, 133, 158, 289
Authorized representatives, 36, 39, 40–41
Auto insurance policy, 210, 243, 274, 282,
  312

317

D

E

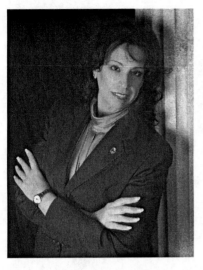

Maria K. Todd, Ph.D., is the leading instructor in managed care and contracted reimbursement worldwide. She has trained more than 50,000 professionals in over 2500 classes since 1989.

Her background includes postgraduate degrees in health administration, experience as an HMO provider relations coordinator, IPA and MSO executive director, contract analyst and negotiator, health law paralegal, and certified mediator. She has a clinical background as an emergengy medical technician (EMT) and surgical technologist. Her professional experience also includes solo and group medical practice IPA, PHO, and MSO development and management and hospital revenue cycle work experience. She is a published author of several professional trade books and hundreds of journal articles and white papers.

In addition to her U.S. consulting activities, she consults internationally in the development of several foreign integrated provider networks to prepare them for the rigors of international accreditation, credentialing, and contracting with and reimbursement from U.S.-based health plans and employers. She also serves as the executive director of the Healthcare Reimbursement Institute and managing partner of Global Health Sources, LLC.

She maintains offices in Denver, New York, Las Vegas, south Florida, and Bangkok, Thailand.